How to Make More Money in the Fitness Industry

"It's time to make more money from fewer members."

Revised and Expanded Edition of
Making Money in the Fitness Business

Thomas Plummer

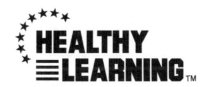

ISBN: 978-1-60679-303-9
Library of Congress Control Number: 2014934026
Cover design: Corey McLenaghan
Book layout: Cheery Sugabo
Illustrations: Jeff Camish

Healthy Learning
P.O. Box 1828
Monterey, CA 93942
www.healthylearning.com

Dedication

This book is dedicated to my long-suffering wife, Susan, who has endured a husband who spends 40 weeks a year on the road still chasing his dream of changing an industry that matters. Living your dream often takes the patience and help of others and nothing I have achieved during the last few decades could have been done without her help and love. Chasing your passion is all that matters in life, but no one can do it alone, so thank you, Susan, for helping me make my dreams possible. For that, I am forever grateful.

Acknowledgments

The acknowledgments section is usually one or two pages no one reads. This is where the author, who you don't know, thanks people you don't know and then he gets on with the book.

I want this section to be a little different because I am a grateful man who has had a wonderful career chasing the things he loves and living life mostly as I wanted to live it and you have to recognize that this doesn't happen without the help of many others.

First of all, thank you, the readers of my work, the followers of my social media, and the more than 150,000 people who have heard me speak during a very long career. Workshops don't go very well if no one shows up, but you, the faithful and gracious supporters, have kept coming to anywhere in the world there is an event organizer crazy enough to book me and you have been doing that for more than three decades. Along the way, I have argued with you about giving up the past, beaten you into listening, and drunk far too much wine with far too many people in far too many countries, but many of you have made money, kept your businesses open, and lived another day in business to chase your dream. Together, we made a good team. My goal was to always give you information that would grow your business and keep you safe and your role was always to become the businessperson you need to be to survive in a tough and competitive field such as fitness. It seemed to work for both sides and I am grateful to all of you who believed.

There would be no books without a publisher and I have had the best in the business my entire career. Jim Peterson, who through his books and teachings is one of the most influential people in modern training, is also a publisher who makes guys like me look good from book to book. Books are necessary if you want to rise in this field, but there would have been nothing on my slate without Jim's support and faith that we could get something out to the fitness public that mattered. Thank you, Jim, and to your entire staff over the years for your help and I am grateful for all you have done for me.

There are also others in the industry who have given me a chance to be heard and to be relevant in areas I would have never been invited without their help. Norm Cates, through his long-running magazine Club Insider, has given me a voice over the years and opened doors to me with his endless list of contacts. Thank you, Norm, for all you have done for me through the years and for your friendship and support.

Chris Poirier, who runs Perform Better, which is the standard for functional equipment sales in the entire country, invited me a number of years ago to be the keynote speaker at Perform Better's Summit Series. His invitation allowed me to fully get immersed into the training side of the industry, which is a totally different segment that few mainstream operators understand or even try to get involved with during their careers, although any owner must if he cares to stay in business in the coming years. Thank you, Chris, for giving me a chance to be part of your team over the years and for all the opportunities you have created for me.

Greg Rose and Dave Phillips, co-founders of the Titleist Performance Institute, have also given me an opportunity in the golf world through their certification process and there is little I have enjoyed as much in the last 10 years as working with those guys, and after my experience within their organization, I believe that Greg Rose is one of the quiet geniuses in the world who never gets nearly the recognition he deserves. Thanks, guys, for the faith and support and thank you, Greg, for the friendship that has gone way beyond the work we do together.

There are also so many people who have taught me things over the years. The problem with this type of list is that eventually someone gets left out that made a difference, but even with that in mind, debts need to be acknowledged and these are just a few people who have given me their time and support through the years and who have made more of a difference in my life than they might ever realize:

- Marian Gurney, who is the only reason our company survived the creative years when vendors failed and the days were a little dark
- Kevin Brochu, for the opportunities he created for me through the last several years
- Chuck Hawkins, who taught me how to live life on your own terms
- Ken Reinig, forever young, forever moving forward, and forever my friend
- Barry Lehane, who taught me how to be creative and think outside the box
- Dick Reed, who taught me you can start poor but you don't have to finish that way
- Bob Riches, who might be the most patient and ethical man I have ever met in my career and taught me about being persistent to get what you want
- Smed Blair, who taught me management and leadership by example

- Shawn Smith, who was a brilliant example of hiring right and leading quietly and always from the front
- Don Coleman, who personified leadership through a quiet expertise
- Robin Dyche, who taught me that if it doesn't kill you, you will come back and be even better than you were before
- Steve Parker, who is the friend I always wanted to be to others
- Meredith Poppler, who championed me to others and opened doors that would have forever been closed
- Sal Pellegrino, who is the epitome of class and integrity in a field that sadly lacks both
- Graham Melstrand, who guided me into a new world of fitness professionals
- Dave Wright, who said, sure, let's do a few gigs in Europe
- Emmett Williams, who opened the door for me to Australia and to one of the most wonderful teaching experiences of my career
- Nigel Champion, who (besides having the coolest name in fitness), along with his partner, Greg Hurst, gave me a chance in Australia without even knowing who I was
- John McCarthy, who gave me great opportunities when he was "the man"
- Heath Debish, for standing with me through some tough times in our company
- Robert Creech and Rick Mayo, partners who will keep the dream going way after I am done

Of course, no list would be complete without mentioning my talented and wonderful daughter, Jillian, who gave me a reason to keep it going when there were so many reasons just to move on in life.

I am also a spiritual person who has been a seeker my entire life. You are who you are because of the gifts you receive and my life has been one constant blessing. I am thankful and grateful to the Almighty, who makes everything possible in my life.

Contents

WHY IS THIS BUSINESS SO HARD?

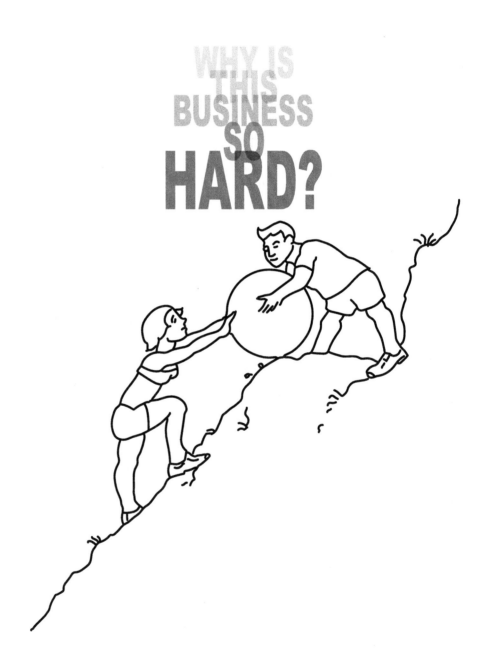

Introduction

When this book was first written back in 1999, it represented everything I really knew about fitness at the time. When I first started in the industry, much of what we did was really all about the owner and little if anything to do with the client. Sales techniques were predatory, the equipment was worthless, few people working in the industry at the time really knew anything about fitness, and getting results for clients and the national image of what we did was horrible. There were still pockets of knowledge out there that resided in the small, physical physique gyms scattered around the country, but the few who understood fitness were buried beneath the hundreds that wanted to exploit the member for everything he owned.

I grew up in fitness in the era of high-pressured sales. We lived, breathed, and failed by learning to sell. The national chains at the time were nothing but repositories of old sales guys who could slam down a dozen a day and then do it again tomorrow. No one thought about or cared about the client, who quickly failed in this system and left. Why care? In those days, the member was easily replaceable and the competition was light. Sell, sell, and sell again.

This is also a system that I learned to hate quickly. The clients then, as they do now, suffered from being overweight, out of shape, and miserable in their personal lives and were looking for us to help them achieve a new level of success. We didn't have the tools, but there were a few of us that tried anyway. Books were scarce and the ones you could find were based on personal experience and ideas with no research or real information to back up the claims and techniques in the books or magazines.

The best thing about this old information was that it predated the bodybuilders. Almost everything you read in those days, which was the late 1970s and early 1980s, was based on a holistic, full-body approach to fitness. You lifted heavy a couple days a week and put a lot of heavy metal up over your head as often as you could. You lifted heavy, lifted often, and worked your full body, and amazingly, it worked for our clients.

At about this same period of time, fitness changed—and changed for the worse. The 1980s was a decade of fixed-plane equipment and the first generation of workout people who chased isolation for the muscle as well as the emergence of the national chains and the end of anyone getting any help unless you paid a trainer to work you out six days a week. This was also the advent of the bodybuilder, which for better or worse chartered a course for the industry that lasted until just the last few years. We went for show in those days and bigger the better, but we also created a generation of false expectations and worthless training knowledge that still permeates the mind-set even today.

My absolute distaste for the early fitness industry still burns my lips today. We lied to the client to get him into the gym and then failed him once he was there. We chased image over health and failed to do any research that would have advanced the industry by several decades. The industry was, for all practical purposes, saved at the turn of this new century by the rise of the functional training mind-set and by solid research that pointed the way. Some of the early functional pioneers, such as Vern Gambetta, Gary Gray, Jim Peterson, Cedric Bryant, Mike Clark, Al Vermeil, and a few others, set the tone for a new generation of trainers and training information. This first wave led to the second and the gurus of change who set the world on fire, such as Mark Verstegen, Gray Cook, Mike Boyle, Dan John, and Carlos Santana, then led again to today's best, such as Alwyn and Rachel Cosgrove, Todd Durkin, Greg Rose, and Pavel Tsatsouline, who have combined to create a new generation of educated professionals who are quickly changing every concept we ever thought to be true in the industry. For once, we had tools that worked and that were validated by educated people who could and would test all the nonsense we had carried for more than five decades.

My mission then, as it still is today, was to change the fitness industry from an image of nasty sales techniques and failed information to one where the client got what he paid for and could trust the gym and the owner he chose to help him fulfill his goals. One workshop, one gym at a time, and one owner until the consumer could look at what we did and trust us instead of fearing us as he did back in the day of the pressured sale in an office.

Writing this first book was a labor of love. It was my chance to spread the word that you could make money in this business and you could do it ethically and professionally and not at the expense of hurting the people who trusted you with their money. There were later books in this long series on the business of fitness, but each new title was only added after I felt I had something new to say, and while I enjoyed the writing process in each and every one, this first one was always my baby that started it all.

At the time this book was written, it seemed so fresh and needed in the industry, but as with everything in the fitness world, time diminishes returns and what was once at the edge of the field and pushing beyond any accepted boundary at the time became dated and no longer the source of vital information that could help an owner understand and master the business side of the fitness industry.

My entire life has been spent going forward. I like living in the "now," and as I have told thousands of clients, you can't change your past and the mistakes you have made, so let's talk about today and what you are going to differently starting tomorrow. Looking backward has never been productive for me—and nor for you—and once something is done in my life, I let it be and keep moving toward tomorrow.

However, being an author is a little like having your own personal time machine. Just one call from my publisher, Jim Peterson—who said "This book is getting dated. How about doing a revised edition?"—led to me firing up the time machine and heading back to 1999. Once a book is finished, there is no going back for me and I truthfully haven't looked through the first edition of this book more than a handful of times in the 14 years since I wrote it.

Picking it up again left me with two impressions. First of all, the material was right for the decade it was written, but it is not very close to how an owner has to think or work to be successful in a market that has changed so dramatically in so few years. Secondly, I was pleasantly surprised that there were still some fundamental truths in the book that have endured over time. For example, building a receivable base is still a fundamental rule that can't be changed even today, short-term debt still can kill a business, and customer service is still an essential.

However, the failings of the original book were glaring. When this book was first published, there were no low-priced gyms, no training gyms that mattered, trainers were clipboard cowboys at best, and the chains that ruled that era have since faded to almost oblivion. Most importantly, back in the day in 1999, competition in most markets was moderate at best, meaning that most gyms could safely operate with little or no competition and the tools of the years that preceded 1999 going back to the 1950s—the era when the gym business started to first rise—were still somewhat valid.

In 1999, gym owners were still pressuring sales in offices, still just selling access to equipment through an inexpensive membership, and still using price-driven marketing to get leads. All these concepts have totally failed in today's market, including the idea that you can be the lowest bidder in the market and simply rent equipment to a consumer who will be gone in a few months.

There is an important rule in the fitness business that no one recognizes but that most everyone is affected by at some time or another. This rule is the 10-year rule and it states that few concepts in fitness will be sustainable for a 10-year period. Every new idea in fitness has pretty much the same curve of growth, but you as the creator or eventual leader get to choose your own ending. For example, in the 1980s, aerobics started a long, slow growth period, got hot and rose to the pinnacle of need, quickly declined in the early 1990s, and then completely disappeared for about a decade.

This pattern is true of most concepts in the fitness industry and it is also why you constantly need to look at what you own and what you're doing and reinvent. This is also why consultants who write books need to go back and question every concept in their older books and ask if that idea is still relevant and if it would work today.

We see this pattern of long, slow grow, followed by a hot "must have it now" pattern, the quick decline, and then oblivion in everything we do and in the real world too. Starbucks® stumbled until its founder stepped back in and reinvented the company. Apple® stumbled until Steve Jobs came back and set it again on its original course and only the future knows if that company can continue to amaze after the death of Jobs.

Great companies in the industry, such as Gold's Gym and World Gym, were the rulers of their decades, but the companies sold and somewhat faded from their once true glory. Gold's Gym was probably the most recognizable fitness name on the planet for several decades, but again, it is a lot easier to get to be number one than stay number one over time. Can these great names be reinvented by their current management and follow the path of Starbucks or will they fade and become just another former success story in the history of the industry?

The difference between long-term sustainable success and oblivion is evolution. Howard Schultz let Starbucks evolve—but only by remaining true to its roots. This sounds contradictory, but under his second-generation direction, the company changed to meet the needs of its continually evolving customer base while never forgetting that it was and always will be about the coffee and the experience.

In the fitness business, creators of new concepts tend to sit on the past and cling to original methods and ideas. This list is long, but how many chains and franchises have you seen rise, become hot, and then fade away over a decade or so because the consumer and market simply grew past the original concept? Curves was a brilliant idea at the time, but a decade or two later and the concept became archaic and a hard sell in the market as the total number of units it operated continued to decline for a number of years. Its method of training—based on a simple circuit concept—was right at the time when it was founded, but compared to the advent of functional training and how the proven methods of training, even for the older woman, has evolved, can this business model be sustained into the future? Everything has to evolve or it dies, and businesses—even wildly successful ones, such as the original Curves franchise model—eventually reach a stage where you grow or fade.

When this introduction was written, there were also a number of other companies that were nearing that vital period where either they evolved into next generation facilities or began the long, slow march to obscurity. Once you reach that pinnacle position of being really hot after the long, slow build, how long can you truly stay hot?

There is another position between hot and the big fall and that is where you operate as a long-term dependable company that keeps its product fresh and service great and is always moving itself ahead. Starbucks is more than 40 years old, but its stores and concepts seem fresh and as if it were a brand-new company. Sears is in the fight now to remain relevant. Montgomery Ward disappeared. Almost all the Curves imitators failed and disappeared. Reinvention is life and whether you grow or you die in the fitness world is driven by your response to the rapid pace of increasing knowledge, better-educated employees—such as the trainers—and much more sophisticated clients who all are pushing the gym owner to grow and adapt or face being ignored and fail.

It will be interesting in the near future to see if such companies as CrossFit, Planet Fitness, Les Mills, Gold's Gym, LA Fitness, and the rest of the current big names or programming giants such as Zumba will continue to evolve and stay relevant or become a victim of the 10-year rule and start that quick slide to where they are rarely discussed and are no longer relevant in the business world of fitness.

Obviously, the first edition of this book was a victim of the 10-year rule and needed reinvention to stay relevant for a next generation of fitness business owners. The business model I have advocated all these years and that has been quite successful for thousands of owners needed to be tweaked and we started the process almost a decade ago. This book now represents all that we know today about running a successful gym as well as validating some of the original concepts that were slightly ahead of the curve.

One of the basic tenets I have always believed in is that going for heavy volume, meaning chasing an endless supply of new clients each month to replace the ones you burned up, was not sustainable over time. The concept was right, but it was also wrong in that it was introduced too early in the market, and going after a higher return per client served was the right idea, but it was hard to sell in the industry when the volume guys were still writing the big sales. In other words, it was the right idea, but we didn't have the tools we needed to get it done back in 1999. But that has changed and now is the time to recognize this principle. And most importantly, owners are listening now because of all the things that have failed in the last 20 years, nothing is more earth shattering than the failure of the volume-based business model.

The missing ingredient all these years was the training component of the business. It seems absurd now, but working people out for money has been a small part of the industry for more than 60 years. We have done nothing since the inception of the industry more than 65 years ago—no matter how this is argued—except sell a membership to a person who pays each month to a gym so he can access or, in other words, rent the gym's equipment.

The statistic that validates this has been constant for several decades. In a typical mainstream fitness center—whether independent or chain—only about 5 percent of the membership work with a trainer on a regular schedule on an annual basis. If you are math challenged, look at it this way: In this gym, 95 percent of the membership gets no help whatsoever and practice some form of do-it-yourself fitness usually regulated to going around a circuit of set equipment that has been proven a hundred different ways not to get the person into shape over time.

The evolutionary key and the premise behind the revision of this book is that the industry cannot last as a rental company for equipment, even at $10 per month. We have to move from a volume approach, where the member is expendable and irrelevant over time, to a training-centric business model where we have to chase the maximum results for the maximum number of clients in the shortest period of time and keep our clients for as long as we can in a hypercompetitive market place.

This revision contains a complete business model to make this happen for you and your business and it doesn't matter if you own a big box mainstream gym or a small training gym on the corner. Everything you need to be financially successful for the coming decades is here, proven by thousands of clients over a 30-year period. We now have the tools, we now have the education, and, for the first time, we now have the clients willing to support a system designed to help them succeed.

There is one thing you have to understand if you want to make the fitness business your life's work. We exist to change lives. We exist to help people who struggle with health and fitness get better. We exist to make a difference in our communities and with the people who trust us with their money. We can do all this and still make more than enough money to take care of our lives and our families. If you are in fitness because you want to make a difference, then this book is for you.

Chase your passion through fitness.

Thomas Plummer
March 2014

Introduction to the First Edition

There just has to be a better way to do business in the fitness industry.

The fitness industry is in a state of change; I am a one-person missionary show, trying to institute this change. After years of business regression and retardation, the industry is finally showing signs of breaking away from its 30-year negative business image and practices—still the standard for doing business today for most owners.

Long-term contracts with high-pressure sales, gas station price war mentalities, and semi-naked models in our advertising that offend most of our women patrons were part of our past and are still part of business as it's done today. Couple this with the trend of building clubs with vast warehouse physical plants that have all the intimacy of standing in the middle of an Arkansas Walmart during a two-for-one long underwear sale, and you have an industry that has stagnated and has been reduced to copying out-of-date and mostly unethical business practices from 30 years ago.

I became part of the fitness industry more than 20 years ago for two reasons. First of all, we offer a product that can make a difference in someone's life. If our product is delivered correctly, then our fitness businesses can initiate positive change in the people we serve. We can obviously change a person's physical shape with what we offer. But we can also subtly change their mental condition by allowing them to become part of something that becomes important in their lives—a place where they are always welcome, where they can make new friends, and a place that offers a social atmosphere linked to their physical conditioning.

Secondly, I realized that I could make a great deal of money doing something I loved, which was being in the fitness business. But sadly I realized that there were no real business principles being applied to this industry. It's almost as if the fitness business were a business backwater that modern concepts such as financial analysis, customer service, low-pressure/high-integrity sales, and advanced marketing concepts had not yet reached.

Basically, it was, and still is for most, an industry that is totally sales-driven. And this lopsided emphasis on sales prevents us from delivering our product, which again is to bring change through the delivery of our service.

Typical fitness facilities today are huge impersonal warehouses of equipment revolving around a sales team. The marketing is also a negative since it is entirely price-driven. This has proved to be totally ineffective in most markets for attracting deconditioned people, people who have had bad experiences at other gyms, or people who have never really been in a fitness facility.

Sales in these facilities are all based on closing the sale on the first visit, a system that is more than 30 years old, and one that most potential members find very repulsive. If this facility is so good, why is the person forced to make a decision during the first visit?

First-visit closes have been an unquestioned part of the industry since it started. But this system drives down the price we should be able to get for our memberships, because in only 30 minutes everything always comes down to price. There is simply nothing, other than the deal of the day, that can be intelligently discussed between a salesperson and a prospective member in just 30 minutes.

As an industry, we haven't changed. Nor have we questioned the dogma that high-pressure/first-visit sales represent a behavior that is still propagated through the national conventions, by most industry magazines, and by industry consultants who are failed owners who are now going to teach you their business systems.

Financially, most of these outdated business systems are self-defeating. For example, the costs of running a fitness facility in the 1990s is two to three times higher than it was in the early 1980s. Yet many owners try to operate their facilities using the same price per member that clubs used 25 years ago. Simply, the volume that can be generated by traditional sales and marketing methods, with outdated pricing, is not enough to ensure clubs' survival.

Traditional fitness marketing is also a representation of the industry's past that leads to a business plan that is doomed to fail before it can ever begin. Price-driven ads with big-haired, big-chested supermodels with 22-inch waists don't work anymore to attract enough potential members, because the ads' appeal is so limited.

Since the club's marketing is ineffective, the club then forces the salespeople to generate their own leads and to pressure prospective members to join on their first visit. Salespeople who are able to do this are expensive and, therefore, take up a disproportionate amount of the staffing budget. Because the salespeople are so overpaid, and the marketing is so expensive, there is no real money left for service people.

Without service people, the current members become frustrated and leave the system, which increases the demand for the salespeople to not only generate new sales, but to also replace the large number of people who drop out. More money has to go into marketing and more pressure is applied to the salespeople, who in turn apply it to the prospective members.

Many people who might be interested in working out in a fitness facility would never even set foot in a typical club, because they already know what is going to happen to them. They will be pressured into a decision, and then receive no help after the sale is closed.

The clubs will be crowded because of the volume approach that goes along with the low prices, and they will also be dirty and filled with broken equipment. Keep in mind that the standard way of doing business in this industry over the past 30 years or more has taught the average consumer this process.

All the large chains based on low pricing and volume marketing in the past 30 years have proved the weaknesses of traditional operating systems by bleeding red ink all over their investors. Even as this is written, the chain of the decade is gobbling up endless clubs by using venture capital, yet the owners are crying over lost revenues in financial magazines.

Their business systems simply don't work anymore. These systems are archaic and provide losses to the owners and investors, and worse yet, do immense damage to the members who bought into the clubs believing that they would get the help and service they rightfully expected. Huge chains with outside capital and lousy business systems, or any operator who follows these systems, also hurt the legitimate owners in the industry—by giving the consumer such a bad buying experience before we ever get a chance to meet them.

This book is about making money in the fitness industry, with the application of real business principles while maintaining your integrity. There is a better way to do business, breaking away from the traditional dogma our industry has been based on during its history, which has always reflected instant financial gratification for the owner at the expense of the consumer. Following are a few of the topics covered in this book that reflect changes from the old style of thinking:

- *Focusing:* You can't be everything to everybody in today's fitness market. Almost every major business or market has evolved from generalist to specialist. Retailing giants like Macy's and Sears have been replaced with retail specialists like Eddie Bauer and Victoria's Secret. Even lawyers and doctors have moved from being general practitioners to very narrowly focused specialists. The fitness industry must do the same to grow and thrive into the next century, yet many owners still practice the one-facility-fits-all theory.

- *Running the business by numbers:* There are formulas and numbers that can be applied to our businesses that can help an owner build a functional business plan. For example, an owner will make much better business decisions if he understands the true yield from a member payment, loss rates, and the expected net from each profit center. There are also important ratios that determine how much of the club's expenses need to be covered by the receivable check and what percentage of a club's income should come from its profit centers in order to decrease the dependency on new sales. By better understanding the financial side of the business, we can better understand how to break out of our old habits.

- *Staffing:* Staffing will be the most difficult issue to deal with in the coming decade. How you hire, train, motivate, and eventually let go of your employees will decide how successful you will be. At some point in time, most gyms will have much of the same equipment and programming. The difference between one club and another will be its focus and the staff that works in the gym. The club with the best staff will win.

- *Service:* We haven't even scratched the surface yet of how we define and deliver member service. Implementing true member service is expensive to maintain and difficult to create because of the entrepreneurial nature of our owners. "Entrepreneurial" is another word for control freak, and the very nature of a typical owner works against letting a member make a suggestion or point out a weakness in the club. To prosper, we need to redefine member service beyond the definition of vast rooms of equipment and free coffee to the members. Member service is not how much free stuff we include with a membership; it's the quality and image of the programs, services, and amenities available to the member.

- *Marketing:* Traditional fitness marketing doesn't work because it has such a limited appeal. It's estimated that 92 percent of the people in this country have never set foot in a health club. Typical fitness marketing only appeals to the other 8 percent who have fitness experience, and it does nothing to develop the other 92 percent as a potential market for our clubs.

The fitness industry as a whole also works off many false assumptions that need to be questioned. This book works hard to uncover these fitness business myths. For example, most owners strongly believe that the typical prospective member only cares about price. Why do they believe that and base their business plan on this assumption, when it is so obviously false?

Some people are driven by price—this is the deciding factor as to what they buy and how they live. There are just as many other people who will pay extra for quality. There are Geo Metros and there are Mercedes. There is Walmart and there is Nordstrom. The problem is that the false assumption most owners follow is that everyone in the world is a Walmart person seeking a discount.

The huge fitness chains demonstrate this assumption in their ads, and the rest of us follow. It's the traditional system of pricing, selling, and marketing that forces the consumer to think price, not the price itself. Because of our belief in this false assumption, pricing in the industry for the majority of the fitness facility owners hasn't really changed in more than 20 years.

In my 20 years as an educator and consultant, I've learned that change is possible and that the false assumptions can be replaced with real business practices. I also know that change hurts. In this and any other industry, change means that you may be leading the charge and going against the rest of the pack. Someone has to do it, and hopefully, it will be the readers of this book who will help bring the fitness industry kicking and screaming into the next millennium.

Thomas Plummer
1999

Important Notice to My Readers

The assumption I made when writing this book is that you will read it in small chunks or use it to train your staff. You will notice that certain key concepts are repeated in different chapters and each chapter was written to stand alone out of the context of the rest of the book. This was done intentionally so you could read and stay focused on the idea at hand rather than try to refer back to a chapter you might not have had time to read yet.

It is also important to note that there are no guarantees in any business and the ideas expressed in this book, while validated in thousands of clubs throughout the years, are going to be only as good as you make them. In other words, use this material at your own risk. Much of what is written here is based upon my experience, my observations, and my opinions and all the content is provided to you as a learning resource to help you understand how the business of fitness works and why, but without a guarantee of success.

In all cases, and especially when it comes to valuing a business, signing leases, hiring and firing, and working with lenders, seek the advice of your local professionals that support you and your business, such as your accountant, attorney, and banker. These professionals can help you make decisions based upon who you are and what your business is doing at the moment, but remember, this information exists so you may have a much more productive conversation with the people you trust.

Neither the author, publisher, nor any party related to the information and development of this book assumes any responsibility or liability for the consequences, whether good or bad, of the application of this material.

You will also note that the chapter dividers are new for this book. The small blurbs separating each chapter are recent Facebook® posts that garnered a lot of views and interest from my readers. I hope you enjoy reading them as much as I did writing each one.

Section 1

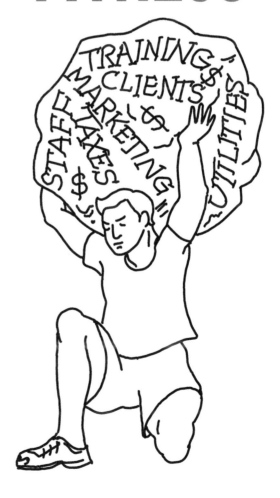

THE
BUSINESS
OF
FITNESS

1

If You're Lost in Your Business, It's Because You're Following the Wrong Path

When you are conceptualizing a new fitness business or re-evaluating an existing one, ask yourself "Why?" Why are you making those specific choices and assumptions? Why are you making those specific plans? Why do you think what you know in your head or, worse, what you think you know because you have seen it in other fitness businesses is the right way to proceed for you and your business?

The fitness business attracts passionate people—ones who are usually getting into the field because they want to change lives and make a difference in the world. Even the new generation, professionally trained businessperson who might open a new gym most likely still has a vision of doing something meaningful and of value to others. However, this passion only goes so far, and at some point, passion has to hit the fan of reality and be translated in a working business concept that can pay the bills and create income and wealth for the owners and investors.

Many times in the fitness industry, a business will fail because it's based on a business plan that never had a chance of working in the first place. This "born to fail" plan is usually based on a version of someone else's patched-together concept or is patched together from ideas copied from other existing businesses without regard to their financial success or without regard to whether what they might be doing could be sustainable into the future. When recreating a business or starting a new one, make sure you follow a path that will give you the highest chance to succeed financially over time and also one that is sustainable into the future. This type of path is based on real business assumptions that have been proven to work over time in more than just a single business.

Over the years, I've visited literally thousands of fitness facilities of all types. A good weekend on the road would always include visiting as many as 20 different gyms, Ys, recreation centers, and any other fitness businesses that could be found listed on the Internet. After a while, the facilities all started looking the same. Ugly front counters, tired circuit equipment outdated by 30 years, poorly trained staff dressed only slightly better than homeless people, gray carpets with some type of black specks, and a general sense that there were very few new and exciting ideas in our industry. And let us not forget those piles of broken equipment in corners, the giant plastic potted plants covered in dust, and the classic but cheap eight-feet mirrors turned sideways in the group rooms. Traditional fitness facilities are locked in the past and today's bigger, shinier, and much more costly models are usually nothing more than the same old brands of equipment set in the same place and the memberships in the gym are still being sold by people whose only goal is to rack up as many scores as they can in a month with little regard for what the client really wants or needs.

One of the major business problems in our industry is too much inbreeding. Everyone steals ideas from everyone else in the fitness business without thought that what you are stealing might be a business plan that is crushing the guy you stole it from in the first place—who actually stole his ideas from the competitor down the street or who is using the plan he learned from his first fitness job 30 years ago. We all do this same type of observation and theft—until it dawns on us that we have to be better than these businesses to win a financial war, not just a poor attempt at being a next generation imitator! Being equal is not the goal. The goal is creating a business that dominates the marketplace and creates a vehicle to provide a needed service to a target population that is willing to continue to pay for it over time.

Most fitness businesses haven't changed their base operating and design concepts in more than 60 years. Cardio equipment—the most in-demand equipment in today's market and still growing—is almost always poorly displayed. Why? Because some brave soul built a mediocre cardio deck in the late 1970s and the next 2,000 people who opened a facility copied the idea and, in many cases, the actual design of the deck itself. We don't invent new in this business. We cling to old, tired ideas that normally would have failed sooner if we had held the industry to a higher standard in the early years. Everyone has heard the old saying "Lucky is better than good" and this helped many a dumb owner survive in the early days of fitness when the demand was high and the competition was nonexistent.

Don't think it works this way? Remember back to the introduction of teal-and-white equipment—a fashion statement in steel from the 1980s. One manufacturer brought some to a trade show, other manufacturers copied the colors, and then for more than a decade you could walk into almost any gym in the country and find teal-and-white equipment—except for the hardcore guys, who all went with red and black. How many hundreds of clubs went with teal and white—without thought to how that choice would impact their total design—because they visited another club and thought it was the new color standard and this guy must know what he is doing because he had more cars in the parking lot?

The training gyms of the past few decades also suffer from this same problem. Some intrepid soul opened a 1,500-square-foot gym back in the 1970s, stuffed it with a full line of equipment similar to the big players, and offered one-on-one training to a few dozen rich white guys who were too fat to go to the Gold's Gym at the time. This gym spawned a thousand more and became the standard for one-on-one fitness: build small, get as much equipment as you can in the room, charge the highest price you can, and call yourself a personal trainer.

Today's training gyms have evolved—and at a faster rate than traditional fitness facilities. New generation training gyms are literally 40 years or more ahead of a traditional mainstream box-chain gym. These new version are open-spaced wonders using that latest research and training tools and usually staffed by trainers who would never consider working in the big boxes and pushing clients to use dated circuit equipment that is guaranteed failure. In fact, these training gyms are the first to realize that we should be in the results-driven business and not in the high-volume chase where the member is considered replaceable once he fails.

By visiting hundreds of poorly designed and weakly managed fitness businesses, you can get pulled down to their level of operation. You visit a few weak gyms, say to yourself "Wow, my place is better than that," and then you fail to develop your business to higher levels because you now settled for beating standards that were too low to begin with when you started your journey. Being the best of the worst doesn't guarantee that you will make money. It only guarantees that you will feel good about yourself as you go out of business: "I was the best in this town, but help me carry my boxes to the truck please." Your mistake is that you are comparing yourself against businesses that are statistically most likely not making money and the only true measure of success over time is whether a business can sustain a profit margin against stiff competition. Anyone can make money in a void. It's the ability to create revenue against a wall of tough competitors trying to put you down that validates your business platform.

Many fitness businesses will fail simply because they follow the wrong business models. For example, many owners still run retro ads featuring seminaked models as artwork. The look of the models changes over time and, of course, the clothes have changed, but the ads are basically the same concept that have been used in the industry since the 1950s: models who are large chested, have exceptionally small waists, and are in full-blown makeup. And, of course, don't forget the perfect hair already damp to illustrate the sweat effect.

Today's version also always has a bare midriff featuring a flat, ripped stomach. Owners justify these pictures as role models for our potential women members, even though the shape most of the models are in is attainable by only a small percentage of a club's members. The scary part is that when these ads are shown to women, more than 90 percent say using pictures of seminaked models is somewhat offensive. Many women flatly state that these pictures would prevent them from responding to any business that feels these pictures are appropriate for their ads.

This intimidation stems from the statement that the pictures actually make to the potential client: If you want to join this gym, you have to be in good shape before they actually let you into the facility. This type of ad creates a barrier that keeps more people out than it does to attract. These ads are a part of the history of this business, but we can't seem to move past this dated tool because of the nature of the owner who always copies whatever the other owners are doing without thought to whether it actually might work. Almost every owner in the country has run this type of ad at some point in his career. They are easy to put together and your ad person can do it in a few minutes by using a stock photo, dropping in some bullet points listing your equipment, throwing in a low-price discount or special, and then emailing you the proof. This type of ad is also a perfect example of following the wrong path in this business.

To build a sustainable business platform that will perform over time, you need to question everything you think you know about the fitness business and question everything you are currently doing. Are you running your business based on principles copied from someone you think is making money? Are you making decisions based on habit because you've always done it that way? And are you using basic business principles that may be outdated by more than 40 years and don't really work anymore in a competitive market? Past success is usually not an indicator that you will continue to be successful in the future using the same tool. Businesses evolve and industries as a whole shift and take new directions. Copying where we were culturally and technologically even five years ago only guarantees that you are now outdated by at least five years from the day you open.

It was easier to make money in the earlier days of our industry. Things that worked in the late 1960s and 1970s, such as discounted renewals, high-pressure sales and long-term contracts, were effective back then because they were perceived as new and fresh tools at the time. In fact, practically everything anyone tried worked back then. Competition was limited and the industry itself was perceived as something new and fresh.

The early fitness consumer was less sophisticated in his sales experiences and hadn't been exposed to nearly the number of sales pitches he is today. Potential members actually believed the old drop-close—that if they didn't sign up today, they would lose money by having to pay more if they signed up tomorrow. Are there any consumers in today's market who haven't heard thousands of pitches for everything from cell phone plans to investment strategies by the time they turn 21? When conceptualizing a fitness business—a new gym or a training center—or recreating an existing facility, the hardest part is breaking away from the accepted norm and from the bad habits we have had for so many years that derived from our early days in fitness.

Setting out on a new path is difficult because so many existing owners claim to be making so much money from copying the old methods of doing business. You visit a national trade show or convention and everyone is rich, everything is working, and the owner is always working on opening his next project. "Yeah, I hired this new guy who used to work for one of the big chains, and man, this guy can sell. He even has an 80 percent closing rate. He's working with my staff and we're signing more contracts now than we have in years."

This owner now claims that high-pressure sales are the answer because he is writing a lot of contracts. The other guy in the conversation thinks his sales are flat, so he needs to copy this method and get himself a high-pressure sales guy if he wants to make money too.

What the second guy and the owner with the new sales guy don't know is this: Does what he is doing really work? What are the losses from such high-pressure sales? Do people sign up with this guy just to get out of the office and then don't pay later? What's happening to the gym's word-of-mouth reputation in the community? No one knows the answers to these questions because the owner doesn't know his business well enough to ask these questions himself, but to an outside owner who has flat sales, this seems like a magical solution. If you are drowning, even a bird feather floating in the water looks like a life raft. This nonsense is not limited to just a sales example. This same owner will buy the latest and greatest equipment, buy a few pieces of functional equipment, and declare himself ready for new generation clients and do whatever price special he hears about in a magazine or online. He is always just one great idea away from turning his business around and he will believe this until someone takes the business away from him.

We know from our own research in this industry that only about 15 percent of all small businesses can obtain a pre-tax net of 20 percent or better on a yearly basis. Despite this reality, the accepted norm is to copy what everyone says at the trade shows or workshops because they all claim they are making money with their ideas. However, the real-life business view is that most of these people aren't really making the money they say they are, so copying their ideas will be counterproductive to your long-term business plan.

Most small businesses of any type usually fall into these general categories. It doesn't matter if you have a flower shop, restaurant, dry cleaning business, or even a fitness facility. The approximate categories generally define everyone in that industry:

- Twenty percent of the industry will be making real money, defined as at least 10 percent pre-tax net or better.
- Sixty percent pay their bills and earn themselves a decent living as a breakeven business.
- Twenty percent would lose a gold brick if you gave it to them and really should have a job working for someone else. Some people should never be in small business, but they keep trying—probably due to being forced out of the real business world and this is the only avenue left to them.

Remember that you seldom hear or read about some owner who is getting his butt kicked in the magazines or online. Every chain claims it is making money whether it is or not because who sits around bragging to his peers that he is a loser without a plan, and besides, you don't get to be on the cover of magazines if you admit you haven't got a clue as to how to change the national dynamics in the fitness industry. There are investors to feed, staff to hire, and competitors waiting at the door, so there is never anything but good times. In a relatively small industry, such as the fitness business, it's easy to get sucked down the wrong path and follow the current trend of the moment—whether it is proven or not in the business.

Another way to get on the wrong business path is to pursue the illogical over the logical. In this business, we seem to follow the illogical. For example, why do most new gyms build sales offices? A sales office in a modern gym is not logical. Few of us are comfortable in an office environment sitting across the desk from someone. The only situation I can think of where you sit across a desk from someone and it's good news is when a lawyer tells you some distant relative died and left you a pile of money. And even then, someone had to die to make the good news happen. In the consumer's mind, most situations where he sits across from someone at a desk is a bad position to be in.

Is sitting across a desk from a car salesperson a pleasant situation? Is sitting in front of a doctor good news? And anytime you're in front of a lawyer, it has to be bad news. No matter what, it's going to cost you something.

Another illogical aspect of a sales office is that it takes consumers out of the environment that excited them in the first place. The colors, the music, the people—all these things excite people to buy memberships. The atmosphere in the facility is a strong part of the buying decision. Why not sign the people up in a centrally located area—right in the middle of the action, such as at the juice bar or at a high cafe table overlooking the action on the floor? We normally put in offices because everyone else has them in their facilities. None of us are comfortable in offices, but we'll make the illogical decision because it's the path everyone else took.

Another example is single-plane, fixed-joint circuit training. We buy a large amount of circuit equipment, give the member a giant workout card that is kept in a file box on the edge of the floor, and then we expect that cold steel to service our members and replace the need for staff attention and interaction. When adding equipment in the club was new and exciting, say in 1985, this worked because no one had seen lines of big, beautifully painted equipment before and this seemingly magical path to being fit had sales and, most importantly, sex appeal.

At that point, most owners abdicated their ability to service people and let the equipment become the central focus in the club. Our sales pitch was no longer how we can help you. It became how much equipment we had and how big the training floor was, so you could now help yourself. Perhaps the most depressing part of this era was that we moved from instruction-based fitness to becoming showrooms for endless lines of equipment.

The last point is our failure to apply proven business principles to the fitness industry. Why is it that good business principles often stop at the gym door? You see it often: A person who was successful in other businesses opens a gym and goes brain dead. Maybe it's the new baggy shorts cut below the knees and minimalist shoes he's now wearing that somehow make the person regress to his pre-business days.

What works in other industries can often be applied to the fitness industry, especially when it comes from other service industries. Instead of studying other fitness businesses, we need to spend more time studying other goods and services businesses. FedEx® is an excellent model for many gyms to study. FedEx does not apologize for its prices, even though it's one of the most expensive overnight carriers. At any time, the company can tell you exactly where your package is and what's happening to it. If you had a very important document to send overnight, who would you trust: a low-priced alternative or would you go with the company that started it all? Keep in mind, FedEx can find any package at anytime and anywhere in the world. Most gyms can't even tell whether the person walking in the door is an active member.

This path of considering ourselves unique and outside the normal operational rules of business is one that our industry has been following for over six decades and it is the wrong path for the coming competitive years. If your business is flat, it may be because the path you chose to follow is not the right one for you or for your business. If you are opening a new gym, spend less time looking at other gyms in your area and more time in businesses that excel in service, design, and atmosphere. But above all, make sure what you do makes good business sense and is not something you do out of habit or because the guy down the street has a full parking lot.

The Fitness Facility of the Future

Bigger or more is always better has been the mantra in the fitness business for the last several decades and your image and chances for success were measured by the size of your workout floor, the number of classes you could offer, and the amount of equipment you could fit into an immense cavern of a workout space.

Most industries evolve and we fail to remember that the fitness industry is only about 65 years old, dating back to the end of World War II, but in reality, most of what we take for granted in today's fitness industry didn't really start until the 1960s, when equipment manufacturers started making standardized equipment available to anyone who had the money and passion to enter the fitness business world.

Prior to that period, much of what was used in clubs was often made locally and designed by the owner himself, who wanted equipment his way. Joe Gold, the almost-forgotten legend who single-handedly changed modern fitness through his creation of Gold's Gym and then World Gym, was still making his own stuff and still stocking the World Gym headquarters gym with equipment he had made in his garage as late as the 1980s.

As noted elsewhere in this book, the peak year for mainstream fitness was about 1995, when the industry enjoyed the magical combination of a growing interest in fitness with limited competitors in the marketplace. This magical time was in many ways the last glory days of the late 1980s, when selling fitness was perhaps as easy as it has ever been in this country.

Based on this success, a new model of club emerged during the 1990s. Space was relatively cheap, bodybuilding ruled the training world, and every major manufacturer in the world was scrambling to invent the perfect line of equipment guaranteed to generate the perfect body.

We often forget the power of the bodybuilding movement and what it did to the fitness business world. The advent of Arnold Schwarzenegger and the acceptance of bodybuilders as the modern standard of fitness that we all needed to emulate led to every club in existence striving to create the perfect bodybuilding environment.

Bodybuilding was the isolation of muscles, with the goal being building size and symmetry. Therefore, there was practically no end to the creativity of the machine designers as they sought to build long lines of equipment that could isolate virtually every muscle in the body. It was not unusual in those days to see five to six different types of benches that were either incline or decline designed to attack the chest from all different angles sitting next to four or more different leg extension machines that all guaranteed a different angle of attack for the quads.

Credibility as a gym was gauged on how much of this stuff you had on the floor. If you were a good gym, you had every piece you could buy all set in perfect lines on your 12,000-square-foot training floor, but if you were a lesser gym, you might have a more limited selection on only 5,000 square feet. National conventions in those days for the big franchises, such as Gold's, were often nothing more than one guy bragging about his new 25,000-square-foot gym—only to be put down by the next guy and his 40,000-square-foot monster that set a new state record for training floor space. More and bigger was the better business and he who had the most toys was usually declared the winner by his fellow owners and the buying public.

There are a number of reasons this business plan no longer works. First of all, the consumer is finally aware enough to at least understand what fitness is not. You could hide in a hut at the Arctic Circle and still not escape the constant flow of information being delivered in all media as to what constitutes modern fitness and what tools the consumer needs to be using to get the job done.

For example, there are at least a dozen magazines on display at any given time in any given grocery store magazine rack touting new fitness breakthroughs and the ultimate workout and there is virtually no end to the information available online in such offerings as the Huffington Post, Slate, the *New York Times*, Yahoo!, Google, and YouTube—all of which offer healthy living sections or fitness videos. There is also the relentless stream of information on TV that includes such perennial favorites as *The Biggest Loser*.

What do all these various outlets have in common? All these feature a constant flow of what modern fitness looks like and how to do it and there is little information out there left that reflects what fitness used to look like compared to what the modern interpretation is.

For example, watch *The Biggest Loser* to see contestants carry buckets of sand up a ramp or watch them smash giant tires with sledge hammers, and if you watch ESPN, there is no doubt you will see athletes training by using ropes, sleds, kettlebells, sandpits, and other protocols that define what fitness is today.

An important side note here is that almost everything the consumer sees or reads is movement and fitness done in groups. Little if any fitness you see in the media focuses on any type of one-on-one training. Everything is done in a group, with even the training of the professional sports teams done with a coach and a group effort.

If you are the consumer at home, you may not know much about fitness, but you do know what it looks like in the magazines and what it looks like when your favorite contestant or athlete is engaged in the pursuit of getting in shape. The important thing to note here is that what fitness looks like highlighted 100 different ways in this myriad of choices is nothing like the fitness options the sales guy is showing you at the local big box fitness facility.

This potential member is inspired and ready for change, but after watching and reading about fitness for a few months and maybe playing with a small kettlebell in the basement, along with the included DVD, he is ready to join a gym. The disconnect happens when the guest follows a salesperson who shows the guy 10 lines of equipment in a row, a few guys doing free weights in the back of the club, and a group exercise class schedule from 1995.

Nowhere is fitness like the magazines and nowhere is there a group of happy people working hard together. If you can do it on your own, join the club and have at it, but if you need help, it is only offered in a one-on-one format at an expensive price that limits who in the club can actually get this help. This disconnect makes for a hard sale, and while the guest may not know how exactly fitness should be, he does know enough to realize that whatever this club is selling is dated and nothing like the way everyone else is doing it these day. The dated clubs that continue to try to sell 1995 technology will find it harder and harder to make money in the coming years because their products will become less and less viable in the marketplace.

Another factor that spells the demise of the big box business plan is the sheer cost of doing one of these projects and then getting it financed. It is not unusual for a 30,000-square-foot Gold's Gym box model go out the door for $4,000,000 or more, and with the increased density of competition in most markets, it is hard to justify this investment for the expected return, especially when small training clubs can generate more than a million dollars a year with a 30 percent or higher pre-tax net. Funding for these big box projects is also getting tougher as investors and banks realize that these monster projects come with an ever-increasing risk factor in today's competitive market and shifting economy.

However, perhaps the biggest threat to the future of the big box is something as small and simple as a kettlebell. The advent of functional training, in conjunction with the rise of the professional trainer, has created efficient fitness that requires little space but that can create massive revenue. The realization that a person can get into better shape standing in a small space using about three kettlebells and a few inexpensive bands than he could using hundreds of thousands of dollars worth of equipment in a box gym is such a harsh reality that most box players just refuse to deal with it and this denial leads to yet another generation of boxes being built that still rely on outdated technology and systems.

There is also a new reality, as mentioned elsewhere in this book, of the small training/performance center that can generate large grosses and nets in small spaces, which is something that very few of the box clubs have ever been able to duplicate in their businesses. The block to the chain clubs and big boxes simply emulating the training-centric model lies in their inability as a business to shift away from the membership-driven model that allocates all resources and focus on just generating as many new memberships as possible each month. The technology and business systems are there for the taking, but the entire philosophy of the business itself would have to change prior to creating big training revenue in those clubs.

The last issue that points toward the difficulty in maintaining the box model is something that most people don't take into account—and that is the shift away from a horizontal business model in the industry to a vertical model. The horizontal model is a legacy from the 1990s and can be defined as virtually every club that was in existence at the time used the same business model and chased the same target market.

There were, of course, other models in existence at the time, such as leftover group exercise studios from the 1980s, early generation hardcore training clubs, martial arts–based fitness, and the random specialty club in the yoga or wellness class, but all these were small in number and the real power in the industry in those days was with the national chains that all emulated each other and sought the same segments in the marketplace.

Horizontal, in this case, refers to the fact that all the clubs could pretty much be grouped in a straight line from left to right and it would be hard to tell the real differences because all were about the same in price, offerings, branding, and services and, most importantly, all were chasing the same potential member. The prime examples of that era were Gold's, World, Powerhouse, and 24 Hour Fitness, which all claimed to be unique, but in reality, if you took the signs down, they virtually all offered the same inside—even in layouts and some design features.

Late in the 1990s and early in the 2000s came the rush of vertical fitness. Vertical means that instead of everyone chasing the same consumer, new generation owners began to open niche or specialty businesses that targeted specific segments of the marketplace. For example, we saw Curves chasing the deconditioned female, Planet Fitness and its target market of the budget beginner, the emergence of the training facility, and the start of the yoga and Pilates businesses. In essence, you could have 10 different facilities in a market and all could claim to be chasing entirely different segments of the marketplace.

The vertical market appeal of this new generation of club works against the "everything to everyone" business model that most of the large boxes are built on. You might have a strong performance center at 6,000 square feet open directly across the street from a box club and thrive because that owner is only chasing about 300 members, which usually represents the top tiers of the box club's membership.

In other words, the training club stripped a vertical segment from the box operator—one of the many he needed to keep his box full of members. Another way to think of this is that the box player depends on a wide variety of members, representing a wide range of segments, to stay in business.

In the fitness business, you don't fail because someone new opened down the street and took all your members. In this business, it is more likely that you ran naked through a field of rose bushes and then died slowly over four years from a thousand small cuts. The cuts in this morbid example are inflicted by a dozen small competitors, which open in your market area and then drain your box of 10 to 20 members at a time by stripping you of your segments. For example, that new small performance center didn't kill you. He just took 30 of your top-end members who want a better training environment.

It is also important to reference again that this 6,000-square-foot club with only 300 members might generate the same revenue or greater than the box player across the street with 2,000 members or more and the smaller training club/performance center can do this with less start-up costs, less monthly expenses, and less risk.

All this leads to a new paradigm in the marketplace where more is determined by less. The strongest analogy is the computer. Most young tech people forget this, but even as recently as the 1960s, a computer that cannot even do most of the functions of a new iPad® was a massive wall of connected units that would fill very large rooms with floor-to-ceiling individual parts that were each the size of the average family refrigerator.

Programmers sat at a console that would be bigger than Donald Trump's ego-driven desk and stuffed thousands of paper cards into the units that told the computer what to do. All the technology we now take for granted—and that can now fit into the palm of our hands—once filled a small house and even then couldn't work as fast or handle any of the tech demands we now assume are a routine part of life.

We are at the same crossroads now in the fitness business. In this case, the large box clubs represents the 1960s computer and functional training represents the state-of-the-art technology that fits into a small space. Put another way and more directly, we can now get better results from more clients by using a third of the space and less than a tenth of the equipment we used to demand. There is simply no need for the big box equipment mind-set anymore. The consumer doesn't need it, trainers don't support it, and the banks hesitate to finance it.

Cardio is the exception here and most current trainers use cardio much more efficiently than we have in the past. Instead of the endlessly long, slow walk to nowhere, most progressive facility owners and their teams are coaching the tread and other key pieces as a tool to support your overall training and most are encouraging some variation of high-intensive interval training as a more effective way to get into shape.

Is equipment, mostly referring to the single-joint, fixed-plane mind-set, going away completely? No, of course not, but what we put into effective clubs now will be totally different from what we have done in the past. There will still be fixed equipment, but most of it will be functional cable-driven tools. There will still be free weights, but most of the isolated bodybuilding equipment will be replaced with rack systems and other tools that allow the client to get a full-body workout.

Everything changes, so why not in the fitness business? The tech we embraced for so many years simply isn't viable anymore for the consumer or the club owner, although the club owner will in most cases be the last person to understand that concept. The box club concept could survive but only if the owners of these chains or individual units start the transformation from a 1995 model to a training-centric, results-driven idea.

The next generation club will be radically different from what we have seen in the past. The following sections present some ideas as to what has to happen in design and concept for the industry to match the needs and the wants of the new generation client.

The new perfect size will be 6,000 to 10,000 square feet, with somewhere between 300 to 900 members.

Everything in this facility will exist to get results for the member. Ideally, there will be a next generation turf area tough enough to push and pull sleds on as well as flip tires and big enough for groups to do dynamic warm-ups. This club will also have a large rubberized area that can handle ball slams and kettlebells, lots of overhead devices and racks for suspension training and pull-ups, open space for large groups and small groups, perhaps a closed area of about 1,200 square feet where you can do large group training and blast music, and two high-end locker rooms.

The next generation of this model will also have to have a top-end design feel. The days of the dungeon concept are gone, and while the club has to feel nice, it also has to have a functional feel on the floor coupled with a little pampering in the support areas. Leading this charge into the next generation is Rudy Fabiano, an architect known through the years for his big box designs but who is now the leading theorist behind the advent of the perfect small club concept.

Larger box clubs—meaning those over 20,000 square feet—will have to "think small."

This means that the mind-set has to shift away from basing your entire business plan on chasing endless volume and working toward seeking a higher return per member. To do this, these operators will have to change virtually everything that goes into the box, such as equipment choices, layout, membership support options, and programming.

The key will be open space. Are these owners willing to eliminate a third of their equipment and replace it with open floor supported by kettlebells, sleds, tires, ropes, and rack systems? Will these owners be willing to take out the giant dumbbells and all the other 1995 free weight equipment that was designed for a generation of members that does not exist anymore or, if you still have this membership, that represents a very small segment of the client population?

The smaller footprint clubs will also change the market.

This class of performance club will have to be at least 3,000 square feet, but it could be a training-centric club, cycle-based, or mind/body. The early generation of training studio is also dying and is no longer a viable business plan. The concept of just shrinking a gym into a small training club by cramming in Smith machines and other leftovers has been replaced with the need to do personal group training and to service members in some sort of group fashion. This new format will be heavily segment driven and can make money on 150 members.

As the definition of fitness changes, all clubs will have to keep evolving.

Eventually—meaning in the coming decade—many of the folks currently supporting the low-priced clubs as members will come to realize that without a strong support system, there are no results. Do-it-yourself fitness isn't going to catch on except for the most dedicated fringe, who have always found their own way and who are most likely responsible for driving change in the industry anyway. For example, many of the best athletes break through at some point because a trainer invents a new way to get more out of the athlete, which eventually spills back to the average training client down the line.

The key here is that the realities of the current world we live in will help force this change. At some point, the culture will shift from the acceptance of 63 percent of the population being obese or overweight to a national demand for change. This is already happening as illustrated by Michelle Obama and her national crusade for health and nutrition during her husband's years as president. Need will drive change and the consumer will seek education and support and, therefore, results, as opposed to just renting a treadmill for a few bucks a month.

We have to move away from the membership and workout mind-set into a lifestyle support system.

One of the biggest mistakes we have made as an industry has been to teach consumers that fitness is an hour at the club and that we don't really care about any other part of their lives. There have, of course, been dedicated owners and trainers who go beyond the membership an hour at a time model, but they are few and far between in the industry as a whole.

For fitness to work and for us to make significant changes in the culture in this country, we need to seek a holistic approach that addresses all aspects of the client's journey. In this case, holistic does not refer to a new age herb-and-mind approach but rather working with the client as a complete entity addressing his fitness, nutrition, and lifestyle.

If we want to make this work, all fitness facilities will have to develop a wider range of tools than we now use. Internally, fitness facilities will have to provide complete nutrition support, probably built into the membership rather than an add-on for pay, along with specialty support, such as smoking cessation, back care, and aging. Many clubs have tried all this for years, but the penetration rate into the membership is always restricted because the clubs depend on the member actually showing up.

Next generation clubs can eliminate this and reach their entire membership by providing all this online as part of the membership. For example, the major nutrition companies in the industry already offer nutrition support online and it is possible to get online access for an entire membership for a flat fee for the club per month. Other support tools, such as cooking demonstrations or a wellness talk, can live on the website and be available to all members as part of their membership at the club.

It is important to note that the standard membership tool that has been so popular for so long in the industry may not be the way to attract the broadest base of members in the future. Short-term extended course format tools, such as a 90-day all-inclusive package based on a theme (such as a loser campaign or a totally fit in 90 days plan), attract people who never respond to any type of regular membership offer. Simply put, people don't want a membership to a gym. They want a solution to a problem.

Smaller clubs that have fewer members but charge more per member will be better able to deliver this newer model than a typical club that depends on memberships and volume as the core of their business plan.

If you have been in the business for a long time, then most of this sounds like science fiction—up there with flying cars and cities under the ocean—but the training performance centers have already set much of this in motion. They have proven as an industry segment that you can generate a big gross, create higher-than-average profits, and make changes in your membership in space that would fit into the locker rooms of the giant box players.

It is important to note that this change is coming from the bottom up. As noted elsewhere in this book, information and technology that used to take years to seep into mainstream fitness is now available within minutes through the Web. This ability to create change in a large number of clients and the business system that drives it is starting as a groundswell in the performance centers and smaller fitness facilities that once depended on memberships as the key to success.

Due to their heavy investment in infrastructure and self-interest in perpetuating their business model, the box players will be the last to change—if they ever do. Predictably, most will fail rather than change. It is a lot like imagining a meeting of the last dinosaurs: "No, really, we are right and don't need to adapt and those silly little creatures covered in skins won't last. How can anything that small hurt monsters like us. Be patient, man, we are coming back." These guys should have asked the same question the chains should today: "If what we are doing isn't working anymore, then what should we be doing to ensure we will survive?"

Applying this material to your business

Consider the following:

- Is your business driven by memberships? Move from the membership model toward the training-centric model.
- If you are expanding, is your business plan based on past success from a different era or based on the reality of the marketplace as it exists now? Make sure your new business reflects the industry as it exists today.
- What can you do in your current facility to start individualizing the process for the member? What can you do to get more members grounded into training somewhere in your model?
- What can you add to your website that offers member support as part of a membership? Retention is involvement and every member who touches your site will often stay longer and pay longer.

Summary

Question everything you do and consider doing in the future. Is it logical? Is it based on real numbers and not a story told to you at a convention or trade show? Does it make sense in today's marketplace with a more sophisticated and aware potential member? If you can't make it work on a spreadsheet, then it probably won't ever work in a real business.

We are also going through a major transition in the industry. Opening a mainstream box club will become a continually more difficult thing in the future due to increased costs and increased and ever-changing competition. The advent of functional training into the clubs, along with the ascension of the trainer, has also forced us to rethink what a club should be.

Most clubs are designed as just newer versions of an already outdated business plan. These "new" clubs are often in reality just a better-painted version of what everyone built in 1995 during the glory years of the fitness business. In the future, the emphasis will shift toward smaller training-centric gyms designed to maximize the results for the maximum amount of members in the system rather than just being a box membership mill designed to turn and burn membership numbers. Low-priced competitors and the sheer volume of new fitness businesses in most markets have ended the easy days in the financial industry, which forces you to run a real business based on forward thinking rather than trying to force your business to be successful using tools that have been outdated for more than 30 years.

January 16, 2014
A good plan now is worth more than a perfect plan never.

Classic overthinkers can kill any good idea by trying to make it perfect, but there is no perfect plan—only your ability to get started and then adapt the plan to the reality at hand. I have seen people trying to open their own businesses spend years thinking about and building the perfect gym on paper and yet this gym is never built. I have also seen someone with a good idea, a decent plan, and a willingness to commit make a million a year chasing the dream. Many of you overthink your career, your businesses, and even your relationships and this overthinking leads to inaction and failure by simply freezing in time. Movement in life is everything and waiting for the perfect time to do anything means most of what you want will never get done. If it is your passion, then chase it until you earn it. If it makes you happy, then you probably should be doing it. If it makes you unhappy, then run away and remember life is too short to waste a day being miserable. Life in many ways isn't complicated. It's avoiding the meaningful decisions in life that makes it seem so much harder than it really is.

December 9, 2013
Absolutely correct can mean absolutely wrong

At some point, being absolutely correct means you are absolutely wrong. Evolving professionally means that at some point, much of what you have spent so much time learning over the last decade just no longer works. Look at the trainers who grew up in the bodybuilding era who laugh and snicker at the "fools" using kettlebells. One day, they were experts and then they couldn't understand why Monday was no longer National Chest Day in every gym in America. This is especially true once you collect a lot of initials after your name. It is hard to admit that the information you learned attending a $2,000 weekend certification three years ago that fired your ass up for months might now be proven out of date and even dangerous. If you want to be a master trainer, you have to know when to let go, and if you ever find yourself laughing at some new method of training, it just might dawn on you that you are now the problem and no longer the solution.

2

Nothing Lasts Forever in the Fitness Industry

There is a natural progression to all business. The new business is created, it grows, and it peaks, and if the owner is any good, this now productive enterprise is recreated and the progression begins again. If the owner isn't any good, the business will peak, the decline begins, and someone's dream fades away.

The catalyst that drives this change is competition. In this country, if what you are doing doesn't work quickly, you die quickly. Other parts of the world have a huge advantage in that the intense competition we see here hasn't hit yet—and the emphasis is on the word yet. Competition forces you to get better in the game or to get out of the game and any small business will usually only be as good as the competition dictates. Fat and happy businesses can survive for years and then fade overnight once a new competitor hits the marketplace. What works in a vacuum for these owners will not always work when you are banging heads against three or four other motivated owners chasing the same potential clients.

For example, in Australia, it is not unusual to only have one or two gyms in a town of 50,000 people and the owners who are competing there will often have the appearance of a "gentlemen's agreement" where each one stakes out a different side of town. In theory, they compete, but in reality, they are far enough apart that both of them can survive over time.

This type of limited competition does not promote change or growth in the product we offer the clients. Why change what you are doing if you don't have any type of financial impetus to do so? As the old saying goes: "If it ain't broke, why fix it?"

Intense competition changes all this. Add four or five new competitors to that same market who open a block away from you and now all hell breaks loose in those old businesses. The old owners now have the immediate choice of either updating their business platform or losing market share and the revenues that go with those lost clients.

Here, it is not uncommon for a single gym to have 20 or more competitors in a five-mile ring around the club and there are markets that exist now that have more than 100 fitness options in a seven-mile competitive ring. You have to question everything you do to survive with this much competition, and if you aren't willing to let go of what doesn't now work and replace those old ideas with ones that do now, your business will not be sustainable over time.

Again, competition forces you to either get good now or get out and leave room for those who are adapting to the new rules of fitness. Remember that old saying "The big eat the small"? This came from doing business in the 1950s in this country and it is no longer accurate, having been replaced with this new truth: "It's not the big that eat the small these days in business. It's the fast that eat the slow."

The problem is that if you ask those existing owners in those noncompetitive markets—who are happily making money prior to the arrival of those new competitors—about their business plan, they will tell you their model is perfect, anyone can do it, and they are business geniuses. It is very important to understand that everyone is a business genius when you have no competition because whatever you are doing will work because you are the only game in town. If you are the only shoe store in a town of 100,000 people, it doesn't matter how bad your service is, how dirty your store is, or how ugly your shoes are. You will sell shoes in this town because there is simply nowhere else to go for shoes.

The fitness industry started on a major upheaval around 2005. There is always a tipping point in any industry—and this industry is no exception to that proven rule of business. The tipping point we faced in this industry happened when the accumulation of a number of powerful drivers added up to the end of the commonly accepted, volume-driven business model we have used in the fitness business since the end of World War II. Simply put, the way the mainstream fitness players (the big box model) did business for more than 50 years just started to fail—not all at once but at a more insidious pace that didn't quite kill this approach to running a gym all at once but just merely wounded it badly and left in on the side of the road to slowly die.

Many owners in the industry don't even realize that their approaches to business stem all the way back to the era when their grandfathers were young men. You open a fitness business, take the system you used at the last place your worked or copy the big chain in town, and off you go. It is important to note that this business model was created in the era where there was very little competition in any market.

For example, in the mid-1960s, it was very common to only have one fitness facility in a town of several hundred thousand residents. All the old tools usually associated with this model, such as pressure sales, lead boxes, and no service, assumed that the client would eventually say: "What the hell—where else am I going to go if I want to join a gym? This is the only option for 20 miles." As stated earlier, the business system only has to rise to the degree of competition in the market, and if there isn't anyone driving you to change, you won't rise too high.

We also shouldn't forget that from 1945 through the mid-1990s were the golden years of growth in the fitness business. For example, owners in the 1980s were doing business in the decade where the average consumer was discovering fitness for the first time in our history and doing so in big numbers. Fitness in those days was newly cool, driven by Arnold Schwarzenegger, Jane Fonda, the dozens of aerobics shows on TV, the advent of the marathon boom, and the arrival in big numbers of the first chains with the California swank, such as Gold's Gym and World Gym. The fitness business was easy in that decade, as ascertained by the advent of so many national chains, the growth of the first big fitness equipment companies after the success of Nautilus, and a national awareness that being in shape, belonging to a gym, and wearing your Gold's T-shirt to the bar were elite things to do and that what was white hot in California must make me cool in Akron.

This business platform, using a volume approach as its basis, is fairly simple to explain. Remember that this method of operation is what most chain clubs and independent owners still use today and have since 1945, although each year is proving harder and harder for the owners and operators to make money using this approach. The following are the key elements you will find in every chain and most of the independent operations in the market. The exception to this model, of course, is the training gym that uses a training-centric business model, which will be discussed heavily throughout this revised edition:

- The standard volume-based business model works under the assumption that the client/member (*client* and *member* will be used interchangeably throughout this book) is replaceable. This is called the volume approach because you constantly have to replace the clients lost through attrition each month and the business model assumes that there is always enough new volume of potential clients to replace the ones that are lost. Keeping members—or member retention—wasn't that important to owners who built their clubs on this model beyond a vague general acknowledgement that they should be doing something in that part of the business because everyone knew that if this member left, he would simply be replaced by a new guy next month. Every operational system in the model was based on a simple progression of sell hard, don't worry if the client ever got any results, let him fail and leave in five to seven months, and then move on to the next sales cycle for the month.

- The return per member is low in this model. For example, a club might show a rate for a single member as $39, but after discounts for students, older clients, families, corporate deals, price specials, and the typical salesperson making deals to just get a new membership that day, the real yield might only be around $27 to $32 per client served. In other words, the price is listed at $39 for a membership, but if you review the last 100 new memberships, you will find that the real average per sale is around $30 or so.

- It is all about the receivable base. There is only one real source of revenue in this model and that is the accumulated number of members paying their payments to the gym each month. Why create other revenue sources when this was all you had to do back in the day to make money? The receivable base—defined as all your members paying dues each month to belong to the club—was sustainable over an extended period of time because there were few competitors in the market to drain that resource. In other words, members would stay longer and pay longer given the fact that there was nowhere else to go. Even if the member drifted away from the gym, he often kept his membership going with the belief that he would eventually return.

- Marketing is always about price and is product driven. This means every ad featured the sale of the day, along with a list of your services. Remember that fitness was new to many people through the end of the last century. If you were newly exposed to fitness and wanted that aerobics class you just read about, clubs advertising classes would draw people. Don't forget the genius theory here stating that any owner who has a business but not competition is always a genius because whatever he does will work. Price ads worked not because they were effective marketing but because the client had limited choices in the market. In other words, we taught ourselves that price-driven specials, such as 50 percent off the joiner's fee, were highly effective tools in our arsenal rather than understanding that any type of ad would work in this time period.

- There were limited other sources of revenue in these businesses. Every club had drink coolers, sold T-shirts, tried tanning, and offered limited personal training, but even the combination of all these done well was a pale comparison to the power of a receivable base built on several thousand members paying $49 a month. Most owners who practice this method of business dabbled in other avenues of revenue, but few mastered any because the focus of the managers and the entire team was to generate as much gross membership sales that month as possible and then do it again next month and every month after that for as long as you can.

- Fitness facilities were defined by the amount of equipment they offered. The more equipment you could cram into a space, the better you were perceived by your competitors and the marketplace.

- The offerings were—and still are—limited. For example, a typical gym based on this model even today really does nothing more than sell a membership, giving access to the equipment or classes it offers. These 1995-model-based businesses—the peak of the fitness era for this type of operation—offer nothing more than equipment rental, called *memberships*, classes that vary according to the current trend, personal training, which has an national penetration rate in all these businesses of about 3 to 6 percent, and the occasional pampering service, including spa or tanning. The stuff in the boxes might be newer and fresher, the equipment might be this year's version, and the classes might reflect this year's hottest trends, but basically, everything being sold today is not much different than gyms in the 1950s or the 1980s. You still pay a monthly fee to practice do-it-yourself fitness unless you pay a little extra for your own coach. The rest is fluff that is supposedly there to make the sale easier and to keep the member around a little longer.

Why Is This Method Now Failing?

There are a number of reasons why this business model is failing in today's market and why it will completely fail in the future at some point, but we will look at the six simplest drivers of change first.

Change is being driven from the bottom up.

In the pre-Internet days in fitness, major changes always came from the top down. If you wanted to learn something new in business or get new ideas, you packed up your stuff and spent several days at a national convention, attending seminars or hanging out in the bar networking. Perhaps the perfect example of this information transfer system was when a major chain of the 1980s sent a speaker to a national trade show and he told the audience of his company's move away from contracts into just open-ended memberships (the members have no contacts obligation and just pay month to month, with a few minor restrictions). The speaker gave a detailed history of why it made this decision and raved about the success it had using this system with members. Imagine being the first to tell the potential member that he wouldn't have to sign a contract to join this club when every other gym in the country was using long-term memberships as its base tool.

The problem was that the speaker and the chain had only been using this system for a relatively short period of time, meaning that all the data and research as to the effectiveness of this system was pretty shallow. However, this didn't stop everyone from copying the move to no contracts. In fact, the years after this debut, there were literally dozens of speakers at the trade shows talking about how to implement this change. It is always important to remember that speakers need something to speak about, and if you don't have depth or real information, the people wanting to make a name—and therefore get consulting contracts—will pound the hottest topic as their own.

Within five years, most of the minor chains and independent clubs had switched to this method, but then five years after that peak, most owners had returned to a combination of contracts (for stability) and open-ended memberships. The information came from the top, was taught at a tradeshow, filtered down into the mainstream, peaked, and then flattened. The entire process from inception to routine took about 7 to 10 years to cycle through the industry.

Some people lead and most others follow and it is easy to get thousands of owners to follow when someone stands on the podium and swears he has the answer to solve all your sales problems. However, the truth was that there was no real advantage to this method at all and you could easily gain any of the supposed advantages by just offering contracts at a slightly lower price than open ended and let the clients decide.

The same path existed in the training world information cycle prior to the Internet. You went to a national show as a strength coach or advanced trainer, someone would present some research on a new training method, you tried it on your people, you presented your results at another show, and off the information went, eventually ending up at the working trainer level, where he would use it on his clients. Again, from inception and presentation at the first show to the daily use by a working trainer could take 7 to 10 years. In both cases, the information came from the top down and took years to disseminate.

Then came the Internet. Now someone can simply post a business concept or new training tip on social media, and by tomorrow, every operator or trainer in every free country in the world has a chance to see the information and implement it into his business the same day.

The important thing to note here in the current era of fitness is that trainers are the ones driving change the fastest. Current training theory is so radically different from what traditional fitness businesses have allowed in their operations during the last several decades that trainers and clients are seeking alternatives outside the commonly accepted norm. In other words, if you just did a group workout with 10 other people running, playing, pulling sleds, shaking ropes, and flipping tires, that old circuit training thing at your local big box gym now looks pretty damn boring.

Keep in mind that the client doesn't even have to actually do this type of working out to begin to hate his gym. He comes home from work, grabs a beer, flips on the sports channel, and catches an interview with his favorite player, who is shown flipping tires, pulling sleds, swinging kettlebells, and doing a hundred other moves not offered unless you pay the big bucks to get access to the special space in the back of the club where all the top secret stuff is kept locked up by the trainers. Even the traditional bodybuilding magazines have grudgingly started to show this type of training and the newer fitness magazines show nothing but functional-based, full-body training.

The issue is that the mainstream clubs are simply too slow to react and lost their edge to the smaller training gyms, which offer nothing but the type of movement and training this generation's clients want. The mainstream players will at some point have to embrace the idea that what they offer to the consumer is outdated by about 40 years, but that change will be slow and many will fail, clinging to old ideas rather than quickly changing the course of their businesses. Change is coming too quickly—and not from the chains that have always liked to dictate change rather than accept it—and this is opening up opportunity for anyone willing to move quickly and away from the traditional training model.

We are leaving the era of emotion and moving into the era of reason.

It is sad to admit, but for decades, almost everything we believed to be true in the business of fitness and the business of training has been based on unproven, emotionally driven information.

On the business side, we used such tools as 24-month contracts for decades, but we really never had the sophistication or business tools, such as advanced computer analysis, that allowed operators to know if this tool was effective and that we should be using it in our businesses. Emotionally and even logically, long-term commitments make sense. If you have to go through the entire sales process, why not sell the guy a long-term commitment and just tie him up in the system longer than just going for a year's membership?

But the industry did progress and now we have the tracking ability and statistical analysis to determine if indeed this is the best tool to be using as the foundation of our pricing and collection system, which in fact we now know that long-term commitments don't track as effective as using 12-month contracts due to the extremely larger loss rates associated with the tool. Owners in the industry felt emotionally for more than four decades that longer was better for the business, but now it can be proven in minutes that the emotional attachment to this business tool will not stand up to reason under scrutiny.

The same is true in the training world. If you want to get in shape, it is no longer what you believe as a trainer that matters nor how emotionally attached to the training you learned in school or when you won that bodybuilding show 20 years ago. It is now about what works and what doesn't and the research is there to prove it either way.

This also relates to the point earlier stating change comes from the bottom up rather than flowing from the top down. The consumer now has the same access to this information through direct access to the coaches themselves who write and post about all the new research the day they read it or create it. This access allows the consumer to demand newer training methods, newer equipment, and a different business approach from the mainstream players.

The mainstream players may fight this change and deny that the industry is moving back to results driven and what works for the consumer, but once you open the Pandora's box of research, there isn't much room left for the emotional baggage of the 1980s. In fairness, an owner who has a million dollars of fixed equipment on the floor or an equipment company that manufactures that circuit line that may not be as effective at making change in the consumer as their catalogues suggest is not going to give up easily, but this doesn't make the reality go away. It just means the fight will take longer than it should.

The cannibals are eating the cannibals.

Every decade brings a new terror to the industry. The first big chains breed fear into every independent operator and yet nothing catastrophic happened to them and life went on in the business. We also had the advent of the circuit clubs and the magazines and pundits at the trade shows spreading the doom and gloom that this was the secret and everyone better get into the 30-minute circuit world or you would be eaten alive by the new megachain. Again, nothing happened beyond a few thousand owners adding cheap circuit lines to their gyms and a few later dumped them and even the mega 30-minute chain that started it all is barely alive these days.

There was also the open-ended business phase as described earlier: the biweekly membership program that allowed you to grab an extra payment a year from your members and let's not forget the enhancement fee—a very sleazy way to grab an extra chunk of money each year from your membership in the name of getting new equipment, but in reality, this one-time-a-year grab usually resulted in nothing more than a new car for the owner. All these can't-live-without ideas came and all failed to radically change the fitness world. It is fair to say that each idea did force a lot of mediocre owners to at least do something in their businesses, but none of these or the others that always overpromised and yet underdeliver changed the nature of the business for an extended period of time.

The hybrid of sequence of the latest and greatest trends was the arrival of the low-price value players or, put more simply, the $10 membership guys who stripped the clubs of most service and amenities and finally admitted that it is really all about renting treads and nothing more.

The reason we can refer to this business approach as a hybrid is that its effect on the business was lasting—but not in any kind of good way. The low-priced players just stood up and screamed the childhood fable loudly enough for everyone to hear: The emperor has no clothes. For those of you who had sheltered childhoods, this fable was about a king who walked around naked proudly, exhibiting the illusion he was wearing clothes. The peasants were so terrified of him that they all agreed that his new clothes were the finest and most amazing in the kingdom. Finally, one brave—or perhaps terminally stupid—subject yells "The emperor has no clothes" and the illusion was shattered for all the rest.

What this loose interpretation of the old tale can teach us is that the low-priced players—just by charging $10 or so a month—were able to finally unveil that despite all the posturing and screaming of unfairness that followed the national rollout of this business concept, it really came down to the fact that for thousands of gyms, all they really did was exactly the same thing for $49 a month that the low-priced guys were now offering for $10. Despite their protests in all the available forums, most mainstream gym owners had enjoyed competition-free years of being able to get away with doing the same thing they now screamed was unfair competition and that was operating for the most part all by offering no real service nor any other advantage for $49 that couldn't be done equally as well at $10.

This did change the market for several years and overall forced prices down into the basement in most major metro areas. But then a funny thing happened on the way to the bank for these players. If you go first and get a huge lead, you can't wreak havoc in the market. For example, if you take an average deconditioned weekend runner and throw him into the Boston Marathon, he can win if he has a 20-mile head start. However, this analogy fails when we take away the finish line. If the race just keeps going, the fast will run down the slow every time if the course is long enough.

In the world of the low-priced players, one chain had a major lead, got all the attention, and had a five-year or so advantage. Success, though, breeds imitators, and when the second wave of $10 operators came, a surprising thing happened: The next generation of cheap gyms didn't really hurt the remaining mainstream players, who mostly had adapted and learned how to compete against the value guys, but the new version of cheap did do a lot to crush the other cheap gyms. In other words, the cannibals that feasted on the weak players in the early days of the cheap gyms were now finding that their business models had spawned their own competitors. The circle was complete and the cannibals were now eating the cannibals.

The industry is still changing from the surge of these clubs, but their true legacy is that the sheer number of low-priced imitators in the market is forcing everyone else to question his own business plan, but the one most people are using is based on the volume-driven, everyone-is-replaceable concept that has been with us for so many years.

Group exercise is declining.

Group exercise is important in the old volume model because you can service a large number of clients rather cheaply while still being able to charge $49 a month or higher in the market. There are two major factors that changed this. First of all, most clubs have either lowered their price or, at the least, not raised it for a number of years. Secondly, as the price for the membership that included group exercise went down, the cost of running a program steadily increases every year.

The decline of group exercise is a derivative of the rise of the low-priced model. Group exercise programs are expensive for most owners to operate and most owners in past years have included all group exercise as part of the gym's base membership. This is a workable system when you are charging $49 per month, but when you try to offer a full program of 60 classes a week or more and then lower your membership price to $29 or less, this gets to be a tougher business venture.

There are exceptions to this rule. For example, there have been a limited number of small chains that offer a modified group programming and yet only charge $19 per month per member. If you operate in dense markets, such as Connecticut or parts of California, you can sometimes make this work.

Keep in mind that the key number to understand about operating a group exercise program is the penetration rate or how many members participate in the group programming each day. The magic number to look for is 20 percent, which means that on a typical Monday at a club with 500 member check-ins, 100 of the 500 attend group exercise of some sort.

Cycling has always been part of the group programming, but at the time this is written, group exercise is re-emerging as a stand-alone offering that better fits a separate classification in the gym. Cycling has always been the renegade child of group exercise. When cycle was first introduced, it was a premium offering that club owners charged extra for in their gyms. Then, it became somewhat of a commodity where it was given to the group exercise people and downgraded to just another class on another given day.

However, cycling has managed to keep coming back due to the group dynamic, the effectiveness of the exercise itself, and serious coaches taking it away from the group exercise people—where the product was diluted—and remaking it as a serious foundational tool for functional training practitioners. Group should have always remained with the coaching staff and perhaps a big mistake the industry made was diluting cycling to the point where you couldn't charge extra for it. All this means is that if traditional group exercise does continue to decline, cycle will most likely end up back where it started as a premium offering for an extra charge.

However, the facts mentioned earlier are still important. What you could charge for group programming dropped while the cost of offering the program went up, making it difficult for many owners to continue to justify offering a full range of classes.

There are also a number of other factors that forced the decline of group exercise nationwide, including the following:

- *There has been a steady decline of usage in many mainstream clubs for a number of years.* The key is that as group personal training/team training has increased—offered either at the owner's own gym or by the competition—the number of participants in group exercise is slowly eroding.

- *The average instructor is aging and becoming harder to replace.* Where oh where have all the old aerobic queens gone? The national average age for instructors is rising simply due to the fact that the skill set acquired by a generation of instructors, who grew up in the glory days of group exercise/ aerobics, is somewhat of a dying art form. Every year, there are fewer instructors still on the circuit with fewer replacements being groomed.

- *The members who do group exercise are usually older too.* We are talking about traditional group exercise in this case and not newer programming, such as yoga. Often, the participants of the group have been doing it for years and will do it until they are too old to go to the gym. Aerobics was their thing. Many most likely lost weight when they were seriously involved and many of the long-term participants just want nothing to do with the rest of the offerings of the gym. The problem with this is that there aren't enough new members coming to this style of programming to replace the older ones who will eventually fade away.

- *The next generation of young women coming into the industry want to be trainers, not group exercise people.* There was a certain status to being a group exercise instructor back in the glory days. Classes in the 1980s and early 1990s were often the centerpiece of the club and the best instructors enjoyed good pay and a strong following of fans. Now there isn't much status left in being a group exercise instructor. Keep in mind that up until around the year 2000, women were mainly seen as second-class citizens in the gyms. If you were female, you worked the counter, were an instructor, or sold memberships, but up until the start of the new century, women were very underrepresented as owners and managers in the business. The status for a female breaking into a traditionally testosterone world was limited to being a super salesperson or being the star group instructor in the gym. Today, the status for many young women is being a trainer and most statistics show that women are almost equal in number to the male trainers in the industry and are putting up serious numbers as owners, breaking way beyond the 3 percent or so of women who owned gyms prior to the year 2000.

- *The return on investment died in group programming.* Group exercise is a hard thing to justify financially as an owner in today's market. Owners are expected to include group exercise as part of the membership and pay the instructors virtually the same in most markets as they do their trainers, and for all this, you are most likely generating less revenue from these added expenses. There is simply no return on investment left in group programming in most markets. Some owners do attempt to fight back. Pricing will be discussed at a much deeper level later in this book, but for now, it is important to note that many owners have destructured their memberships in the hope of offsetting the additional expense of offering programming. In this example, an owner might offer a base membership to the gym, called simple access, where a client would pay $19 for the right to use the cardio and weight equipment but have access to nothing else. If this person wants group exercise and the owner who does this is trying to maintain that 20 percent group usage rate by his membership, then the client might pay $39 for access to group exercise, effectively passing some of the increased cost of the program to the clients who use it regularly. (Note that it is either $19 or $39, not $19 plus $39.)

The decline of group exercise invokes changes from several angles. First of all, group exercise used to be a tool that separated clubs from one another. If an owner had a strong group program, he had a strong differentiator in the marketplace. Now group has very limited strength as something that will vastly separate you from the other owners offering group exercise. Keep in mind the fact that there are fewer instructors in the market and many clubs in a market actually share instructors who work at all the clubs in their areas that offer programming. How different can one club's program be from another if both have the same instructors doing the teaching?

Secondly, group exercise just isn't the bait for memberships that it once was. As the penetration rates slip below 20 percent for most clubs, it becomes much more expensive to continue to market and support programs that more than 80 percent of your membership doesn't use or want. These factors are forcing owners to take a different look at what once used to be a foundational tool for any mainstream fitness business.

Traditional one-on-one training has flatlined.

Anything you offer to a client in your business that is only accepted by 3 to 6 percent of your customers is hard to declare as a success and any normal businessperson would question the value of that product over time and either try to improve the number of clients who use it or change the price structure and hope more people buy into it. In the fitness business, personal training is this product, and after more than 60 years of trying, the national average of people paying for personal training in a mainstream box gym is only 3 to 6 percent of the club's total membership. In other words, after more than six decades of promoting this product, we still can't get over 6 percent of a gym's membership to pay for help we all know they need.

Club owners have tried just about everything to drive up the percentage of members paying for training, but nothing has worked consistently across the board for the majority of clubs. Owners have tried to lower the price based on the number of sessions the client buys, which proved a great way to devalue the trainer. Is the trainer a $75-an-hour trainer or is he really a $50-an-hour trainer if you buy five sessions at $250 or maybe he is really a $40-an-hour trainer if you buy 10 sessions at $400? The product couldn't be sold at the regular price, so the owners, not realizing that the goal is to create a team of highly skilled professional trainers, simply lowered the price in hopes that discounting would attract a wider range of clients. It didn't move the needle beyond the 3 to 6 percent national average.

Other owners tried to cut the time—and therefore the price—to make it more attractive and the 30-minute training session was born. If you can't sell an hour at a reasonable price, then cut the time and price and hope there is a new clientele out there that was just waiting for this version. This did not work either and the national average stayed at about 3 to 6 percent of the club's membership paying for training.

The real issue is that the product itself is flawed. There are simply not enough members in any mainstream club who want to buy this product. The following are three reasons it is a hard sell:

- *Personal training is too much of an elite product.* Price is relative to the marketplace. You might see training sold for $30 an hour in Iowa and $150 per hour in New York, but in reality, the price is the same in both markets and mainstream gyms using personal training as their primary training solution will still stall their numbers at 3 to 6 percent of the membership base. Personal training based on hourly rates only appeals to a limited number of wealthy people in a given community. The price in this case—be it $30 or $150—is really the same price because it is based on the maximum a gym can charge for the product based on the affluence matrix in the market. The affluence matrix is just a nice way of saying there are a lot more people who don't make enough money to afford nice watches, big houses, and sleek European cars than there are ones who can buy these images of wealth and the top money people in any market is still a smaller number of the total population as a whole. Personal training in most markets is a display of wealth because we are not just looking at $150 per hour in New York for training, but we are looking at the fact that the client is paying more than $1,000 per month if he trains a couple times a week. It is not the hourly rate that is the barrier in training. It is the total sum of money it takes to be with a trainer for the month that is the absolute limiter of how much training can be sold in any market.

- *Personal training is boring.* If someone spends a year training with the same trainer, you have usually moved beyond a trainer/client relationship into a modified friendship. This client has heard every story the trainer has and the trainer knows more about this person's life than he ever really wanted to know. Training becomes boring because the intensity drops, as it does in almost any relationship, and as the intensity drops, so do the results in many cases. Even master trainers who strive to do the right thing every time with a client will have a difficult time keeping up the needed intensity for any given period of time. The result is that as the intensity drops, the results drop, and as the results drop, the client moves on. Yes, there are cases where clients stay with trainers for years, but overall, the long-term keep rate of any trainer will fade the longer he is with the same clients.

- *People want and thrive with a group dynamic.* Doing fitness in groups drives higher results. Group workouts give you a sense of light competition or heavy depending on the coach and system and more energy from the synergy of the participants and, most importantly, group situations allows the participants to build relationships among themselves, which is a key to long-term member retention.

The key financial aspect of a flatlined personal training component in a gym is that the training fees really haven't risen much in a decade, whereas the cost of the trainer has continually inched higher. Owners in the past could count on an approximate 40 percent or so net from their training revenues, but this number is often less than 20 percent net in many mainstream clubs. This slow erosion of profits from personal training has led to owners just farming out their entire training department to outside training companies, therefore giving up an chance of profits, or the owners turn to alleged independent contracts who pay rent or give splits of the fees to the club.

One-on-one training just can't be fixed and there isn't much that can be done to drive up those numbers after so much history of trying, but what if the 3 to 6 percent is correct and the owners just need to add a wider variety of products to the offering sheet that offer more price points and appeal to a wider target market? This is the premise of the training-centric business model that will be discussed throughout this book.

The microgym has become more popular.

Microgyms are the strongest parts of a typical gym done separately. For example, cycle studios, mind and body, and personal training are all usually strong parts of a mainstream box gym, but the trend now is to open stand-alone studios in the marketplace specializing in each one of these activities.

Microgyms were big in the 1980s, with the first-generation aerobics studios and eventually the first stand-alone cycle gyms. As aerobics faded in the early 1990s—to be replaced with the birth of group exercise around 2000—the microgym faded away temporarily. Personal training gyms were out there in that decade, but they were usually small and very ineffective because at the time, those businesses were nothing more than shrunken mainstream gyms. Functional training, accompanied by new generation functional equipment, hadn't yet arrived. Therefore, the early generation training gyms were small, cramped places based on a very limited one-on-one clientele.

The microgym trend is here to stay this time for many reasons. Most importantly, there are just too many different types now to fade as a group. Besides cycle and traditional mind/body, you can now add the small franchise gyms (again, just shrunken mainstream gyms), martial arts–based gyms, boxing gyms, a dozen variations of yoga, rock climbing gyms, and even free running academies. There is now a huge range of possible options, and even if one or two die, there are just too many to kill them all off.

The jewel of this crown is the hybrid training gym, which at about 6,000 to 7,500 square feet is probably the highest return per square foot in the industry. These are relatively cheap to build, fit into space the mainstream guys can't take, and return a profit of about 40 percent pre-tax. Why build a $4,000,000 mainstream box in rental space when you can build spend $400,000 to open a training gym and net the same amount of money? There will be much more on this model later in this book.

The microgyms are driving change in the traditional business model through the taking of the clients from the mainstream gyms. Members in the 24 to 40 age bracket are bored with mainstream gyms and would much prefer to be doing large group team training using functional equipment and were the first ones out the door when such gyms as CrossFit entered the market. The 35- to 55-year-old client started to leave a little later as traditional training gyms mastered the art of small group training and came to understand that a lot of people out there would like to share the cost of the trainer rather than get stuck in the endless cycle of one-on-one training.

In other words, all the microgyms started to drain off the better members in the gym, meaning the ones who usually paid more for the additional offerings.

Pareto's Principle and What It Means to the Fitness Industry

In 1906, Vilfredo Pareto, an Italian engineer, noted that 80 percent of the property in Italy was owned by 20 percent of the people. Later in the century, a business management consultant named Joseph Juran coined the term Pareto's Principle, or, as it is also known, the Law of the Vital Few.

Everyone probably knows this principle as the 80/20 Rule and there isn't probably anyone over 21 years old who hasn't had someone tell him that "80 percent of your sales income will come from 20 percent of your clients." This rule has become so common and applied to so many different ideas that it has almost become a nonsensical term that people just throw out in a conversation because it sounds good. However, this principle still has a lot of life to it and the Law of the Vital Few definitely applies to what is happening in the fitness industry today.

The Law of the Vital Few is a way of saying that a small segment of people in any population are statistically likely to have larger influence than the rest of the group. For example, at a country club, there might be 600 members, but there is always that group of 20 or so core members who drive the events, complain the most about the services, sit on all the committees, and, in general, exert far more control at the club than their small number would logically dictate.

This is also true in mainstream fitness facilities. The Law of the Vital Few applied in that type of business states that there is a small number of clients who contribute a very large portion of the club's monthly revenue. For example, a typical box chain gym might have 3,000 members, but only 5 percent of this total population would pay for personal training. You could also add in another 5 percent or so of the total group, giving you a working total of 10 percent, or 300 clients, who support additional cost programming, such as Pilates, massage, yoga, or other specialty workouts or services.

The average member in this type of club might pay $39 per month to be a member and buy one or two shakes a month and maybe a T-shirt. In other words, this guy might have a total revenue contribution of $75, which is most likely on the high end because so many of the members in this type of business just do their workout thing and go home, spending nothing beyond the basic membership.

Now look at the 10 percent who really drive the revenue. A typical member in that group might do eight training sessions a month at $400 (8 x $50), buy a shake each time she is in the gym, bring a guest, pay $69 extra for a boot camp weekend, and spend money on other extras, such as a spa or a massage. This client might spend $600 or more a month in the gym and will stay longer, pay longer, and contribute more over time than the regular member who is just there to do his own thing.

If this 10 percent of the membership, which is estimated in this example as 300 clients, only paid an average of $300 per month per member, then this group would contribute about $90,000 to the total revenue of this gym. If this gym has 3,000 clients and those clients each pay $39, then the total of all membership revenue would be $105,300 (2,700 clients paying $39 equals $105,300 per month not adjusted for losses).

Comparing the two categories, the 300-member group might spend $90,000 per month, with their $39 per month membership included, as opposed to the regular membership group of 2,700, who would only generate $105,300 in dues. Even giving this regular membership group the benefit of the doubt and adjusting their monthly contribution to $60 per member per month rather than just $39, we still only end up with $162,000 (2,700 x $60 per member spent per month).

Put another way, 300 clients spend $90,000 per month in this gym and the 2,700 regular clients might spend $162,000, assuming that every one of them is buying something extra each month, which in reality doesn't happen. This is a perfect example of the Law of the Vital Few in effect, where a small group of the entire population has a greater impact on the business than their numbers would logically dictate.

When the low-priced players entered the market, those type of facilities might take 3 to 7 percent of this sample gym's membership, which, while irritating, was not death inducing because that 3 to 7 percent came from the regular membership pile and even a full 7 percent might only account for a loss of revenue of $11,340 (2,700 x .07 = 189; 189 x $60 = $11,340). Again, $11,000 might be irritating, but it wouldn't take down this chain gym.

But what if a microgym, such as a 6,000-square-foot training gym, opened across the street and drained the 300 core members representing the Law of the Vital Few? This style of training gym appeals to the affluent, who want advanced training and are willing to pay for it. This type of gym also can do about $1,200,000 a year in gross revenue, with a net of 35-to 40 percent pretax, based on only 300 clients at maturity around the 18th month of operation. Thus, what happens if this new gym drains the core revenue producers from this mainstream box?

This is what is happening to this generation's chain or large independent player, and mostly, they don't know how to fight back. Remember that it is never one thing that takes down a business plan. It is a combination of different factors that come together to form the perfect storm. When things don't work in a business plan, most owners try to place the blame on only one particular factor rather than stepping back and questioning the entire plan.

For example, let's say that a national chain of 350 gyms starts recording a consistent downturn of 30 percent in sales leads compared to the same periods last year. The management might punish the sales teams in the clubs for not doing enough cold calls or pushing hard enough for buddy referrals. This same management team might also fire its national marketing company or marketing vice president because whatever marketing the company is running obviously isn't working.

This process might be correct and there might be issues in these two areas. It could happen that there isn't enough sales training going on in the gyms and it could also be true that the current marketing isn't efficient. However, both of these approaches assume one common denominator: They assume that the business plan is correct and it is just an execution issue.

All the six factors listed earlier defined through Pareto's Principle point to another issue and that problem is that the business plan this type of fitness facility has been using for decades might be broken. The real problem in the chain example listed earlier is not marketing or sales training but rather the fact that no one wants to buy a pager in the era of the smartphone.

The chains could change the product they sell, how they sell it, and how they market it, but most likely, that will only happen after the beating occurs through the effect of all these combined factors. Put bluntly, the business model we have come to accept as standard issue for the industry is failing and it will take some time before the mainstream players realize what screaming truck ran over their dogs.

What Does the Next Generation Business Model Look Like?

Figure 2-1 represents the annual revenue from a typical mainstream metropolitan fitness facility that is about 10 years old. The business is profitable and does about an 8 percent pre-tax net, which is not great, but considering this unit has approximately 20 competitors in less than six miles, it is still holding its own. The owner does reinvest and the gym is decently maintained. This business also offers the usual mainstream programming, including group exercise.

Membership Revenue	Training Revenue
$960,000 a year in net membership income	$84,000 a year in training income
($80,000 x 12)	($7,000 x 12)

Figure 2-1. Annual revenue from a typical 10-year-old mainstream metropolitan fitness facility

This particular gym has about 2,200 members and has approximately 27,000 square feet. The numbers on the left represent the monthly membership revenue generated by those 2,200 members, which averages about $36 per month per member. The numbers on the right represent the training revenue generated by the portion of membership that participates in the gym's traditional one-on-one training model.

There are three important questions that need to be asked about the numbers on the left side of this chart. In other words, what does the $960,000 annual membership revenue really mean to this owner? Consider the following:

- *How much can you grow this number after 10 years of being in business?* If this owner did everything he could possibly do to grow this number, such as heavy marketing and advanced and intense sales training, how much could he really change the $960,000? If he were outrageously successful, he probably couldn't change it more than 5 percent in a year, which would take the $960,000 to $1,008,000 and the $80,000 per month gross membership revenue would increase to $84,000. Five percent represents a substantial increase, but over a year's period of time, this increase would only add about $50,000 to the total revenue of the gym. If you are locked into the high volume/low return per client business model, then chasing that $50,000 is your only option.

- *Can you sustain this number over time in a market that is still adding new competitors and currently has 20 other fitness options within six miles?* The owner has to go into his business with the realization that if there are 20 in the market now, there will be more coming later. The microgyms will find any major metro market, and while these businesses don't take huge numbers from your gym, a bunch of them can slowly erode your membership over time. It is important to note that if the $960,000 per year in membership revenue either flatlines or perhaps decreases, the gym owner's operating expenses will do the complete opposite and continue to rise by at least 3 percent per year. If the money to keep paying your bills doesn't come from the membership, which as we can tell from the chart is the gym's only major source of income, then where will it come from after the owner cuts the expenses as bare as he can?

- *Does this number represent the ceiling for membership in this gym and in this market?* Most gym owners fail to see the bus coming that eventually runs over them. If the $960,000 is the ceiling for this gym, you have to assume that it just won't be a static number forever. In reality, many owners see a trend developing but tend to ignore using a strong rationalization process. "Yes, my membership income did drop a little this month, but it was raining a lot and no one was getting out" or "Yes, my membership income did drop a little this month, but it was really sunny, so everyone was outside." Rain or shine, the reality here is that the number dropped. The basic rule you should always remember is:

> Any trend that lasts three months or longer
> is not a trend—it is your new reality.

If the membership revenue for this business trends downward for three months, the gym owner needs to react now, not at the end of the year while he waits to see if it comes back. Business reality here states that if the number trends down for three months, then it is not a trend but your new reality and this means that what you are doing is failing and you need to attack the business rather than wait it out to see if conditions change without your effort.

The harsh reality is that this simple chart represents a lot that is wrong with the current business model most of the mainstream fitness businesses use. This chart tells the owner that he depends too much on just one source of revenue and that he needs a constant stream of new members to replace the normal attrition rate most mainstream box players face.

Normal attrition in a metro area for a gym such as this, especially in a heavily competitive market, could be 60 percent or higher. This means that 12 months from now, this owner will lose 60 percent of his 2,200 members and will need to constantly replace them each month. Again, this was a good theory in the 1980s when this gym might have only had a single competitor, but in today's market and with 20 different fitness businesses fighting for a potential client's attention in this particular area, the chances this owner can continually replace lost members will get smaller each year.

Many owners in this situation attempt to add other profit centers, which a gym should have, but these extra sources of income will not offset the potential losses that occur if the membership revenue declines by a few points. For example, this gym should have a high-quality recovery shake bar; cooler drinks, including premium waters; specialty programming that adds additional monthly revenue, such as advanced cycle or yoga; and maybe a few spa services, including massage.

Even if the owner had all these additional revenue sources in his gym and was good at managing and promoting them, all combined, the added revenue is still short of what the owner will need to survive in a highly competitive market and with a most likely shrinking membership revenue base.

The Law of the Vital Few still applies in this situation: No matter what you add, there will still always be a limited number of clients who spend a large percentage of money on additional offerings. If this owner can broad-base the offerings and adds everything listed here, there will still be probably less than 10 percent of the entire membership who will spend additional money on a regular basis. Remember that these are add-on extras that are not vital to having a successful membership. While offering these in the gym will increase the return per member, because these particular profit centers are not fundamental to success in a gym from the client's viewpoint, there will always be fewer people who support the amenities or niceties that are offered.

Thus, where is the potential in this gym hiding and what should this owner do if he wants to shift from the old volume-based business model to a more competitive platform? Figure 2-2 simply represents where the only real potential left in a mainstream fitness facility lies. Keep in mind that the training-centric microgyms have already discovered this, which is why you see small 6,000-square-foot training gyms generating $1.2 million a year or more with a high net and with only 300 to 350 members.

Membership Revenue	Training Revenue
$960,000 annual net membership revenue	$960,000 annual training revenue (net of 35 to 40%)

Figure 2-2. Your goal within 12 to 18 months is to increase your training revenue to the point where it equals what you generate each month in membership dues.

The potential in any future fitness facility will not be in the ability to generate a high volume of members that will eventually have to be replaced as they are lost each month. The next generation business model is very simple: You need to learn to make more money from fewer members. In other words:

We have to learn to generate a higher return per client served.

The only real revenue potential in any gym is through training. For more than 60 years, we have been in the membership/equipment rental business and we now have to evolve into the results-driven/return per client era.

Figure 2-2 represents several important things:
- In approximately 12 to 18 months, any mainstream fitness facility should be able to match the monthly membership revenue through training revenue if the training model is completely renovated.
- The number on the right does respect the Law of the Vital Few and is based on only a 40 percent penetration rate into the gym's membership base.
- If the number on the right is achieved and this gym can generate as much money in training revenue each month as it does in membership, it will

become less vulnerable to competition and more sustainable over time because it is generating such a large amount of its income from members already in the system.

- The profit potential is much larger through training revenue than through membership.
- Traditional one-on-one training would represent less than 15 percent of that total number on the right. The complete pricing structure needed to create this revenue stream will be explained several times throughout this book.

The business of fitness has changed during the last decade, but as an industry, we are living in denial. The drivers of change, such as the rise of the microgym and the challenges in pricing that derive from the low-price players in the market, are forcing all owners to look at their business platforms and evaluate their effectiveness.

Bluntly stated: What we have been doing for more than six decades just does not work in the heavily competitive markets we now all live in. You cannot now and you will not in the future be able to run an effective business based on heavy volume and using the assumption that every client you get is easily replaced.

December 23, 2013
Being grateful

Being grateful for what you have and being aware of how you achieved what you have are often lost at this time of the year. No one—no matter how big your ego—got to be anyone without a hand that reached out and helped you at some point. The following are a few people you need to remember with something a little more touching than a text or a Facebook post this year:

- If you have clients who pay you—and that pay allows you to do what you love—then buy a bottle of wine, hand out Starbucks cards, or do something besides mumble as they leave the gym. You exist because they pay and it is time to be grateful.
- If you work for someone and the job doesn't suck, then say thank you for the opportunity with a small gift. You work because he pays you and it is time to be grateful.
- If you have a mentor that patiently opened a door for you and you are a better person because of that person, then say thank you. You achieve because someone else believed in you and it is time to be grateful.
- Don't forget the family. If someone sacrificed something in his life to make yours better, then you owe him and that debt can never really be repaid. You had a start because someone in your family gave his time and energy to you and it is time to be grateful. The universe is a funny place: The more you give, the more you get back and there are a lot of you who owe a big debt because of the talent and gifts you have been given. Acknowledge that debt this year and surprise the hell out of everyone by remembering who you are and where you came from.

December 6, 2013
The fitness industry has changed (women).

The fitness industry has changed for the positive more in the last five years than it has since the 1970s. We now know how to get results and train effectively and gyms are no longer just man caves for the underdressed and overmuscled.

One of the biggest drivers for change that is never talked about is the new generation of fitness women. In the past, women were all but banned from most weight rooms and told to go down the hall and dance. Or if they lifted weights, they were all pink, chrome, and two pounds. If a woman worked in a gym, she was front counter, child care, or an aerobic queen.

Today's fitness women are educated, in better shape than most bodybuilders ever could dream of in the 1980s, and are training equals in every sense of the word. The industry has changed, and as usual, it has taken a bunch of dedicated kick-ass women to get it done. Welcome to the dance. I wish you would have shown up earlier—we really need the help out here. And thank you for pushing for change. Hanging out with just a bunch of sweaty guys has really been boring.

3

Building an Effective Business Platform

Just about every small business works the same. You create a product, you figure out what it costs you and what you have to sell it for to make a little money, you create a way to get it to the public—either through opening a store or online—and then you deal with sales and marketing. If you're really good at small business, you also figure out a way to track your progress each month using all the key indicators of your business, and if you are really good, you spend a lot of time on customer service and trying to get those new customers to stay loyal and keep buying what you have to sell again and again. All these steps and processes could be called building a business platform.

However, it is impossible to build a working business platform if you aren't sure what you are trying to accomplish in your business or what a business platform really represents.

First of all, in the fitness industry, a business platform is not a training methodology. For example, many fitness facility owners become confused because they equate training protocols, such as CrossFit, boot camps, or kettlebell certifications, as a potential business solution to a specific problem. In the case of most of the chains and independent mainstream fitness business owners, the problem they are currently trying to solve is the erosion of their client base lost to training gyms and other single-purpose microgyms.

All the samples mentioned in the previous paragraph are merely systems offering a method of how to physically train people but do not in any way represent how to charge for the product, market it to the public, pay staff, or build an effective business using CrossFit, advanced kettlebell certifications, suspension training, or any of the literally dozens of training protocols as the core of your business.

The perfect example of failure that results from this confusion in the owner's head is when he says: "Yeah, we have functional training and CrossFit and we do it in a separate room in the back of the gym and the members pay extra for it." This owner is assuming that by just adding a method of training and tossing it in the spare room in the back of the gym will now make him competitive in the training-centric business market. In other words, he is assuming that adding a different way to train clients is going to also solve his business issue, which it won't or can't do.

This owner will fail with this method in several areas. In this example, he did not change his price structure or dependency on membership with this addition. In fact, he is going to kill his attempt at reaching a deeper penetration of his membership into training beyond the traditional 3 to 6 percent usually achieved by just offering one-on-one training alone. This owner doesn't build this type of training into core offerings of the club, but rather he attempts to sell it as a simple add-on that can be purchased at the front desk along with a smoothie, T-shirt, or tanning package.

He will also fail in that he did not change the culture in the gym. The culture has to be defined as your approach to business and your belief in how to get it done. Current mainstream gyms are based on a culture of do-it-yourself fitness, which is apparent through every single thing the club does or offers.

For example, the gym's ad is based on a deal of the week with the focus on just price to gain access, not about getting help or getting results. Walk into this club and your first experience will be with a salesperson whose sole goal in life is to sell you a membership today. If you buy a membership, you are turned over to a trainer who only has one goal and that is to find out if you have enough money to buy one-on-one training from him. If you do not buy, you are deemed lower class and you are shown a circuit and left to do fitness on your own. Yes, this club does have all the current training tools this member read about in the current fitness magazine, but because he won't pay extra for one-on-one training, he is stuck using the 1970s circuit equipment that covers all available floor space in the gym.

This gym owner is in the membership business and the entire culture of the gym, which is represented by the combination of everything the owner does and offers, was created to do nothing but support the sales team's effort to consistently sell memberships over time. In fact, this gym only really has two products: You either rent equipment, including attending group exercise, or you pay more for one-on-one training, which only about 5 percent of a typical box club's members do.

Despite adding a few different ways to train, this business is still what it was prior to the addition of this training method, and despite the claim in the ads that "we now offer functional training," the members will view the room in the back as just another way the gym owner is using to get them to spend a little extra money. This owner didn't change his business platform. He just added what he hopes is a small profit center that allows him to change his marketing somewhat and claim he now offers what he believes the competitors are using to kill him.

Your business platform is the combination of all the systems in your gym you use to generate revenue, train your staff, market to the consumer, and retain your clients. Most importantly, your business platform also has to represent your business philosophy, such as the culture in the gym and your values. The following are the key areas every business approach must include if that business is to be successful and sustainable over time:

- *You have to clearly define your product.* What exactly are you trying to sell to the client?
- *You have to create a clearly defined business platform.* How will you price this product, what is the culture that allows for the delivery of the product, are there other products you have to sell to support your main product, is your idea of opening a new business doable in this market, and do you have the money to get it done? Other considerations at this stage that should be considered include is there a market for this idea, how is it different from all the other similar businesses in town, and can you compete in an already crowded or competitive market? We also can't forget staffing and the ongoing training issues associated being able to deliver a consistent product over time.
- *The actual delivery system also has to be defined.* In our case, the delivery system is a brick-and-mortar building and the delivery system has to reflect the product you are trying to sell the consumer.
- *You have to establish a sustainable method of marketing your product to the potential buyer.* Brands are built slowly over time and many owners never take into account that marketing has to last as long as you are in business. And good marketing—retro (such as ads in the newspaper) and electronic (including such factors as social media)—has to be done every week and every month for as long as the business is open.
- *There has to be an effective sales system.* If the marketing works, then potential clients will come to your business and then you have to have an effective method established, allowing you to convert as many potential clients as possible into buyers of what you offer.
- *There has to be an established system of benchmarks.* Benchmarks done correctly track your progress, but most importantly, benchmarking keeps you on track and points you to the weaknesses of the business.
- *There has to be a system of retention in place that keeps the customer buying from you again and again.*

Perhaps the best way to understand the concept of a business platform is to directly apply it to several types of businesses. First of all, let's look at an elementary example of a weekend barbecue king and the world's greatest hamburger as an example that should help define the keys components of a working business platform.

Joe, your neighbor, is passionate about barbecuing and his specialty is creating the perfect hamburger. Joe gets so many raves about his burgers that he is inspired to open a restaurant and start selling his burgers to the public. The following are the questions and steps Joe should work through to turn his dream into a business reality:

- *What is Joe's product?* He creates a world-class burger.

- *What is Joe's business platform?* What is the culture that allows for the delivery of the perfect burger, are there other products he has to sell to support the burger as his centerpiece, is his idea of moving from the backyard to a restaurant scalable, and does he have the money to get it done? Other considerations for Joe at this stage include is there a market for this idea, how is it different from all the other burger guys in town, and can he compete in an already crowded burger market?

- *What is Joe going to use for a delivery system?* Should Joe open a restaurant, a food cart, get a mobile kitchen in a truck, or find another way to get this burger to the burger-buying public? Joe also needs to figure out a pricing system and sales strategy for his burgers. And somewhere in his thoughts, he needs to figure out his unique selling point. Why is this burger different, keeping in mind that everyone in the world that makes burgers claims to offer the world's best, and what sets his effort apart as unique to the burger client?

- *How will Joe market this new entry into the gourmet burger field?* Remember, Joe can't market a product until he understands what his product truly represents and what its unique selling point is going to be. This is where so many businesses go wrong. Products are created, but no one can simply explain what makes this product different or unique in just one sentence. If you can't define your product in only one sentence and clearly state why this product is different, then you will never be able to market it to the public because you will not be able to design marketing that reflects the true nature of your creation. Keep in mind that there are no such things as "better," "higher quality," or "best" in the real business world. These are all nonwords or phrases that mean nothing to anyone, along with "quality," "state of the art," "cutting edge" and "great service." For example, would you really run to a business that claims in its ads "We are the best restaurant in town and our people offer the best customer service of any restaurant in the area" or have you hear this tired old claim so many times that you are now immune?

- *How will Joe sell this product in his business?* Will his servers match his vision or will he forget about this and just hire anyone once he gets it opened? Look at most of the mainstream fitness businesses in any market and you will see a great example of how we forget that our people are part of our delivery system. We build mainstream gyms for $4,000,000 and then dress the staff in cheap T-shirts or badly fitting golf shirts. In small business, as Joes should remember, everything counts and his new staff, especially his sales team, which would most likely be his wait staff, have to dress to fit the system and be trained to clearly explain and support the product.

- *How will Joe benchmark this business?* For example, the key number in a restaurant is food cost. Food costs were never important to Joe in the past because his burgers were made for friends and family on the weekends and he was more concerned about the total quality rather than the actual costs. Joe is getting into business driven by his passion for burgers and the success he has achieved by cooking for his friends and family. But now he wants to create a business that has to make a profit if he wants to keep it going. This is an important transition for Joe: He has to move from a passionate amateur with little if any accountability to a professional who has to pay bills, borrow money, hire staff, and bring in a profit to keep the entire concept going. Benchmarking, or key number tracking, will be one of the key ideas Joe has to learn if he wants to build a financially successful business that allows him to live his dreams.

The same is true of a trainer who loves training and opens his first training gym. Most of the people who make this move have some type of experience, which drives this dream. The problem for these potential owners is the same Joe has: You simply don't know what you don't know. This means that being a great trainer in a garage with 10 clients or being the king of the backyard grill really has nothing to do with running a real business. Passion may be the foundation for a great idea, but it takes another level of business sophistication if you want to move from the backyard or garage to owning and operating your own business and that first level of understanding always has to be centered on mastering the key indicators of your business.

How will Joe create the repeat client? Getting a potential client into your business the first time is always fairly easy. Getting the client to keep coming back is one of the hardest challenges in small business. Retention is always based on a very simple principle: Did the client get what he paid for in his experience with you? In Joe's case, how good was the experience wrapped around the food? Good food sets the tone, but it's service that keeps someone coming back. In other words, is Joe able to create the total experience in his business?

The same is true in the fitness industry. Most clients don't leave unless they are driven out of a business. Bad service, lousy staff that is undertrained, a dirty gym, and traditionally being ignored after the sale all leads to a client who stays for a few months and then quietly leaves. Most importantly, clients leave because there is no mechanism in place that leads to them getting results. People who get results from their gym experience will stay longer and pay longer than those who don't. Results are the core we seek. The experience of your gym is the vehicle that makes me want to come back again and again.

Joe and his quest for the delivery of the perfect burger is a simple analogy, but who does this well in the real world? Look no further than Starbucks for a perfect example of perfect:

- *You have to clearly define your product:* Coffee—just coffee—and everything else supports coffee.
- *You have to create a definable business platform:* Coffee is the product. How Starbucks supports the sale of its product is the business platform. The goal was to create a European-style coffee experience in a country where everyone is in perpetual motion. Starbucks was the first and it mastered making the server a professional, along with a sophisticated pricing structure that resulted in being able to charge almost double what everyone else in the market was able to do.

- *You have to create a delivery system:* Walk into most any Starbucks in the world and the menus, smell, atmosphere, baristas, and overall feel just makes you want to buy something.
- *You have to create sustainable marketing:* Its marketing has evolved over time to the point that it doesn't have to market. Its locations are its marketing and is there anyone living on this planet in any civilized country that can't tell you what the green circle means?
- *You have to create a sales system:* Starbucks replaced the old-style, bad-tempered waitress model with an entire generation of nicely dressed and polished coffee professionals, which might be the true secret of their success. If you work for Starbucks, you aren't just a person working in a coffee shop. You are a barista who has advanced training in all the coffees it serves and who wears a professional uniform to prove it.
- *You have to benchmark:* There probably isn't any business in the world that can furnish more data on same stores sales than Starbucks
- *Retention is in the experience:* You stay, you linger, you drink, and you come back tomorrow and repeat. Consistency of product and service has created a company with almost 20,000 stores worldwide.

Understanding that a business platform does exist and applies to what you are doing allows you to increase the odds that you can build a financially successful business that is sustainable over time. The fitness industry, represented by any fitness business, is not the exception to the rule as so many past owners have declared. Business is business, and if you can't create a product someone wants, price this product for the market, and figure out a way to get it to the public so people want to buy again and again, you will fail.

The important thing to note is that whatever business platform you use has to be changed and updated over time. Business models are created for the times they were born in and what worked even just 10 years ago doesn't always work today. For example, whatever happened to phone booths, 24-photo development stores, full-sized computers, and the traditional old school department stores, such as Montgomery Ward and Woolworth's? (Look these up if you are too young to remember.)

All these business ideas were created for what was happening at the time in the culture and in the business world and all these failed and went away because each idea was either overrun by new technology or the company failed to update and meet the needs of a changing market. Again, why would this not happen in the fitness industry?

Let's contrast the traditional business platform discussed in the last chapter, which was created in the 1950s, with a new generation model that was devised to meet the needs of today's consumer and owner/operator.

The following are the basic components of the traditional volume business model used today by most mainstream fitness facilities of any type in the industry:
- The product is memberships.
- The business platform is based on the need for continual new volume. The customer is assumed to be replaceable. The prices generally range between

$9 to $49 in most mainstream fitness businesses. The assumption is the lower the price, the higher the volume. The business concept is sales driven, with most owners putting the bulk of payroll dollars into building a sales team that can maintain the needed volume to support this model. Revenue is generally limited to just one source, which is memberships. The most important part of the platform to understand is that these clubs charge a monthly membership that does nothing but give you access to equipment and services and in no way does the majority of memberships sold give you any help or support as a member. Based on the premise of just selling access, it is easy to see that this business system is designed to generate a low return per client over time but with the goal to sell as many memberships as you can cram into your box.

- The delivery system is a traditional big box primarily filled with fixed-plane, single-joint equipment (circuit machines), along with cardio pieces. Most mainstream fitness facilities have group exercise of some type and a number of current clubs have started to offer some version of functional training based on a group or team training concept. All the other components of these gyms are designed to attract and support membership sales. The focus is not on results for the client in this type of box but rather creating a system where the majority of the clients can be serviced with the lowest possible costs.

- The marketing for this type of facility, which represents all the major chains, most of the large independent chains, and the majority of all independent mainstream fitness facilities, is price driven. Price driven is defined as putting the membership offered by the business on sale, such as offering 50 percent off a membership fee.

- Sales are the primary driver for this type of business. The sales team and sales management generate most of the payroll expense. Some of these facilities do have a fairly large number of trainers servicing the membership using traditional one-on-one training and this can also be a high revenue expense, but in a volume-based business, sales are everything and all the real money has to go to keep the sales team selling enough new members to replace the ones lost each month.

- Benchmarking is usually done well in most chain clubs, with the emphasis on sales numbers, including year-to-year comparisons, closing rates for each salesperson, number of leads through the door, number of salesperson-generated leads and referrals, and other numbers that give management a way to evaluate the sales team's performance.

- Retention is basically a nonentity in these businesses beyond a simple acknowledgement. Talk is cheap in this industry, and while everyone talks a good story on chasing retention in his business, the true retention numbers of clients staying year to year is dismal. Most mainstream fitness businesses will lose 60 percent or more of their current membership during the next 12 months, which again highlights the fact that volume drives these businesses, not the longevity of the individual member.

As noted in the first chapter, this business platform was created in a time where there wasn't much competition in the industry. Volume businesses work if you are the only gym in a town of 300,000 people, but the system fails when there are another 100 gyms in that same market all chasing the same need for volume to keep their doors open.

If this system doesn't work in today's market, then what will? The forces that drive business today are moving us away from the volume approach. We mentioned a number of these movers in the first chapter, but the real big dog that is forcing change is competition: There are simply too many gyms in any market all doing the same exact thing and chasing the same exact potential client. If we can't do volume and support the endless progression of "sell, lose, sell, lose," then we have to find a new way to run these facilities.

The only choice we have left if we can't keep selling the big numbers is to switch away from volume and start seeking a higher return per client served. Remember, when you are trying to fix a business that isn't performing well, you only have three approaches to go after the problem:

- You can sell more of your product—either through sales improvement or by lowering the price and increasing the number of units you sell.
- You can cut expenses.
- You can make more money from clients already in the system through extra services or offerings.

Increasing Sales

How do you increase sales when you have other hungry competitors opening every day in your market? The derivative of this approach is to cut your price, which is supposedly going to increase the number of buyers. This approach does work in the short term. Go to a market, drop the price to $10, and your sales will increase, but at some point, you will run out of potential buyers in the market who are willing to pay even $10. With any product, except perhaps sales of water and food, there are only a limited number of people who want to buy anything.

You can also improve the way you do sales within your company. For example, if your current sales team only closes 40 percent of all leads through the door and you have the potential to close 65 percent, which would be a solid number for a mainstream fitness club, then intense training and hiring a more efficient team might make a difference. The flaw here, of course, is that you are assuming there are enough leads coming through the door in the first place and that price-driven marketing will bring you in as many potential clients as you need, but again, we are now back to the effect of too much competition in the market, which limits your ability to keep marketing prices low and drive leads to the business.

What if You Can't Increase Sales?

If you can't increase sales, you cut expenses. The problem here is that there just isn't that much slop factor in most gym businesses. If you can save 5 percent of expenses, you would be doing well in most clubs. The big variable, of course, is payroll, and once a gym owner starts running out of money, he whacks this category right after he cuts marketing out completely and then stops all reinvestment in the gym.

Cutting marketing is like telling a hungry guy not to buy food. Leads are the nutrition a gym needs to live. Cut your marketing and you are in fact cutting the lifeblood of the business, which is the generation of potential buyers of your product. But if your marketing fails due to intense competition—all of which are running price specials and price-driven ads and lowering their prices in order to steal members from existing gyms—then running a monthly campaign isn't helping much anyway.

The rule here to remember is:

You can't save yourself *into* profitability.

Reinvestment is also an issue. Big boxes wear out fairly quickly, and if you want to stay current—at least with the other box players in your market—you need to constantly keep the gym updated and clean, the equipment fresh and repaired, and your programming reactive to the demands of the market. However, when gym owners get into financial trouble, the second thing usually cut after marketing is buying equipment and services you need to keep the membership you do own.

What if You Can't Cut Enough Expense to Stay Financially Healthy?

If you can't increase sales and you can't cut expenses, then all you have left to choose from in your mission to fix this ailing business is seeking a higher return per client served. If you can't sell a lot more of your product, then you are going to have to figure out a way to get more money from every client you do sell to.

This system is the foundational tool for a modern training gym. Those owners understand return per client far better than almost any mainstream players. Training gym owners will happily open a 6,000-square-foot gym just down the street from a $10-a-month gym with the understanding that they only need about 250 clients paying an average of a $150 per month or higher to make a workable profit and to sustain this business over time.

There was a famous quote from a police officer that circulated for years on the Internet. He pulled over a car for speeding and the driver admitted he was indeed speeding but then claimed that so was everyone else on the road and he was just following along with all the other traffic:

The officer responded: Sir, have you ever gone fishing?

The speeder responded back: Well, yes, sir, I have. What does this have to do with fishing?

The officer: Sir, when you went fishing did you ever expect to catch all the fish?

The idea behind this story is that if you own a gym business based on the traditional volume business platform, then you are fishing with an expectation of catching all the fish. This plan goes wrong when other fishermen find your spot and now you have 20 boats all fishing for the same fish.

New generation training gyms understand that they are only looking for a few specific fish who don't mind paying a little extra to get out of the mainstream fitness fish pond. They don't need all the fish, as a volume club does. They just need a few fish that want a different product and are willing to pay for it.

Mainstream fitness facilities can switch from a sheer volume approach to seeking a higher return from the clients they do serve. The solution is fairly simple and the price structure you would use to create this system is highlighted in the next chapter. First of all, let's look at the components of the higher return per client served business model and compare these points to the traditional volume system defined earlier.

The Higher Return per Client Business Platform

The product

The clearly defined product for this shift in business philosophy is results. Instead of selling the most memberships and then replacing the lost business each month, you now seek the maximum results, for the maximum number of clients, in the shortest period of time. People who get results from interaction with your business will stay longer, will pay longer, and will pay more for memberships. Your goal using this business platform is to generate the highest amount of revenue possible from a fewer number of clients.

The business platform

The entire pricing structure will be discussed in the next chapter. In this example, we need to establish several key principles that are part of the entire approach we would use with this method of doing business. If we are focusing on maximum results for the maximum number of clients, then we need to change how we charge for help and guidance. In traditional mainstream fitness facilities, the only ones who get help are the 5 percent who buy one-on-one training. Everyone else who is working out in the gym—with the exception of those who attend group exercise—practices do-it-yourself fitness.

If we want to get results for a higher number of clients, we need to establish a wider range of products, offer a wider range of support for the clients, and get help to the largest number of clients we can reach. In the volume method, there are only two products: You either pay for access to the gym so you can use the stuff or you pay more for one-on-one training.

In a results-driven model, we have to create a layered structure that allows almost any client—at any age and within any budget—to get help because the goal is to generate a higher return per client served instead of seeking the highest number of new clients possible with the assumption that those who do get help will stay longer and pay longer.

The delivery system

This would be a generational leap in fitness facility design. The 1995 gym design model is based on large space, tightly packed rows of equipment, free weights stacked against the wall and as many group rooms as you can handle. If you chase volume, you need lots of equipment in case everyone shows up at once, which they all do for about six consecutive weeks starting in mid-February.

The theory is that if the gym's staff isn't able to deliver any help to the client beyond the group exercise instruction and coaching with the one-on-one clients, then you have to throw enough equipment on the floor so the members can entertain themselves. This worked several decades ago when the limited amount of competition any owner would face limited the options for the member to pick up and head somewhere else or if the member did quit, then no one really cared because he would be replaced in next month's sales numbers.

Next generation fitness facilities will be smaller and cheaper to build because the emphasis is now focused on getting results for a smaller group of patrons who are paying more money for the coaching and leadership. Instead of a hundred pieces of fixed equipment targeting individual muscle groups, you will have piles of functional equipment, which is obviously substantially cheaper, that works the client's entire body. More done with less is the new theme in building a next generation gym.

Open space is an asset hard to find in today's mainstream gyms. Owners just can't stand having a big space in the club and have the primal need to kill it instantly by stuffing the latest and greatest equipment into every square inch with the premise that no member will ever leave this gym because we didn't have … (fill in this week's hot, must-have perfect piece).

In the newer delivery systems, space is the big draw because this is where all the action is in the group team training. The sea of equipment has been replaced with 1,500 square feet of open space used by 20 clients and a coach all screaming, pushing sleds, hanging on racks, and flipping tires. Instead of servicing just a few members at a time throughout the day, you can now service a large pile of them at a low cost with minimal equipment, such as kettlebells and suspension training tools.

There will still be a need for cardio and certain pieces of selectorized equipment but not in rows, running $500,000 per gym to replicate. There will always be members who enjoy a long walk or good run on a decent tread and that isn't going to change, but the need to fill rooms with the stuff will as the client changes his expectations about how and why he trains.

Next generation delivery systems will also have to be more narrowly based. If you are looking for a client willing to pay a little more for help versus chasing a client who is only concerned about the cost of renting a tread each month, then what you offer in the gym will be aimed more at getting results for people who come to the gym to get it done and get out instead of targeting people who are less intent on results and who will leave you for a gym down the street that is a few dollars less a month.

Marketing

Holistic functional training is outside the experience range for many of the potential clients who will be coming to the gyms in the coming years. Virtually every young male in the country has bench-pressed something at least once, but how many potential clients have experience on 50-foot ropes or pulling sleds? Traditional marketing, based on the price discount and special of the week, will not overcome this inexperience. You simply can't build a marketing concept based on a single visit and expect the client to understand something complicated after only one try.

There are only two ways to bring a potential client into a gym: You offer a price slash or you allow the client to try the product first and then buy. The first one is based on price; the second one is based on exposure.

Price marketing is based on the premise that there are millions of people in the market already interested in your product and who are just waiting for a chance to buy it if it goes on sale. For example, cut the price of a top-end Mercedes to half and see what happens at the dealership that day. There are millions of people already familiar with the quality of the car and know the brand and they would most likely stampede through the streets if they could buy that quality of car for half price.

But what happens if the client isn't familiar with the product? Selling smartphones to the older population in this country is a perfect example of no matter what price the phone is offered at, you are just not going to sell many phones. Put another way, there has to be prior interest in a product or it doesn't matter what price you list it at because nothing will happen in sales.

Older people didn't grow up with smartphones, and while a few adapt to modern technology, there are many still carrying old flip phones or those special senior phones with the giant numbers that do nothing but make calls. You could offer the highest-end smartphone in the world with all the extras at a tenth of the price, but if the client doesn't understand what it is or how to use the product, then there will be no sale.

Traditional circuit training never had this problem and there probably aren't too many people left in America who haven't tried a seated chest press. Price marketing works when the client understands he needs fitness and has a working knowledge of what will happen to him in the gym. The marketing for this person can be price driven because every gym offers the same equipment and it all comes down to how much to rent this stuff for.

However, traditional marketing fails when you pitch price to a person with no prior fitness experience. As of this writing, 83 percent of the people in this country do not belong to any type of fitness facility, leaving only 17 percent who are actively involved in gyms. Price may work with the experienced gym goer, who also knows that every mainstream fitness facility—despite the claims—sells the same products to the same clients. The question then becomes, how do you market to the other 83 percent who don't belong to gyms and are now faced with joining gyms that use tools they have no familiarity with and have only seen in magazines or on TV?

Exposure marketing means you try before you buy. This concept will be discussed in depth throughout this book, but for now, we have to understand that exposure marketing means that we allow the client to experience the gym and, most importantly, the team that runs this gym prior to being forced to make a buying decision. Next generation training-centric businesses would most likely use a 30-day paid trial that allows the client to get a full experience using every service the gym offers before having to commit.

Sales

If the marketing changes in the new business model, then the sales process also has to change. Price marketing is based on driving a potential client into a gym, where the sales staff has one shot to close by applying leverage—either through offering yet a better deal or by old-fashioned techniques, such as using a sales office and high-pressure tactics.

The combination of traditional price marketing and traditional fitness center sales tactics leads to one outcome: Everything has to happen during the potential client's first visit. The system fails in that if the client doesn't buy during the first visit—when he was most likely given an even better deal than the ad—why would he ever come back again? The sales team tried and it failed and there isn't much hope of retrieving this guy after he walks away.

Marketing and sales have to have a different expected outcome in a training-centric business model. Your goal is to get a potential client into the system and keep him there while he gains experience and confidence with the product. The most important point to understand is that someone who has tried the product for a few weeks or even up to a month will not be fighting over price when he makes his decision to buy. The determiner will shift away from price and instead be focused on service, the products offered, the total experience, and accessibility.

It is also important to note that who sells the memberships has to shift in a training-centric business. In the past, salespeople seldom had any training experience and didn't need any because the product they had to present wasn't results-based training but just a membership to gain access through the front door of the club.

Today, the members have grown more sophisticated in their demands and most want to talk to someone about training and not just salespeople pushing a membership. We will discuss at length in the following chapters how fitness has to be sold in a next generation fitness facility.

Benchmarking

The major shift in how we track progress is a move away from volume toward a return per contract generated.

In a traditional gym, the return per sale for the gym owner is usually lower than the offered rate for a single user. For example, a gym salesperson might present a monthly rate of $39 for a single member, but if you average the last 100 memberships sold in that gym and split the couples or divided the group memberships down to an individual rate, the true number per client sold would be at least 20 percent less than the $39—somewhere in the $27 to $31 range.

This happens because almost every client sold is discounted for some reason. For example, it would be a rare gym owner who didn't discount for the second member of the family, senior citizens, students, older members, and just about any corporate situation where more than two people joined at the same time. This gym might present $39 as the rate, but it would usually average $30 or less per membership sold.

The complete opposite is true in a training-centric business. The gym's sales team might show $39 as the single rate, but as will be discussed in future chapters, it will charge more per month for group exercise, team training, small group intensive coaching, and traditional one-on-one training. All these layered prices would still be offered monthly, and if the targeted 40 percent of the members in a traditional mainstream gym signed up for one of the more expensive memberships, the gym could present $39 as the base fee but perhaps get as much as $59 or higher per month as the average per membership. Training gyms would of course have a much higher return per client served and it isn't unusual for a training gym to average $300 to $400 per month per client on 12-month agreements.

Retention

In the old model, the member is replaceable. In the newer model, people who get results, as proven for decades in training gyms, stay longer and pay longer. Strong retention lowers the cost of operation. Your commissions are lower, your marketing is cheaper, your start-up expense per new client drops, and your general service costs also drop because you aren't constantly turning over memberships and solving those issues.

Conclusion

The fitness industry has been mainstream for almost 70 years and any business expert would probably doubt the success rate if, as an industry, you can only claim to penetrate 17 percent of your target market. In other words, we live in one of the most obese countries in the world and our fitness industry only touches 17 percent of the people who live here.

The question to ask is whether this failure is due to people just hating fitness and not being aware that they need to get fit or is the issue with our product, how we build fitness businesses, and with the product we sell? It is hard to live anywhere without picking up an article or hearing a news blast on obesity or health. And keep in mind that there are more than 300,000,000 people in this country and we only have about 51,000,000 in our businesses. How good do we have to be to make a difference? Just adding 3 percent, or another 9,000,000, would overload every fitness option in this country with new members if distributed equally.

In summary, what we have been doing in the fitness industry has gotten us this far, but we now have to realize that this same business system is what is now holding us back from continued growth in the future. The training gyms, along with all the other smaller next generation players who will be discussed in detail in this book, have figured this out, but if we want to grow this industry, we can't patch a broken model. We really have to get in there and break it apart.

November 24, 2013
Creating magic

Just heard the "Somewhere Over the Rainbow/What a Wonderful World" medley by Israel Kamakawiwo'ole on satellite radio—the one with the ukulele and slow, steady beat. The song was released in 1993 and the singer died in 1997. I wonder what was in his head when he recorded that song? Did he know at that moment that he created something magical that would last more than 20 years past his death? Consider any classic song, book, or work of art. Does any great writer or artist realize at that moment that he has mastered his craft and that the work at that moment is perfect? I believe most people never live up to their potential because they don't chase the magic in what they choose to do with their lives. Everyone can be a true artist in what he does and somewhere out there is the perfect workout, the perfect class in school, the perfect presentation, and the perfect day in your life where you finally achieve mastery in your work through your passion, and when mastery occurs, there is always magic. Mastery simply means that for a few minutes on a given day, all your insanely hard work paid off, and for a brief time, you were the best that has ever been. Seek the passion this week and see if you can create some magic that will be remembered forever.

January 6, 2014
For many people, talent isn't a gift—it is a burden.

Embracing or living up to your talent should be your life's work, but so many people I see spend so much time running from or denying their gifts that they accomplish little of importance in their life. There is always an epiphany moment for someone who gets life going in the right direction and that is when you get up one morning, look into the mirror, and acknowledge that you have talent and that if you don't get off your ass and do something with it now your life will be lost. I believe God has a weird sense of humor. He won't show you home videos someday of everything you did stupid in your life, but He will ask you one basic question: "I gave you a lot of talent—what the hell did you do with it?" That question holds true now. You have talent and gifts, but what are doing with that gift and will you live up to your potential or just be known as that person who "could have been somebody if only …"?

4

Next Generation Gyms Are the Future of the Business

One of the hardest challenges you'll face in the coming years is learning to focus or "niche" your business in relation to your community, your personal expectations of the business, and your competition. In this era of maximum competition, learning to narrow and focus the scope of your business will give you a key competitive edge in the marketplace.

The industry is currently going through perhaps the most abrupt period of change since the dawn of the modern fitness era in 1945. Much of this change is fueled by the decline of many of the practices and habits owners have counted on through the years as the foundational tools they use to build clubs and generate revenue. What worked prior is now failing, and for most owners who have a history in the industry—coupled with a limited imagination to see the future—this caused a great deal of trauma to an industry that hasn't really changed that much in decades.

The driver behind all this is a simple concept: Markets are maturing and the relatively moderate competition of the last century was replaced with an intense struggle to survive due to an almost limitless surge of new players in the game. These new players caused damage because they ventured out of the traditional horizontal approach to competition in the industry into vertical tracks that wreaked havoc in the markets.

The 1990s were in many ways the golden age of fitness for many owners and operators. Competition was at best moderate, most of the players knew each other, and many had an almost gentlemen's agreement not to open a club too close. Even the major chains of the era picked territory carefully and seldom declared war on each other. Pricing was also relatively tame, with most of the chains and franchises offering prices at around the $39 per month per member rate.

Horizontal positioning is the sign of an immature market. When a player goes horizontal, it means he opened a business similar to the other players in the market, emulating the type of equipment, the average price, and most of the standard offerings that everyone else in the market was doing. In the 1990s, there wasn't a lot of difference between a Gold's Gym, a World Gym, a 24 Hour Fitness, or a Bally Total Fitness. All were large boxes with big workout floors covered with the latest equipment, big free weight areas, group programming, and a price in the $39 range. They were all different, but in many ways, they were all the same.

The reason many fitness businesses stayed horizontal so long was there wasn't enough competition to drive innovation. If there are enough members to go around, then there is no need to differentiate from your competitors. Do what has always worked, update it a little to make it appear current, and keep doing what you have always done. For example, sales in that era were done the same way they had been done since the late 1940s: dedicated salespeople doing tours and then ending up in an office to apply the high pressure needed to get someone to buy today. The best salespeople of that era were actually the worst in the sense that the more you sold, the more skilled you probably were at using all the old sales tricks that have given this industry such a bad image. The tricks and systems were nothing new—just techniques passed down from generation to generation.

Vertical positioning is the direct result of intense competition applied over time. During the late 1990s and into the early 2000s, there was a burst of growth in the industry that was unprecedented. Markets matured, meaning that more clubs were opening in your direct and immediate market and these clubs now tried to distinguish themselves by going for a different segment.

Perhaps the best example of maturing market and segment erosion in the country is Baton Rouge, Louisiana. The oldest club in town was opened in the early 1960s and was sold to an employee who eventually expanded to another club across town. One of the owner's friends was a real estate developer and speculator who owned another nine clubs in town. In approximately 1995, there were about 15 to 18 clubs in town and two friends owned 11 of them. Baton Rouge at the time was a city that listed about 250,000 residents, but perhaps a third of the market would have been considered too poor to join a fitness facility.

Fifteen years later, the owner of the oldest club in town was still in business and had added a third club to his family's business. However, he now had more than 100 competitors offering some type of fitness alternative within seven miles of his main location. These competitors couldn't have gotten into the market as horizontal players all trying to offer the same things. There are simply not enough members to feed the ever-growing pig. Fitness facilities need a constant source of new members or they will die, and if you had 80 owners fighting for the same market share, then most would fail quickly.

The majority of these survive because they embraced the concept of vertical positioning illustrated by their ability to target segments. Targeting segments means that the owner goes after narrowly defined populations in the market and he builds a facility primarily to service this limited group. For example, when CrossFit first entered the market, the better operators in that organization were able to build viable businesses around a group of clients not serviced by the mainstream box fitness facilities.

A CrossFit member at the time was someone who wanted the group dynamic, who wanted a challenge and to be pushed a little, and who wanted new and exciting methods of training—all of which virtually none of the mainstream chains clubs offered and in fact few offer still today. In other words, the CrossFit operator found a segment that was underserved, created a business specifically for that segment, and was able to survive and even thrive opening directly across the street from established clubs that had been in business for decades.

However, over time, this segmentation started to have a dramatic effect on all the operators in the industry. If you were an operator of a typical mainstream fitness facility in that 25,000- to 60,000-square-foot category, you at first noticed a slight decline in small segments of your current membership. For example, you might notice that you aren't signing up as many younger members in that 24- to 44-year-old range (gone to CrossFit) or that some of your reliable one-on-one training clients left (gone to Fitness Together, a franchise that specialized in just one-on-one training in that era but has since also expanded into group offerings) or even that you aren't getting as many first-time experience members (left for the surge of circuit clubs in that era, such as Curves).

In the fitness business, you don't die from a bullet to the head, meaning that one new competitor can crush you overnight. Death—defined as the loss of your business—is a much more insidious experience in this industry. Imagine running through a field naked and falling right in the middle of a flock of hungry chickens. These chickens slowly just peck you to death one small bite at a time and it takes about four years for the chickens to slowly drain you.

This strange but efficient analogy means that most clubs fail in the business because they lose small segments of members over time to competitors who only drain 20 members here or 10 members there. You don't lose your business in one big swoop but rather over a number of years as you slowly lose the variety of members that comprised your membership.

Once vertical, though, you can't go back. There is no retreat to the safety of the 1990s. Segmentation, or the advent of the target-specific club, is here to stay due to the sheer number of competitors trying to find a way to market themselves as unique and to fight for enough market share to stay in business.

The result of this trend is that the era of just selling memberships is dying and being replaced by the next generation of fitness facility that is focused on getting sustainable results for its memberships. In the past, most of these big box, everything-to-everybody facilities sold just one product and that was a membership. While called fitness centers, no one really sold fitness. In these facilities, you weren't paid as a sales guy to help people get into shape. You were paid and promoted by the number of memberships you could turn each month. In fact, the entire fitness business was—and mostly still is—designed to do nothing but turn as many new memberships as possible and then replace the lost members who leave the system months down the road.

The chaos caused by the new segment players, the advent of functional training that allows trainers to get more results for more clients, new tools (such as group personal training), and the enormous cost of building the big boxes have led to the perfect storm in the industry. When all these factors collide, you have destruction for some, such as those who cling to the way it has always been done, and opportunity for others who are not only willing to change but who are also actively seeking change.

For example, look at the chaos in the record industry with the advent of digital music. The establishment on the record company side tried everything it could to stop digital downloads, but in the end, we saw the end of an era as the great records stores, such as Tower Records and Virgin Megastore, faded into the past and iTunes® arose as the next generation music source. Chaos and disarray for some means there is opportunity for others who are willing to let go of the past.

Chaos is reflected in the fitness industry by the current approach to try virtually everything at once. This broad-based approach is a direct result of too much pressure to change at one time.

Perhaps the biggest example of this was the price wars that started in the early 2000s. A relatively new player in the game, Planet Fitness, started a franchise based on an approximately $20 down membership and $10 per month. The premise behind this change was that there wasn't any real place for beginners to go in mainstream fitness and that most people just want to come walk on the treadmill anyway or use some equipment, so there was no need for these people to pay real high prices to just rent equipment.

While low-priced memberships are nothing new in the industry—you can find chains charging under $9 in the 1970s—the reaction in the industry this time around was sheer panic. Was it just the price that caused the trauma in the industry or was it a combination of intense segment-driven competition, a changing training culture based on results-driven functional training, or a faltering economy and a more educated consumer who was tired of being told that going around in a circle on circuit training three times per week was fitness?

The combination of all these factors forced many of the operators with businesses based on old school systems to rapidly update or fail—and many failed because they simply couldn't change fast enough to adapt. Mature markets flooded with low-priced competition force everyone to find different ways to compete because there just aren't enough potential members to feed dozens of clubs who depend on sheer volume to survive. When all you have to sell is price and someone takes that away from you by going even lower, you have nothing left to compete with in the market.

We Are at the End of the Membership Era and the Start of the Training-Centric Club Model

Low-price concepts, large, impersonal physical plants, no support systems for the majority of the members, nonexistent member service, and a too young, too dumb, undertrained staff were all part of the large chain approach to fitness in the latter part of the 1990s. These old-style operating methods were also parts of our past—aspects of the business that have worked against clubs over the years because they were so negative in the consumer's mind.

This business plan, based on the "Be everything to everybody concept," has had serious adverse effects on the entire industry. The problem with this plan is the need for heavy volume, meaning that the typical club has to generate an almost endless supply of new memberships each month.

The fitness business is at an unusual crossroads in its history. On one hand, we have the implosion of the box club concept as mainstream fitness centers struggle to stay relevant in a hyper-change business environment and where for decades the club's equipment has been the star at the expense of the member. On the other hand, the evolution of the training-centric model that puts the client back into the center of the business plan is putting pressure on how we do business and who in the fitness business will survive in the coming years.

The rise of the mainstream chain-style club during the 1980s also directly corresponded to the demise of most of what has passed as member service for the last 20 years in the industry. Chain clubs, along with the independent operators who emulate that business model, exist for one reason and only one reason and that is to sell as many new memberships as possible each month. Membership revenue in these clubs is often 85 percent or more of the businesses' total deposit each month, and if there isn't heavy volume in the form of new memberships, there is no business. The problem is that volume and creating a training-centric business are mutually exclusive.

The rise of a training-centric, results-driven business model will perhaps be the most important breakthrough in the last 60 years of fitness. While this statement seems simplistic, it does not negate the power of what is happening in the industry. We are currently witnessing the end of the membership-driven model while simultaneously watching the return of the client-centered business—a concept mastered in the first-generation modern fitness facilities in the late 1940s and 1950s but lost in the era of "Bigger is better" box clubs.

Simply stated, today's fitness business owners have to figure out how to get the most results for the most clients or eventually fail because the cannibalistic nature of the bottom-feeders is that the cheap eat the cheap, leaving little room to exist on volume alone. Another way to look at this is that most markets can handle one low-price player with a membership that is $19 a month per member or lower, but if you add several clubs in that class, the cannibals eat the cannibals because there is only so much volume that can be generated in any given market.

The average consumer has also grown too sophisticated for just the price-driven concepts and is expecting more from today's fitness facility. Does today's potential member really expect great service from a high-pressure sales factory using sales concepts dating from the insurance industry in the 1950s? Do consumers really expect great help from a 19-year-old front counter kid who is in her first job? The answer is "Definitely not," but many of today's businesses are still trying to sell these dated concepts rather than adjusting to the changing business environment and the evolution of the client.

This clinging to the habits of our past highlights a major problem in the gym business, which is that we don't really understand what clients are buying when they make an investment in our businesses. Most owners think members buy the possibility of fitness—a place to work out or the concept of just renting equipment for a low price.

Worse yet, many old school operators still think a person's final buying decision is based on your facility having the ultimate line of equipment that can attack the outer part of your quads three inches above your knee from 82 known and three previously unknown positions. Yes, there was one bodybuilder in 1982 who was overly concerned about those three inches and who made his buying decision based on those choices. But if you base your business plan on this nonsense or once-in-a million situations, you'll make the same mistake that many other club owners make in their business plans: You'll fill your facility with endless equipment stacked row after row, line up as much cardio equipment as you can get, make all the support services and amenities (such as locker rooms and service staff) minimal, and then pressure people into buying because you have more stuff than the other guy offered at the lowest price on the street.

Successful owners understand what they are really selling: the client who gets results will stay longer and pay longer than one that doesn't. If you want to change your thinking away from the volume model, start with one simple thought in your head: "What if the clients I have now are not replaceable?" In other words, what if you had to survive on just the clients you have now in your club and couldn't replace them with next month's new memberships? What would you do different in your business and how would you train and support the members you do have?

The results-driven business plan means that the consumer wants and demands more from the gym of his choice. He wants equipment, but he also wants a great deal of help learning to use it. He wants to work out in a well-lit, exceptionally clean facility, surrounded by a slightly older than expected communicative staff. If he needs help with his diet, he expects it to be available. If he needs training help and advice, he expects to get it. He may pay extra for some of these things, but he still expects the club to have them available and not just limited to the 3 to 6 percent of a typical club's membership that can afford personal training.

This concept is the edge that the small training clubs have in the game. If you have 300 or so members who agree to the following three things, you will keep members longer than a typical club that can't deliver on these points:

- You will have a coach—either one-on-one or in a group training situation—every time you are here pushing and guiding you.
- You will be coached on food and the staff will help you find an effective way of eating for you that keeps you healthy but also losing a few pounds.
- You will take supplements as part of a growth and recovery program (for those of you who believe and endorse supplements).

Getting your clients to stick to these three pillars of success almost guarantees that the client will get results, and if he does, he will stay longer and pay longer, saving the cost of replacing him in the marketplace. Comparably speaking, few clubs that have more than 500 members are able to live within these tenets with their membership. In the past, the restriction of just offering one-on-one training keeps the number of clients you can service per month limited in most club models.

However, the advent of newer tools based on a functional training approach has changed the rules of the game substantially. For example, the group personal training/boot camp model allows a large number of clients to access a coach each time they work out for a much lower cost than the typical one-on-one model allows. This means that this larger group of people will become more involved through the group dynamics they share with the rest of the group and through the fact that they are still getting guidance from a skilled trainer/coach during each workout. The more touches you have with a person, the longer the person will stay and pay.

It's not enough in a highly competitive industry to just have the best equipment, the most stuff, or the biggest facility. Equipment is only part of the experience and even the type of equipment we have depended on for so long as the star in the game, such as lines of circuit equipment, is being replaced by "functional tools," such as medicine balls and kettlebells. And these large, impersonal, and unfocused facilities work against the gyms in today's market because the next generation member doesn't associate the biggest with the best and most intimate service.

The key to the member's perception of the fitness experience is the atmosphere in which these elements are delivered. Think of a good restaurant. Great restaurants are not huge. They are not usually overcrowded unless they have a planned 15- to 30-minute delay that keeps customers in the bar working on drinks while they wait for a table.

The lighting in a good restaurant is warm and inviting, the guests can linger over wine or cocktails after the meal, and the service is supportive of an excellent dining experience. Even if the food is just average, an excellent dining experience can make it seem better than it is. Guests are buying a dining experience, not just food, which they could have bought at a drive-through window on the way home.

Good service in the restaurant business is almost always associated with the word *intimate*, as is service from an attorney, financial advisor, or golf pro. For example, take a golf lesson with four other people and you will automatically expect more help and better service than you would at a golf camp where you and 20 others are banging balls on the range with one professional.

The restaurant and fitness fields are service businesses. If they are good, both try to sell an experience that surrounds the product they are delivering. If they are bad, they sell the product itself—much like an all-you-can-eat buffet that has no atmosphere or service but simply offers cheap food that if eaten may keep you alive. Training-centric fitness businesses are the move away from the buffet approach we have used for so long in the business and where now there seems to be a "buffet fitness" place on every corner toward a fine dining experience where every client gets better service and a better result from the experience.

This is also why positioning, as it's called in the business books, is so important to owners who are trying to conceptualize their businesses to stay competitive into the future. Positioning has many definitions, but the most important for us is how your business relates to other fitness offerings in the area and to the rest of the industry. It also means how you define the business and the product it offers. But for our use, we define positioning as the ability to focus the business from a "one size fits all" concept to a narrowly defined, very specific business plan that specializes in one single aspect of the fitness business.

The one-size-fits-all, volume-driven approach makes it very difficult to provide a salable fitness experience to the consumer that the experience becomes so impersonal unless the impetus for the sale is just price. If there is no act, atmosphere, or service to support the fitness experience the consumer is seeking and no evidence that the business has any understanding of his specific needs, then the only thing you have to sell is how cheap you can go compared to the other fitness businesses in the area. This system fails, of course, if the guy down the street matches your low price or even goes lower. When price is the only thing you sell, then it will be the key factor your competition chases, and again—as you will note throughout this book—if too many clubs go low in any given market, there is only so much volume available for those players in that category.

However, most club owners believe they are already focused and that their service and ability to get results is the niche they already own in the market. In fact, every human being that has ever owned a fitness business has claimed to have the best service in town and his club is the only one that has the equipment to get you into the shape of your life.

Talking to this owner is kind of like talking to 30 different parents at a school function. Every parent brags about his kid being above average and really special in school. Someone is lying. Who owns the average and below-average kids we read about in the papers? Which one of these parents owns the school idiot who blows up toilets, spits on the school nerd, and is always in trouble?

Most mainstream clubs only really touch a relatively small percentage of their members. For example, look at the following breakdown of a typical box club. Assume here that these numbers are for every 100 members in the club:

- Twenty percent or so just won't change (read: too stupid to change). These members do the same workout they did 20 years ago or read about in a magazine and simply won't change.
- Twenty percent or so—depending on the club's penetration rate into its membership—will do group exercise. Being in group exercise is a good thing because the participants develop relationships with each other and the instructor, resulting in a relationship that leads to higher retention numbers.
- Roughly 5 percent will pay for one-on-one training in a typical box. Some clubs do a little better than this, but it is the extremely rare club that approaches even 10 percent.
- This means that 55 percent of this club's members get no help whatsoever after the initial one workout and then solo routine.

Service and workout support as a whole in this industry suck. It's so bad that "suck" is the only word to describe it. For example, you can't buy a cold nonworkout drink in more than 50 percent of the gyms in this country. Only a small handful of gyms in this country will actually let you try the facility for more than one workout before you have to make a buying decision. Very few offer amenities in the locker rooms. Most have no training advice available unless you pay for one-on-one and it is not unusual for a club to have private areas where all the newest and most desirable equipment is restricted to the elite training clients. Guest policies are still left over from the 1960s, when the guest has to fill out two to three pages of worthless information and go on a two-hour tour before he can actually join his friend.

The sad thing is that most clubs believe they have covered the service niche because they have a trainer or two on the floor and because they have more equipment than their competitors. Most of the clubs that fall into this trap of believing they have excellent service really don't because they are comparing their service against other clubs in the industry.

In other words, they are comparing themselves against an already low standard. It's like being a kid and calling your friend names. "Hey, you're stupid," you yell. She answers: "Well, I may be stupid, but at least I'm not ugly." Who really won here and is stupid really better than ugly?

Service in the fitness industry is sort of the same. As a whole, it is so bad that you can offer above-average service according to the industry standard and still stink. You are better than the other guy but still not really much better off. You're stupid, but he is still ugly.

The standards we operate against haven't really changed in 30 years. For example, 30 years ago, the salesperson would take the prospect into an office and pressure the person into a sale. Thirty years later, most of the large chains are still using sales offices—something the average consumer feels extremely negative about due to the intimidation factor when he visits a gym.

Thirty years ago, the main way to advertise was to run price specials (sales) and then work to close the prospect during the first visit. This is still the same operational procedure in most clubs today and especially by the chain players.

Thirty years ago, you had to bring your own lock, shower in questionable locker rooms, and bring your own towel. Except in a limited number of clubs, you still have to bring your own lock, shower in death-defying conditions, and bring your own towel. The clubs are bigger, the equipment shinier, but still everything is different but the same.

One final comparison to note is that 30 years ago, a trainer would set you up on a program and then turn you loose after one to three workouts—whether you understood it or not and regardless of whether this program is really the one you should be doing. Thirty years later, most clubs will still set you up on a simple circuit workout and then force you out on your own after one or two laps with a trainer whether you are ready or not.

Nothing has changed much. The industry's perception of getting results is still about the same. A lot of the things we do out of habit today are based on things done at facilities that were mostly unfocused in their positioning and that operated under the concept that their facilities met the service needs of every single type of consumer.

The problem with assuming you already have a results-driven focus—based on your perception of service—is that you often aren't really giving consumers what they want. Many business plans are based on assumptions that are no longer true or relevant in the gym business, meaning that the focus of the business is either too broad or too outdated.

For example, it was extremely hard to make money with child care, group exercise, and racquet sports for most of the 1990s. Child care is based on too small of a population in the gym, but by maintaining too broad of a focus with our business plans, we felt we had to have child care to compete. Aerobics/ group exercise faded away in many clubs, as discussed in other chapters, but owners were still developing new projects that included $75,000 aerobics rooms—something the majority of members would rather had seen replaced with extended cardio presentations. Owners offered their own version of what a club should be that often had no relationship to what a member from that era wanted.

In today's markets, some members still want child care and some pockets of the country are still hot with group training. But do enough of these people really want it and will enough pay for it to make it profitable for the club? Is the club offering these programs because it might make money or because the owner's perception of service and quality includes these concepts, which might no longer be important to the majority of members? And would this owner be better to cut back classes, eliminate child care, and expand his functional group personal training?

Quality is also a focus that many clubs believe they already own. Advertising that you're the best club in the area is irrelevant to the average consumer. Everyone says they have the best gym. Have you ever heard an owner say "Well, my gym really sucks compared to everyone else's. I have a really ugly and pathetic staff comprised of my in-laws and we don't really clean often, but we still manage to hang in there."

The problem for the owner who believes his club is already focused in the quality niche is that probably nine times out of 10, the average consumer with little experience can't tell the difference between a good gym and a weak gym during just one visit. This changes, of course, if the individual is involved in the club for some relevant period of time and those who have spent years in a club know right away if you have what it takes to get their money.

Another problem with the quality focus is that while most clubs seek quality, they tend to ignore the member's perception of real quality. In general, the club owner applies his own definition of quality to the club regardless of what the member really wants.

For example, at one club, the owner set up a program where every new member had to go through a fitness analysis before he was allowed to work out. The analysis included a strength test, a body fat test, and a complete functional movement screen. The owner thought this was a wonderful competitive edge against the competitors who were not doing any initial workups. This was all done during the sales process and mostly prior to the client becoming an actual member.

However, the majority of the members—in response to a verbal survey—had no real interest in the analysis as a group. The majority preferred more intense and patient help with their initial programs instead of being turned loose too soon. Many of the members were older than 35, had limited gym experience, and felt they needed more help understanding their programs instead of getting analysis in areas they didn't feel were really relevant for novices.

Put another way, the potential member already knows he has issues. You don't really need to take a fat guy who already feels bad about his shape and then do a body composition on him during his first workout, especially if he isn't yet a member. He already knows he is fat, which is why he is there, and he probably doesn't need to know an exact number as to how fat he really is.

Most analysis is better used to establish a baseline for someone who is already in the system and not for a potential client who is already scared to death and hasn't been in a club for two decades. Fat is fat and he doesn't need to know that he has 35 percent body fat, which is the fattest guy you tested this week.

The owner in this example was providing a costly and labor-intensive service because he felt it gave the club a quality edge in the marketplace. However, the members felt that the club wasn't really meeting their needs as a group and they wanted more help and guidance during their first 30 days rather than testing that did nothing for them prior to starting. While the owner's attempt to apply quality as the club's focus was a good idea, the applied definition was wrong.

The perception of quality is what people buy, and although your facility may be truly better than your competitors', a potential member may not perceive it as such. The sad truth is that most potential members feel that all gyms and fitness facilities are somewhat the same. And when you look at a typical grouping of clubs from almost any marketplace, they are basically the same.

For example, consider the staff. Most gyms have the same configurations. The front counter people are typically young women who are constantly being replaced by other very young women, as the current position holder leaves for another job. Many of these women are too young and too inexperienced to have acquired the communication skills necessary to effectively deliver member service to a large range of members at the front counter.

The trainers and other support staff are also mostly very young folks who are willing to work for pretty low wages. The problem with a staff of mostly very young employees is that due to the somewhat unstructured nature of the fitness business, it takes some maturity and intensive training to learn to give great member service.

We have to remember that we are not serving endless trays of hamburgers. In the fitness business, an employee may be responsible for a variety of tasks throughout the day that aren't necessarily covered by a simple member service strategy.

The only real adult people working in most clubs are the salespeople and managers—folks who seldom come into contact with as many members as the junior staff. These folks may know and be able to deliver member service, but it's the lower-level staff who are responsible for the daily image of the club.

The potential members who visit more than one club see this. All the staffs seem somewhat the same, all the equipment looks alike, and most of the club's programs and offerings are simply duplicates of a competitor's. The owners may say: "Hey, wait a minute—our cycle program is twice as good as the guy's across the street. How can you compare us to them?" They can— and do—because both programs look just alike to the consumer. The bikes are about the same, the room is about the same, and even the color of the schedule is like the competitor's. In other words, there is no difference in the perception of quality between the two programs.

Quality and the Perception of Quality

Can you truly stand out in a competitive marketplace with better quality or can you increase your quality and the perception of quality and really be different?

When you focus the business, you improve perception of quality. When you let the business become unfocused, the perception of quality in the member's mind goes down. Everything you do should increase the perception of quality and narrow the focus of the business.

For most fitness businesses, there are only two mantras that have to be repeated daily in your head:

- This member is not replaceable. What can I do to keep him?
- What can I do to get the maximum number of members the best results at a reasonable cost to them and a profit for me?

Consider the following scenario and try to evaluate the focus and perception of quality from the member's viewpoint. We have a 40,000-square-foot facility that offers everything. The club has weight equipment, aerobics, cycle programs, cardio equipment, children's programming, senior programming, basketball on a half court, weight loss, personal trainers, and a small pro shop and juice counter. Let's look at some typical questions a potential member might ask about the club and the problems these questions could raise for the owner.

Who is this gym for?

It's a multipurpose club that's for everyone. Without a specific focus, such as a family recreation center, this club would have a hard time even putting together a marketing piece. Who would the piece target? How could you put together a piece that goes after absolutely everyone in the community?

What kind of personal attention can a gym of this size offer me?

The club may claim a lot of personal attention, but in reality, how much real attention can a club of this size give the individual member in most markets? The exception might be rural markets where the cost of delivering service is cheaper. But in most markets, this club would need to do a lot of sales—probably between a minimum of 75 to 150 per month and as high as 250 or more a month depending on the market if it is a low-price player—to stay in business. That situation usually doesn't lend itself to the delivery of great member service. The club could indeed give decent service if the circumstances were right, but the feel of such a large facility works against the owner. It just doesn't feel that such a large business could give great personal service.

Without a specific target market, such as a family recreation center or an upscale adult facility, this club would have a hard time even putting together a marketing piece.

How would the member mix work?

A club with such a broad focus would have trouble mixing such a wide range of members. Do small children and serious lifters work together? Do high-energy folks in their late 20s work well with a daytime senior population? Most clubs that operate without a specific target market try to segregate the different populations by either time or into separate areas in the club—neither of which works well.

For example, a serious cardio person who stops by the facility during his lunch hour will be frustrated when faced with a herd of little old ladies on the treadmills walking at one mile an hour and watching soaps. The mix is bad because the focus is bad.

Keep in mind that it's not the club's size that doesn't work. It's the lack of focus toward a specific market segment and the member's perception of quality. Clubs this size that are narrowly focused can and do work, but the owners face problems that smaller, more intimate facilities don't. However, common sense tells you that the bigger club should make more money because it's bigger and can hold more members. Be everything to everyone seems logical, but a club like this could probably make more money by going after a narrower niche, such as becoming a family recreation center or a corporate club.

Also keep in mind that in today's market, progressive training clubs are now doing the total deposits that these big boxes once did with a substantially smaller start-up costs and monthly operating expenses. The burden on the operator of this club would be how could he turn this into a training-centric club that might penetrate as high as 33 percent or more in some form of training, such as group personal training or semiprivate group training, rather than the typical 3 to 6 percent one-on-one training?

From the member's perspective, how can a club so big give any kind of personal service? If you want service, don't you usually go to the small, personalized specialty stores? And how can a club this size really specialize and service so many different groups of people? The club may have a little bit of everything, but nothing is complete. A good example of this is the new breed of recreation centers going up around the country. They're big and well capitalized and are built to serve the entire community.

The argument made for the big clubs usually cites the Nordstrom model. In this model, a large box retailer can provide legendary service known throughout the industry and best of class, so why can't we? However, this argument breaks down when you take into account the volume that this store would service at any given time. Most of the encounters are limited engagements between a customer and a sales clerk that involve a little guidance, leading them to the right area of the store and then ringing them up.

This sales encounter takes a lot less time than it does to set a person up on a new workout—one that he will forget in the car on the way home—and the client is now coming back on a recurring basis as part of a large group during primetime. In the fitness business, that lucky member who can work out at 2 p.m. gets a lot of help compared to the one out of 400 in the club during primetime.

But these new types of recreation facilities mentioned seldom work financially or meet the member's expectations of quality. For example, two facilities were built a short distance apart near the ski areas in central Colorado. They were built as community recreation centers and both enjoy a great tax base for support. The clubs have some of everything related to fitness, but nothing is really done right.

For example, each facility has weight equipment, but because the facilities are trying to offer so many different programs to so many different people, neither is really a complete weight room. Both facilities have rooms that are small, cramped, and dangerous to the user and have low-end equipment furnished by the lowest bidder. There is enough equipment for basic workouts but not enough for quality workouts. The average person or novice could enjoy the rooms, but anyone with any higher expectations wouldn't be happy very long.

Both facilities also have running tracks that are used by a small percentage of the members. But both facilities have lousy cardio presentations—the equipment most desired and expected by members all around the country—probably in part due to the commitment to the track. They have cardio but just a representation and not enough to satisfy the needs of most of the facilities' clients.

If your business has too broad a focus with the dream of being everything to everyone in your community, you end up like these recreation facilities, where you end up nothing more than big, impersonal boxes resembling warehouses. You have a representation of everything somewhere in the building, but nothing is complete or focused toward any specific group. This leaves the users of those areas frustrated because those areas or that equipment really doesn't satisfy the need. If you have to wait for a treadmill because there are only three or four, it's very frustrating if that's the reason you joined in the first place. It's like saying "We'll put a little of everything in this place and try to make as many people as possible happy." It just doesn't work because the offerings never really satisfy any specific group.

How can an owner focus a business? He needs to start by understanding the word *category*. Category means you are picking one specific niche to make your own from the broader category of fitness facility. Your goal is to choose, develop, and then own the specific niche in that category for your market.

Keep in mind that the goal is to focus the category down to one very specific point. For example, a large category may be full retail, such as a Walmart store that carries one of just about everything on the planet. It would be hard to open a Walmart-style store across the street because it owns that category.

However, a businessperson could open a specialty retail clothing store right next door and still do well. Walmart might sell a few similar lines of clothes, but the offerings are usually somewhat limited. If you wanted a basic dress shirt, you may go to Walmart. But if you wanted a nicer shirt and tie, you would most likely end up next door in the retail shop.

Also keep in mind that in the fitness business, you can't be everything to everyone. In fact, trying to appeal to every single person in the market is impossible. For example, consider price. There is no one price that appeals to every consumer. If the price is too high, it may limit folks looking just for cheap rates. If the price is too low, the perception of quality won't be there and folks looking for a full-service, top-end club won't respond.

Another practical example is the karate school business. It makes sense to have a karate school open to all students of all ages. But this is not the way to maximize the business in most markets. For example, several martial arts organizations have experimented with children-only facilities and have experienced great success. By being open to just children, you are sending the message that you specialize in children, that your children will be safe here because they don't have to interact with adults, and that the entire staff and facility are geared toward the needs of kids.

Most fitness businesses that wish to get focused need to follow this example and learn to subtract. Many facilities simply offer too many different types of programs that try to appeal to too many different types of people.

Keep in mind that backward common sense tells you to offer as many things as possible so your business will appeal to as many different types of people as possible. But common sense doesn't always work in the real business world when faced with the reality of the marketplace.

In the karate school example, the business that specialized in kids prospered because parents who would not have considered the regular schools would take a chance on a kids-only school. The generalist didn't appeal, whereas the specialist did.

Looking again at the recreation facilities in Colorado, a fitness facility that specializes in adults between 24 and 45 years old could successfully compete against the target-challenged recreation centers. This type of adult center could specialize in adult training needs, nutritional guidance and music that is more specific for this age group and could plan and decorate the facility for an adult population. For example, locker rooms could be several levels better than those offered by a recreation center that services large groups of kids whose idea of a great Saturday is trashing the lockers.

Niches, or areas of focus, that are possible in the fitness business include but are not necessarily limited to the following:

- The 3,000- to 7,500-square-foot functional based training gym
- The 7,500- to 12-000-square-foot training-centric club with a target of at least 40 percent of all members involved in some type of personal training
- The sport-performance training center with a highlight on the athletes in the area, especially the children who want to learn about agility, strength, and quickness prior to learning the actual skills of their chosen sport
- The 12,000- to 15,000-square-foot training-centric club with group exercise
- The women-only, training-centric club. It is important to note that most women-only clubs are based on a very outdated model and in fact are nothing more than mainstream box clubs that are shrunken. This type of business plan will not be sustainable in the future and the days of telling women they can't sweat or use a kettlebell are gone. This club works, but you train the female clients exactly as you would any athlete, except you might use lighter or small tools.
- The high-energy, athletic-based facility. These clubs would work better in towns where a bigger part of the population works out, such as Colorado, and the basis for this club is emulating the athletic lifestyle. This is what the franchise clubs in the 1990s used to be like before following the mainstream box model.
- The very serious or hardcore niche club, such as a kettlebell club
- The corporate niche. Due to the newer emphasis on functional equipment, it can be built for a cheaper cost in a smaller footprint.

- The neighborhood or community niche. This niche is appropriate in more rural areas and is more of a full-service club, but it still has to be training-centric, focusing on a higher return per member through targeting at least 33 percent of its members involved in some type of training.
- The family center niche. This niche still works in some areas, especially the South, but the cost of building these big boxes and the difficulty in getting financing for them will limit their growth in the coming years. These clubs are simply too big to build and too expensive to service.

These are all niches that might work in a variety of areas around the country. There are also a large number of new fitness concepts that are out there, such as free running academies, urban fitness facilities that use the environment as the equipment, and even the reappearance of group exercise–only facilities again. The important thing to note is that the new operator, along with the new consumer, is redefining what a fitness business should be and most of what will be will not resemble the 100,000-square-foot box that now represents state of the art for so many owners.

A final point to note is that when you are selling a service, which in our case is a results-driven membership, we are ultimately selling a relationship. By seeking a narrower target market, you will be able to build a club that allows you to create a stronger and more long-term relationship with the customers who eventually choose your business.

This will happen because your gym will be filled with folks who chose your business because it matched them and their perceptions of the fitness business, as opposed to your building a business around whoever happens to join. In fact, we are learning to seek a very specific member group instead of trying to match our business concept to whoever shows up at the door.

This selection process allows you as an owner to be more proactive in the running and decision-making process of your business. By planning a business that targets a specific clientele, we can better serve our customers, better prepare for their needs, and build better relationships because we specialize in their individual needs.

The trend in the industry is toward unfocused, impersonal facilities that attempt to appeal to an exceptionally wide range of clients. This type of owner doesn't really seem to understand what the consumer is buying. Members don't buy endless rows of equipment and workouts. They do and will buy the fitness experience with the ultimate goal of getting sustainable results over time.

Part of the fitness experience is developing a perception of quality in the business. Your gym may really be better than everyone else's in town, but the member may not perceive the difference in quality. All your marketing and business planning should be centered on developing this perception in the member's mind.

Many clubs can't develop or improve this perception of quality because of the fuzziness of their focus. Trying to be everything to everybody does not increase your potential business but rather limits it because there is no specific appeal for any one group. To be successful in the coming years, you need to learn to focus by limiting or narrowing your concept. A functional training gym or women-only center is an excellent example of a business that has a narrow and specific focus under the general category of a fitness facility.

December 4, 2013
Forgetting the ones you love

Days pass quickly when you are busy in your life and time can pass so fast you simply lose the ones you love. Refuse to do this. If you find people you care about and want to keep in your life, reach out to them often and never let go of those you love. And as rare as it is now—and will be even more so in the coming years—actually talking to someone for even a few minutes is so much more powerful than a few lines of text delivered impersonally through whatever device you have at hand. An evening with friends—filled with conversation and perhaps a glass of wine and plenty of laughter—is in many ways the essence of life and is something that isn't determined by how much money you have or where you live. Friends are life and the good ones are worth effort and whatever it might take to keep them close to your side. Keep this thought close this month. Sometimes, we forget that there is more to life than just getting it done today.

January 21, 2014
Generalists eat last.

Generalists are people who try to do everything well, but in reality, they end up doing everything—at best—at an average level. Specialists are those who niche themselves in the market and who focus their education and training on working with groups that fascinate them. If you are a women-only specialist, sports performance in golf, or maybe fitness after 50, people will drive past the average "I do everybody" trainer to work with one who understands their needs and problems. Find an area you are passionate about and then kill it by being the master of that niche. When you focus your energy in mastering a specific segment, it doesn't take long to be the expert—and experts eat while generalists fade away. Three years from today, you could be the best there is in the world in your chosen niche, and if you want to be the leader, the writer, the front of the room presenter, and the expert, then declare that niche and go crazy mastering everything it takes to be that person.

5

If Your Financial Foundation Is Right, You Can Make a Lot of Mistakes and Still Stay in Business

How you charge your members and collect their dues is the most important decision you make as an owner. If the financial foundation is right, you can make a lot of mistakes and still stay in business. If the financial foundation is wrong, there is nothing you can do to save your business. It is like real life in the fitness world: You can't out-train a bad diet, but in this case, all the membership sales in the fitness universe won't overcome a bad financial foundation.

Fitness businesspeople, especially trainers, seldom ever agree on anything in the business, but there is one universal truth: The goal of any fitness business is to be profitable. We all talk about it and everyone seeks it, but just what is "profitable" in the fitness business? In other words, how does an owner know if his profit is enough or if this profit keeps the business on track for future growth?

If you're losing money, that's pretty much bad form in the industry and it also answers the question about profitability. One seldom hears "Yeah, I could have made money last month, but I decided to take a $10,000 loss instead." Losses—or brackets on the old financial statements—are not considered desirable. But when your business does break through on the plus side, how much profit is enough profit?

In the fitness industry, almost all numbers and ratios are easier to comprehend and relate to if these numbers are looked at on a monthly basis instead of annually. Keep this in mind: Fewer than 15 percent of the clubs in the country net 20 percent on a monthly basis. For example, if the club's base operating expense is $80,000, which includes debt, utilities, salaries, and other general operating expenses, then less that 15 percent of gyms in the country would deposit $96,000 or more per month. This is also true internationally, and in fact, in many countries, it is harder to sustain a profit over time due to tax restrictions, although there are still a few magical places to do business where the competition is thin and owners can enjoy a profit using tools that would otherwise not work in heavy competition areas.

This is, of course, on a pre-tax basis and the cost of operation includes the owner's salary at a fixed rate and adjusted to reflect a manager's working salary. In another example, a profitable 6,000-square-foot training-centric club in the Northeast might have an overhead of $40,000 per month and deposit on the average $46,000 to $75,000 per month. To live and operate in the more expensive markets, such as Connecticut, a profitable 12,000-square-foot club might cost $80,000 to $100,000 to operate on a monthly basis, with a deposit of $120,000 to $130,000. Both of these examples demonstrate variable profitability in the 15 to 20 percent range or higher on a monthly basis.

Parts of the South and the Midwest also show steady profitability, but that's often because of lower rent factors. A facility in Alabama or Iowa that is the same size as one in the Northeast might have a 30 percent smaller operating expense. This decrease in expense is due to lower rents and much lower payroll expenses.

For example, a 12,000-square-foot club in certain parts of the Midwest might only cost $35,000 to $40,000 to operate and might deposit $50,000 a month. The operating costs are lower and the club deposits less, but the 20 percent net is still intact.

The other 85 percent of club owners operating traditional fitness businesses in the country don't net 20 percent on a monthly basis. Many of them are at best month-to-month operations with little or no profits. However, the era of endlessly low returns is starting to change in the industry, as real businesspeople create new fitness businesses or invest in existing clubs and with the advent of the training gym, which generates a consistent profit in the 30 to 40 percent range. Real is defined as people who understand business and who run their facilities with the idea of making a profit—something a lot of rookie owners don't forecast in their business plans nor is long-term profit a motive for many of the old school owners who look for the quick hit and then move on to something else as they find that their operating techniques don't allow for a sustainable business plan.

The percentage of owners in the 20 percent range should not be discouraging. It's not just our industry but most small business in general. Most small businesses in the country, such as mom-and-pop dry cleaners, flower shops, gift shops, or independently owned restaurants, are really just month-to-month businesses. The difference is that you can start a flower shop or card shop for a lot less than a full-blown fitness facility.

This is also changing in the business. After the recession in the first decade of this century, there were fewer openings of the bigger box-style facilities. Lenders were skeptical, the money needed was too big, and the overall economy was starting to damage many of the major chain players.

This was also coupled with the advent of the smaller, more financially efficient training model. For example, new generation owners who might have once been people who would have opened a Gold's Gym were no longer looking at the big box model and instead started opening the smaller training-centric hybrid clubs. Hybrid means that this style business model was really a modified training facility but with an additional layer of open membership being added. These clubs could be opened for $400,000 or less, which included full build-out and equipment and can generate more total revenue than many of the dying box clubs at a much lower overall risk.

The difference between the owners who consistently make money and the rest of the players in the game—or looking at it in different words, the difference between the business-centric people and the passionate people who often bring energy but far less business skill to the industry—is often how they develop and handle their most important asset: their receivables base.

While there are a few small exceptions, most of the profitable clubs' business basics are the same. For example, most club owners who make money over time—defined as those who net 20 percent or better—put more emphasis on mastering the training component, understand member service, hire an older and more mature staff, and have several other thriving multiple profit centers. These clubs also use 12-month contracts, price their monthly memberships aggressively for the market, and have a strong receivables base that allows them to project their business into the future.

The key to the fitness business is receivables. The strength of the receivables base drives the business. Without strong receivables, the business might be healthy in the short run due to cash flow from an intense sales period, but it will most likely never be profitable in the long run because the business really has no secure financial foundation.

Before going further, let's define what a receivables base really is. Simply put, it means people owe you money you hope to collect sometime in the future. A more specific definition that fits our industry is this: If you never sold another new membership at your facility, how much money could you count on collecting in the next 12 months?

The following is a simple way to understand what a receivable base is and how one works. Let's say you have a very, very small club with only four members. We're talking a really elite business here. The club has payments of $40 per month and uses the preferable tool for gym memberships: the 12-month contract. For example:

- Bill is a new member and owes 12 payments: 12 x $40 = $480.
- Ann has been at the club for six months and still owes six more payments: 6 x $40 = $240.
- Joe has only three payments left on his membership: 3 x $40 = $120.
- Kristen has been around for a full membership and owes only one payment: 1 x $40.

The total outstanding payments this owner could collect if everyone paid as promised is $880.

This club's total receivables base, meaning all the money it could hope to collect during the next year if it never sold another membership, would be $880—the total of all outstanding member payments yet to be paid.

Why are receivables so important to a fitness business? Each month, the business receives a check from the member payments that affects the stability and the profitability of the business. Once this check gets strong enough, the business is less vulnerable to outside forces (such as competition) and variable factors (such as weather or short-term economic damage in the market) and becomes able to grow to the next level. The next level for most owners is reinvestment in the physical plant and stronger growth in the future through the maintenance of the membership base, which translates to increased renewals of existing members.

New generation business models do not just depend on the strength of their membership receivable base as the older-style clubs had in the past. In prior business models, the receivable base check might represent more than 80 percent of the club's total monthly income. This style club constantly has to generate a constant flow of new members each month to replace losses (the volume approach) and to keep new cash arriving each month through down payments and other immediate membership transactions.

These clubs usually did a little training revenue, which was seldom profitable and might have a few other small profit centers, such as cooler drinks or a tanning bed or two. In this example, the club has a total monthly deposit of $75,000 and the income might arrive like this:
- $61,500 as a net membership receivable ($75,000 x .82*)
- $7,500 as new membership cash, including daily fees and down payments
- $4,000 in personal training
- $2,000 in snack bars, cooler drinks, tanning, or other minor revenue sources

In a more modern business model, smart owners are chasing both sides of the formula. For example, look at this more extended breakdown of the previous example projected out over a year:

Membership revenue: $61,500 x 12 = $738,000

Training revenue: $4,000 x 12 = $48,000

In the past, the only number that counted was the $738,000. If you wanted to make more money, you simply tried harder to add more memberships and you could in the earlier days of the fitness industry because there were far fewer competitors fighting for a limited market share. However, this doesn't work anymore due to the severe increase in competition, the advent of the low-priced players who depend on sheer volume, and a decrease in new available memberships that isn't keeping up with the increase in new clubs.

The owner sometimes forgets that there are really only three ways to make money in a business:

---

*The national average net membership receivable for mainstream gyms is 82 percent of the club's total revenue. In other words, on average, only 18 percent of a club's revenue comes from other sources besides memberships.

- Get more new clients and/or add more new business by increasing sales or lowering the price of the product offered and go for volume.
- Cut expenses and/or lower operating costs.
- Make more money from the clients you already have and increase the return per client.

When competition is low, you only have to live with the first one on the list. Sell fast, run hard, and let the new sales cover any increased cost of doing business. This is the model the fitness industry was built on, but it is also a model that no longer works. Selling more memberships often becomes impossible in markets where you have a saturation of competition. This is when owners drop their price and go for volume, hoping to undersell their competitors and take away their clients. Once you burn up that market of people willing to change brands for a lower price, which is never as big as anyone really hopes because members are often just too lazy to switch for just a few dollars a month, price then becomes irrelevant because raising it or lowering it fails in a price-driven market.

The negative here is that owners who start their business with a heavy volume approach don't know what to do when times get tough. The newer business model that began appearing during the price wars driven by the declining economy was based on a healthy mix of all three rather than just totally depending on just volume alone. This new trend was also a direct derivative of the advent of functional training delivered through newer tools the owner could sell to the consumer, such as group personal training, small group semiprivate training, and boot camps.

The same club that deposited $75,000 a month might now have a higher deposit despite the owner still doing the same membership-driven revenue. For example, let's look at the club turned into a training-centric business model with a deposit now of $100,000:

- $61,500 as net membership receivable income
- $10,000 in new sales cash
- $26,500 in training revenue
- $2,000 in other small profit center income

This is still a weak business club in today's business world, but this owner is shifting in the right direction. In this case, he is now decreasing his need for sheer volume by tapping into the membership base he already has, which is shown by the increase in training revenue. In other words, he is making more money from clients already in the system.

This is also assuming that this owner has stopped the old practice of just selling sessions and packages to the clients, such as 10 workouts with a trainer for $500, and instead moved into the business model where all training is done on 12-month contracts and tracked separately each month, with the goal at some point being having the total training revenue in the club equal to the total net membership receivable check.

This shift also reflects that the membership-driven business model is failing in the industry and being replaced by a model that emphasizes return per member and membership but with the recognition that there is only so much membership to go around in any given market.

What Does a Healthy Business Look Like?

For a business to be healthy and stable, a certain percentage of the club's base operating expense (BOE) should be covered by the monthly receivables. The BOE is defined as what it takes the business to pay its monthly expenses minus the owner's salary. Rent or mortgage, payroll, utilities, advertising, debt service, and general operating expenses are all included in the BOE.

The goal for a healthy business is to get a minimum 70 percent coverage of the BOE by the net monthly receivable check. For example, a club's BOE is $80,000 per month and the monthly check from the member payments from the receivables is $56,000.

$$\$56,000/\$80,000 = .70$$

(in this case, the club owner has 70 percent
of his monthly expense covered)

This coverage is one of the first and most important financial indicators an owner should master as an analysis tool in his business. A new business just starting out can hit this ratio at about the 13th month of operation, which is the first level of maturity a club business goes through due to the first influx of renewals. Training gyms can achieve this number in as little as six months and often 100 percent of their operating expense will be covered by the net receivable base by the end of the first year.

It's possible to do better than 70 percent coverage of the BOE. In fact, about 5 to 8 percent of the mainstream businesses in the industry achieve 100 percent coverage and this can happen beginning around the 25th month of operation, which is the second level of maturity a club passes through as the second round of member renewals occurs.

How important is this ratio? It might be the most important number to watch in your business. If your club's receivables ever achieve this percentage of the BOE, you can make a lot of mistakes and still survive. You could also last in a fight against a new or existing competitor because at this point, you have income that can be counted on for at least five months before it starts to deteriorate, even if new sales slow down. This should give you plenty of time to react and revise your business plan without having to make major mistakes because you're rushed.

A second ratio to look at is the relationship between your total outstanding receivables and your monthly BOE. The desirable ratio is 5 to 1, meaning your outstanding receivables are five times greater than your monthly operating expenses. For example, Club Workout has a $50,000-a-month BOE and a $300,000 outstanding receivables base:

$$\$300,000/50,000 = 6$$

In this example, Club Workout has a 6 to 1 ratio of outstanding receivables to its BOE.

In a second example, Club Fitness has a $48,000-a-month BOE and a $210,000 outstanding receivables base:

$$\$210,000/48,000 = 4.4$$

In the second example, Club Fitness has a 4.4 to 1 ratio of outstanding receivables to its monthly BOE.

If achieved, a 5 to 1 ratio greatly decreases a club's vulnerability in the marketplace. If the owner had to step away from the business due to illness or family matters (and remember that most owners are the key person in their organizations), the business's income could dramatically decline. Or if a tough competitor opened and you needed time to rebuild or if there was simply a downturn in the local economy, the club could count on a reasonable amount of income projected into the future.

Without a 5 to 1 ratio, Club Fitness and its 4.4 ratio would not have sufficient reserves if any of these things stressing things happened to the owner and his business. The owner might have to scramble to survive, which leads to mistakes, such as the severe discounting of new memberships, which makes existing members who paid more furious. Other scrambling-style mistakes are offering cash specials, which immediately decrease the return per member and will destroy a club in the long run, or other short-term solutions that eventually weaken and then destroy a business plan.

Note that the Club Workout and Club Fitness examples are based on 12-month contracts. Long-term contracts, meaning they are two years or longer in length, have extremely high loss rates, which will be discussed later in this chapter. If you are currently using 24-month contracts, simply divide by two and then apply the formula.

If you use strictly open-ended memberships, which are also called month-to-month memberships, you have cash flow but no usable ratio and no real long-term stability in the business. The cash flow obviously has value each month to the owner, but this delicate and inconsistent source of revenue can very easily be disrupted because there is no established obligation on the member's part.

Obligation and Method of Payment

When working to establish a receivables base, you have to learn to recognize the difference between obligation and method of payment, which are often confused by even experienced fitness business owners.

Obligation is the time commitment the member agrees to when he joins the club. This commitment may be one week, one month, six months, or even three years if the member is crazy enough to join a club that has its business plan rooted in the 1960s and is willing to commit to a service business for the next three years of his life.

Members in today's market have been known to become extremely distrustful when their memberships last longer than their car leases or marriages. These clubs need to wake up and realize that Elvis is dead (maybe), TVs now have color, and the members are much more sophisticated than we give them credit for when it comes to making business decisions.

Method of payment is how the member elects to make his payment each month, meaning he has a choice instead of being forced into a specific payment method. We're still talking about making payments each month at this point and not about cash or paid-in-full memberships. Paid-in-full memberships will be briefly discussed here and covered in depth later in this section.

Method of payment is also where the confusion arises for many owners and their staffs because of the advent of electronic funds transfer (EFT) that has been a steadily increasing part of the industry since the mid-1980s. EFT means that the member authorizes the club to make a monthly deduction from a checking account, savings account, or credit card. Because of some of the ad campaigns run over the years by some of the EFT companies in the industry, many owners confuse obligations—or the contractual time a member commits to through the membership—with EFT, or the automatic deduction of funds.

Setting a member up on EFT does not mean the member guarantees to pay. It just means he is allowing the club to deduct the monthly payment until the member says stop. EFT does not imply obligation. Obligation has to be established first and method of payment is the secondary concern.

Some of the EFT companies make such claims as "Collect all the money from all the members every month automatically." The implied claim is that the member no longer has to make a decision each month to write a check and that the money would be drafted from the member's account or credit card automatically without any interference from the member.

This is not only not true but also actually misleading to club owners because these owners are expecting the system to be somewhat bonehead proof and that the burden of collecting the money from the members each month shifts away from the club owner to the EFT company. Due to this, these owners are not usually ready to handle common EFT problems that arise in every club's account, such as closed accounts, nonsufficient funds, or bank routing problems. When these problems do occur, the EFT company often charges the owner a number of additional fees, but eventually, the owner will find the burden of the collection will ultimately revert back to him and his stressed-out staff. This scenario is only true for EFT companies that are mere processors and does not apply to the more sophisticated third-party financial service companies that provide EFT as a part of their total collection and service efforts.

The club owner should first focus on establishing an obligation with the member and then allow the member to choose the method of payment.

Keep in mind that the development of an outstanding receivables base, which should be every owner's goal, is based on a time obligation commitment from the member. Twelve-month memberships are the tool of choice for obligation because they have traditionally lower loss rates, which will be discussed later in this chapter.

Although EFT does perform slightly better than allowing members to write checks each month—usually about 5 to 7 percent better on the average—there are still some major problems when using it exclusively or, worse, forcing it on members as their only method of payment.

For example, let's look at Figure 5-1, which is a simple and somewhat stereotypical representation of a club's total membership.

10	Wealthy person, great watch, real car, spends money in the club, probably in his late 40s
9	Not quite as wealthy but is still above average in income
8	A solid citizen, a family person, has a good job, good income, and is a regular member
7	On a starting career track, has a new family, real house payment, and is just now getting to the point where there is a little discretionary income
6	Acquiring his first assets, maybe his first nice home and corresponding payment, has a lot of credit card debt but is on the right track
5	A young executive or manager, maybe is renting or owns a small condo, in credit card debt but having a great time. The club owner should first focus on establishing an obligation with the member and then allow the member to choose the method of payment.
4	On his second or third step in a new career, has a new car, has a bigger apartment, and is leveraged to just above the eyes in credit and consumer debt but doesn't care because he is having a great time in life and he'll deal with it later
3	Your basic solid lower-paid, blue-collar type, living check to check, but pays his bills on time and still lives within his means
2	First real job, first steady income, and always spends just a little more than he makes
1	Has his hat on backward, no checking account or savings account, and couldn't get a credit card if his life depended on it. Don't forget his cutoff jean shorts and combat boots. Paying bills on time for this guy? What does that mean and why would he care? He is just looking for a place to work out.

Figure 5-1. Range of a club's total membership

Again, this is a crude illustration of a range of members that might belong to a typical club. Each member is different and those differences mean that not every member would accept the same system or method of payment. There is no one size fits all when it comes to pricing and charging your membership.

Despite the hype about its ease of use and growing acceptance through the years, EFT is still not totally accepted by all consumers, although it is inevitable that ultimately everything will be electronically driven and tools from the last century, such as checks, will be museum pieces, but for now, there is still a certain population that needs a choice when it comes to paying you for a membership.

The people in the 8, 9, and 10 slots are those who seldom bounce checks, may be more sophisticated when it comes to money, and may choose to use

EFT as a method of payment because they understand it and are comfortable with it. They will let you tap their checking account or, most likely, a credit card for their monthly payment

On the other hand, these folks might also be your slightly older folks in the club who did not grow up with EFT and who prefer to pay with a method of payment they are more used to, such as writing a check for their membership each month or using electronic banking. In other words, the people in these slots would probably agree to a 12-month membership but may or may not allow an EFT draft depending on their age and personal experience with the method.

Slots 4, 5, 6, and 7 are usually people who are a little older than the lower slots, meaning mid-20s to early 40s, involved in a career, but are often check-to-check folks. They may agree to EFT, but they often prefer to write a check because of float in their accounts. Clubs that force EFT may get some of these folks in this group, but these are often where the account problems occur due to such things as closed accounts or insufficient funds.

Many of the people in this group would also not join a club that forces EFT because of the lack of control on when the money is taken from their accounts, although this barrier is also decreasing. The obligation is not the problem. It's how they get to pay that matters to them. Some clubs claim they have no problems forcing EFT on the people who come into the club to buy a membership and they are correct about this group of dedicated buyers already in the business, but it's the people who don't come in because the club only has EFT that are the problem, and in this case, the system is limiting the business potential of the club.

The bottom echelon—slots 1, 2, and 3 and even stretching into 4 a little—is the people who don't even get to play in most club's memberships systems unless the club is charging $10 or less and then you might sign these people up as members, but you then open all kinds of new problems trying to collect from this category. Clubs that force EFT eliminate these folks altogether, which is bad business because of two reasons. First of all, clubs are still the best social outlets in a community. For $19 to $39 per month in most markets, a member can come every day, stay as long as he likes, take a shower, meet his friends, and generally hang out and work out. Clubs are still the best entertainment buy around no matter what the economy is doing.

For many people in the lower slots on the chart, the club becomes one of the most important aspects of their life. A lot of sacrifices will be made when it comes to paying other bills just so the person can keep that membership going if the member is treated correctly and can join using a payment system he is comfortable using.

The second reason it's bad business to eliminate these folks is actually the other side of the same reason most clubs force EFT: to keep these folks out in the first place. Some of these people are horrible bill-payers. They don't have checking accounts and the concept of credit cards is only something they dream about at night. But these people may actually pay for a while, which is money the gym owner wouldn't have had if it hadn't allowed these people to try.

No owner should ever expect to collect all the money from all the members. It's just a wild fitness fantasy to expect to come up with a 100 percent perfect collection system. But losing money is frustrating, and when a member stiffs you as an owner, you vow to never let it happen again. A lot of financial vendors in the industry, such as the EFT companies, capitalize well on this emotional response to getting stiffed. Often, it's not the members but the system the club is using for charging and collecting memberships that's the problem.

You can't expect to collect all the money. It's not reality in virtually any business and it is definitely not the reality where a discretionary money option is involved, meaning that the person will always pay for his car, house, food, and other necessities before he will make a payment that is more of an option than a need. However, the reality is that whoever collects the most money from the most members in this industry wins. Every pricing and collection decision you make when it comes to building a financial foundation should be based on collecting the most money from the most members over time.

That's why 24-month contracts are no good. The losses are too high and you don't collect as much money as you should per member. That's why discounting for cash is no good either. It lowers the return per member too much and will eventually evolve to less than $200 per year. And that's why forcing EFT as a method of payment and confusing it with an obligation is not workable either. It eliminates potential members, creates losses the club does not have the staff to handle daily (such as closed accounts), and forces a system that many people still haven't totally accepted as part of their personal financial lives.

The final point when it comes to obligation and method of payment is that the club establishes the desired obligation it seeks from its members. As we'll discuss later, 12-month contracts, with variations as needed, are the heart of your membership system because this tool allows the club to build up a strong receivables base with minimum losses.

Once the member agrees to the obligation, he should have the choice of method of payment. Some people will seek EFT, some will pay by check each month (as they do their other bills), and a few might pay for their year all at once. EFT is cheaper to have serviced by a third-party financial service provider and checks are usually a little more expensive to process, which is passed along to the owner.

Due to the higher cost of processing and collecting member checks, some clubs do charge members who want to write checks each month up to $5 more a month over their EFT rate. For example, a club's monthly EFT rate might be $34 and it might charge $39 for these same folks who want to write a check instead of agreeing to a draft. This is a dated system and not recommended. You have a new member who is trying to pay you each month using the system he is most comfortable with, so take the money any way he wants to pay you, especially because he is paying you and not your competitor. Keep in mind that what seems best for the owners is not necessarily what's best for the members when it comes to member service.

Eventually, every member will pay you monthly by some form of electronic transfer, but until we get to that point, keep your system open enough to collect the most money from the most clients you can get.

Increased Yield

By choosing a financial system that increases return per member and by making choices that depend on loss rates and membership collectables, we are ultimately trying to drive up the yield. Simply defined, the *yield* is what's really left over from the member's monthly payment after certain adjustments are made. The higher the yield, the stronger the receivables base and the more money the club actually has to work with each month.

For example, many novice owners build business projections based on a certain payment amount, such as $40 per month per member, but never adjust for loss rates, cancellation rates, cost of collection, or the impact of "free" services—all of which affect the final yield from that payment.

Freebies, such as free child care, free coffee, free towel service, and other giveaways, in the name of member service or beating the competition all work to lower the yield. It's true that the cost of these services is shown on the expense side of the financial statements as part of doing business, but there is no quantifiable co-entry on the revenue side. In other words, these free services decrease the yield without demonstrating any corresponding increase on the revenue side.

One of the free services creating the largest drain in a modern mainstream box gym is group exercise/aerobics. In recent years, overall membership prices have actually dropped in the industry. With the advent of the low-price players, many club owners dropped their simple access fee—defined as the fee a member would pay to just use the equipment and cardio—in order to appear competitive in a price-sensitive market. However, many of these clubs have continued to include group exercise as a base offering. Group exercise as defined here is not to be confused with group personal or team training, but rather, *group exercise* is defined as the old-style aerobics classes.

What makes this so hard on the business plan is that the group exercise part of the business is declining due to the rising popularity of the group training, the increasing age and difficulty of finding instructors, and the migration of the young women entering the industry into the training realm rather than the group exercise field. Due to the scarcity of instructors, the ones who are left are demanding more money to teach and are getting it, increasing the cost to the owners of running a competitive program.

In other words, group exercise has traditionally been included in most club's base offerings as part of the membership, but with rising costs for running the program—coupled with a decline in what the club can actually charge as a membership fee—many owners are realizing that it is no longer feasible to give this away as part of the membership.

One other factor that is also affecting this "free" aspect of the club is that many owners who add group personal training to their club's offerings are finding they can charge additional monthly fees for this program while paying the coach the equivalent of what it costs to pay a group exercise instructor on the other side. Put another way, why pay a group exercise instructor $40 a class that is included as part of the membership when you can pay a coach $40 to lead a group personal training where the participants pay more than the basic membership?

As the membership prices tend to stay volatile, owners are now forced to question every service or program that is included in the basic membership and many are starting to strip away anything that is considered free that lowers the return generated against the average membership return.

To better understand yield, let's start with a payment amount of $40 and work through each factor that affects the ultimate yield from this payment. Again, the major factors are loss rates, cancellation rates, cost of collection, and the impact of free services.

Loss Rates

It is impossible to collect all the money from all the members—a point we've already established. Your goal, then, is to collect the most money from the most members.

Simply defined, money is lost when someone who contracted to pay you doesn't pay—for whatever reason. For example, a member who dies is a loss because the contract was signed by someone, but this obligation doesn't get paid because the member is gone. We track loss by figuring out how much we can expect to collect from the contracts written with the members who take a chance on our clubs compared against what we thought we would collect in a perfect, "Everyone pays" world.

Each tool we use to obligate members has its own verifiable loss rate that can be tracked on a monthly basis. The largest and most credible financial service companies in the industry have been tracking loss rates since the early 1970s. Many owners hurt their receivables base and, therefore, their businesses by choosing the wrong membership tool as their primary membership agreement to establish obligation. An analysis of each tool currently in use in the industry and its loss rate shows how the receivables base and, ultimately, the final yield are affected.

Open-Ended, Month-to-Month, and Pay-as-You-Go Memberships

Open-ended, month-to-month, and pay-as-you-go memberships are all different names for the same tool. Each means that the member has a very short obligation to the club. They commit to the end of the current month and can quit at any time with some type of formal notice to the club. If the member is being drafted on EFT, by law, that member can notify his bank and have the draft immediately cancelled. Therefore, in many cases, he can circumvent the club's cancellation policy.

Loss rates for this tool are about 3 to 4 percent monthly or about 36 to 48 percent annually. Losing 3 to 4 percent of your members each month *doesn't sound* too scary for most owners, but compounded over 12 months, it can add up to losing 36 to 48 out of every 100 members the club has. Keep this simple concept in mind: Losses are figured monthly but compounded annually.

For example, if you use open-ended contracts and sign up 100 people in January, by the end of December of the same year, you will only have between 52 to 64 people still left as members who are still paying.

The big picture here is that the club incurred the cost of advertising to get the members, paid commissions to sign them up, paid staffing costs to get them started on their programs, and suffered the wear and tear on the club from members who didn't stick around.

It's not a good business plan if you only keep half the members you sign up over a year's time. If the club can't keep the members it enrolls because of no-obligation memberships, all the club's resources—key staff and payroll dollars—have to be dedicated to replacing those members.

Open-ended memberships can be part of a club's financial system if they are used as a more expensive alternative to a 12-month contract. For example, if a club has a monthly price of $39 per month per member, it could offer an open-ended membership at $46 to $48 per month. If the club is located in a heavily competitive market, it could still offer an open-ended membership, but the majority of members would most likely choose the 12-month plan because of the price advantage. This, then, strengthens the receivables base because the member not only had a choice of taking a membership that best fit him, but about 80 percent or more take the 12-month option, which is the most collectable of all the membership tools. Simply put, most gyms of any type only need two options: You can sign up for 12 months or you can go month to month at about a 20 percent higher premium.

As to yield, if a club lost 40 percent on every dollar of the membership dues, a $40 payment would already be reduced to $24 ($40 x 60 percent = $24). Therefore, because of its extreme loss rate and effect on the yield, an open-ended membership is not a good tool for most clubs because it is not collectable over time and returns a lesser amount of money to the club.

24-Month Contracts

Two-year or 24-month contracts have been an ugly habit in the industry for most of its history, but we are finally seeing this tool completely disappear. The use of long-term contracts—those 24 months or longer—have been traced back, depending on who you believe, to the early life insurance guys in the

1950s who were some of the industry's first salespeople or to the Arthur Murray dance studios from the same era who were at that time nationwide in scope and who had years of experience establishing long-term membership options. You could learn to dance, but you had to sign up for the next five years of your life and only then did your receive a perceived discount.

The 24-month contract has been a standard for years in the industry, but it is a hard sell to a more sophisticated clientele and this tool is much more difficult to collect than most other membership tools. It's interesting to note that all major failures in the history of the fitness industry as well as some large chains that are still in business posting losses year after year all used or use a 24-month contract as their base membership tool. This anecdotal evidence does support the fact that every business in this category used the hardest tool to sell and collect, which ultimately led to failure for each of the players.

The loss rate for 24-month contracts is about 3 to 5 percent a month or 36 to 60 percent per year on a national average. There are exceptions to every rule and there have been a very small handful of clubs that have used 24-month contracts and survived for a reasonable length of time. Most have not. This tool is also losing any traction in today's market because the more sophisticated consumer refuses to have anything to do with a two-year commitment with a fitness business and one seldom sees longer-term memberships being offered anywhere except in the old-style chains that are still barely alive in the market.

Loss rates are also the most important number that affects yield and the receivables base, but most owners don't track this vital statistic and the drastic effect it can have on their businesses.

If you have 100 members and you lose two each month for nonpayment, you have a loss rate of 2 percent or a 24 percent annual loss rate. Don't count members that move or cancellations as part of your loss rate formula.

Those numbers are tracked separately under the cancellation rate and have their own unique loss rate of about 1 percent per month or 12 percent annually.

Let's look at a typical membership that was being sold in many major metro markets about 10 years ago and see the results of using a 24-month contract. This is also a representation of a membership that has been sold in the industry for more than 30 years.

This club offered a floating membership fee, meaning the salesperson had the discretion to give a potential member virtually anything he wanted as long as the salesperson got some type of membership sale. The club actually listed a membership fee of $150, but only the dumbest human beings on the planet ever really paid that much down. The old adage "Start really high and settle for half" was the rule of thumb for decades in the industry and most players would take less than half if pushed.

The monthly dues for that club, which is how much each member paid each month, was $20 (actually $19.95 but rounded off here for ease of calculation) for a two-year contractual membership.

Some form of a two-year, $20-a-month membership has been used for years in the industry. Salespeople love this membership because it was supposedly easier to sell than a simpler but more expensive one-year membership. The contract amount was also bigger at $20 per month x 24 months = $480 and led to bigger commissions for the salesperson.

However, the reality is that the more salesmanship and pressure it takes to get a member to sign up, the bigger the losses will be from the total amount of memberships sold. Salespeople usually don't care or understand about losses. All they know is their job, which is that they are supposed to write a lot of "gross," which results from the sale of two-year contracts. The salespeople don't have to look at the end result, which in this case is that the product they sell may not be very collectable over time for the business. Therefore, it yields a far lower return per member sold.

Because two-year memberships really don't make sense to a potential member anymore, it's a harder product to sell. Because it's also a harder concept to sell by a typically younger and more fitness orientated staff, you need a much more sophisticated sales system in place to get it done, which means a more expensive sale and a more expensive salesperson that emulated the old "sales dog" mentality of the earlier years of the industry.

Because a lot of the club's staffing budget has to be dedicated to sales to make this system work, service suffers. And lousy service, coupled with a tool that has at least a 36 percent loss rate, leads to a lot of missing members who either left because of no help or balked at the long-term, 24-month contract. At this point, the club's income drops on the back end as members disappear, there is no multiple profit center income, and the owners do the only thing they usually know how to do: They pressure the sales staff to write more gross.

Salespeople working in an old-style system selling two-year contracts have a stinky job. Cold-calling people who are eating dinner at their homes and trying to set appointments out of lead boxes always make for a good time at the gym job. And don't forget harassing members for the names of their buddies or slamming people foolish enough to actually walk in because the salesperson has to make quota or lose his job.

It is interesting to note that many of today's chains also suffer from a version of this business mistake. When chain clubs started posting a declining membership base, most of them blame their sales teams and then add a great deal of pressure to the teams to drive up sales. If the teams fail, they are replaced and the cycle starts again. The truth is that the system itself used by the chains is the problem and that no one can post solid numbers over time because the methods they are using in the form of pressure sales, drop closing, and big end-of-the-month closeouts simply don't work in today's market where the client is so much more mature than in previous decades.

All these negatives are all part of a typical day in a high-pressure, sales-driven system that leads, in the short run, to very highly paid employees. Those who do manage to temporarily survive in this pressure earn pretty big money for this industry—often $4,000 to $5,000 or more a month. This is good for them but bad for the club because a simpler system could have led to lower-cost employees and a lower cost per sale.

You still need to sell, but you also need to create a system that only needs one strong sales trainer and which functions on a much simpler basis with fewer old sales dog types of people.

Your first hint that you have old sales dogs on your staff is when your top three salespeople used to sell used cars or cell phones at the mall or worked as cold callers for car insurance companies.

What causes so much pressure in this type of system? No one has ever really stepped back and looked at the system itself. The owners provide more sales training, more marketing, more lead boxes, and more pressure on the salespeople to drive results when the numbers drop, but no one looks at the 24-month contract itself or the actual sales system as the culprit.

The 24-month contract simply can't be collected at a high enough rate, which causes all the other problems that then follow. Look at the actual yield after losses and you can see where the problem begins. For example:

$20 x 24 months = $480 in gross contract sales to be
collected over two years

$480 x .64 percent (36 percent annual loss rate) = $307.20

The club can expect a yield of about $307 from a $480 contract. This is before club cancellations, cost of collection, or the effect of free services. The insurmountable problem with this amount is that the money arrives over two years. Another way to look at it is that the $20 payment becomes $12.80.

Another side problem with 24-month contracts is when the losses occur. The losses are not spread out over the full two-year period proportionately but happen disproportionately during the first month, third month, and again around the sixth month.

Buyer's regret—where the consumer has severe second thoughts about the purchase he just made (perhaps as an impulse)—happens frequently at the one-month point. The person just starts working out, is not yet in a routine, and then misses a few workouts. The person also realizes he is not going to get any real service from a sales-driven club, and unless he pays heavily for one-on-one training, there is no help available. In fact, in most turn-and-burn volume clubs, he has been there a month and no one even knows his name.

Then, while he is reading his bank statement and notices the payment was taken out, he realizes there are still 23 more payments to be made on that impulse contract he felt forced into from a high-pressure salesperson. This is the type of person that defaults on that contract early and may not even make that first payment at all. Many of the current players in the market try to hide this fact by lowering the price to just $9 per month in hopes the client will say "Hey, it is just $9, so I will keep paying and I will start again next month." Good theory, but in reality, $9 is still $9, and while the member might use this mental game for a couple months at some point, the reality of not using the club will cancel any perceived illusion that the member is going back and he will cancel the membership.

At the third month, a person who defaults might be one who comes into the club expecting to change himself in a short period of time. Around the third month, reality hits. Working out is not an overnight commitment and getting in shape will take a long and consistent approach. A sales-driven club focusing on 24-month contracts or using other high-pressure sales tactics adds to the member's frustration because almost any service and direction might have led to some early results, which would have kept the person motivated and in the system.

In the person's mind, he still has two years left on that membership, which can be overwhelming, and he walks away from the membership. The same people—coming to the same realization—will often pay a 12-month contract to term because there are only eight to nine payments left instead of 20 to 21. Without service, the person may not train, but he is more likely to finish the 12-month commitment instead of the 24-month commitment. The older-style clubs using 36-month contracts—which are not legal anymore in a number of states—compounded this problem in their collection efforts by the sheer length of the commitment that members had to make to even join the club.

Six months is when the lack of service and the physical plant start to strangle the average member. The person may be working out faithfully on his own but not getting any results because he is just winging it by doing an old high school workout or trying to learn from books and magazines. This—coupled with the fact that many sales-driven clubs fail to reinvest in their physical plants because of the ongoing cost of the sales effort—costs clubs members at this stage. Coming in to work out and finding four treadmills out of order and the rest in use can wear a member down over a six-month period and he takes it out on the club by defaulting on the contract.

Keep in mind that it's a lot easier for most consumers to walk away from a fitness facility membership than it used to be. Many credit agencies and other credit providers don't recognize a health club contract as a real obligation because of the reputation the high-pressure, sales-driven fitness clubs have given the industry.

Because of the high loss rates and low yields and because of the actual yield arriving over a two-year period, the 24-month contract is an extremely hard tool to make money with as a club owner. In the end, it doesn't matter how good your sales force is if your basic membership tool doesn't allow you to collect enough money from enough members.

12-Month Contracts

A 12-month contract, with its low loss rates, high rate of collection, and easier appeal to members, is the ideal foundational tool for clubs to use to establish obligation.

As mentioned earlier, a sample club from the same era as that mentioned earlier was offering a membership at $20 for 24 months, or $480. This membership only yielded the club $307.

Loss rates for 12-month memberships are only about 8 to 12 percent per year on a national average and traditionally average less than 10 percent if you are using a strong third-party financial service company. How the membership is sold still leads to a higher loss rate even for someone using the 12-month contract as his primary membership tool. Remember, the higher the pressure at the point of sale, the higher the loss rate.

The same club in the example was offering a $30 per month 12-month membership, equaling $360, using this tool for those potential members who balked at the 24-month commitment. The club and its sales force, though, worked hard to force the 24-month contract onto its potential members, mainly because of the larger gross sale at $480, which led to higher commissions.

But what is the real net result to the club from a 12-month membership? First of all, the gross is obviously smaller at $360 compared to $480. But the final yield is surprisingly strong. For example, let's figure the loss rate at the midrange, or 10 percent, and apply it to the 12-month membership:

$$\$360 \times .90 \text{ (10 percent loss rate)} = \$324$$

The club can expect a return of about $324 from every $360 membership it sells. Again, this is before club cancellations, cost of collection, or the effect of the free services, but when compared to the two-year membership, this is still a surprisingly high return.

However, the key here is when the money arrives. In the 24-month example, $307 arrives over a two-year period. In the 12-month membership illustration, $324 arrives over only a 12-month period. Which tool would be more effective to maintain cash flow in a fitness facility: a membership that supplies $307 of income over 24 months or one that supplies $324 over 12 months?

This should be an easy choice, but it goes against all human—and salespeople's—nature to believe that the smaller gross gives a higher yield for the business.

The One-Time Membership Fee

The one-time membership fee is money the club gets in addition to the monthly membership payments. In the previous membership example, the club was asking for $65 in addition to 12 payments of $39. That makes the entire gross membership worth $533 to the club before losses and other adjustments.

The membership fee can change throughout the year depending on seasonal or current market conditions, but the monthly dues have to stay the same or go up. No new member can ever pay less than a member who has joined before he joined.

However, the club does always have to offer at least one membership with a one-time fee of less than $90, and in most cases, the club would be in a better sales position if it restricted the total money it gets up front from a new member during the sale to $79 or less. Again, studies conducted over the years by people who study consumer buying habits show that any money outlay over $90 becomes a family decision that has to be discussed with significant others. If a person is a nonfamily person, laying out more than $90 often forces the person to stop, go home, and think about the decision before the money is spent. Even clubs that cater to an elite clientele should have one of their joining choices below $90 as a getting-started amount for a member.

We are striving for the impulse sale here. Making the first step easy logically increases your ability to add new clients to your business. Note here that the membership fee is a separate fee that the club uses to offset some of the cost of getting the new client started, but it should not be so high that it restricts sales.

The goal of a fitness business is to create a business that has a large receivable base that projects the business into the future. As noted elsewhere in this book, if a lot of members sign membership agreements (contracts) and promise to make these payments into the future, you can now project your business forward because you are creating a recurring income stream of payments over time.

When it comes to the one-time membership fee, you must separate it from the monthly payments. For example, many club owners want to get the membership fee and the first month's payment at the point of sale. There are two problems with this. First of all, the total will almost always be larger than $79 to $90, therefore restricting new sales by killing the impulse nature. Secondly, you are reducing your recurring income stream, or the receivable base, by 8.3 percent (1/12 of the outstanding membership payments). You will be much safer as a business operator if you get a smaller down payment and go for the 12 payments instead of trying to get the additional payment today.

Keep in mind that we are really talking semantics here. What you are really doing—no matter what you call it—is to get one chunk of money today and a bunch of chunks in the future. You can call it a membership fee or whatever else makes you happy, but even if you get a small chunk today or a bigger chunk by asking for the membership fee and the first month's payment together, you are still trying to get a new client started as easily as possible and then create the largest receivable base you can to protect your business over time.

The membership fee is important to the club because most of the labor and administrative costs a club incurs for a new member happen during the first 30 days of membership. Sales commissions and marketing costs should also be somewhat defrayed by the membership fee.

Another important consideration we've discovered over the years is that a great majority of members make the decision to pay their memberships to term and eventually renew during their first 30 days as a member. Therefore, the member has to experience the best service possible, with the best staff and training support, during the first 30 days. This costs money—money that should be delivered in the form of a membership fee.

Another factor connected to the membership fee is that members are more likely to continue paying for their membership if they have to make an initial investment. In the case of a 12-month membership at $40 per month, or $480, the member should put down a minimum of 10 percent, or $48, as a membership fee. This lowers the loss rate and increases how collectable the contract will be over time.

Creating a Membership Structure for Your Business

This section is designed to help you start thinking about what it takes to create a membership system that will help make your business more financially successful over time. The information is divided into two parts: one for mainstream clubs and a second section designed for training-centric businesses, which are the fastest-emerging clubs in the industry.

The key concept we are trying to create is that of a layered pricing system offering a variety of entry points for a wide range of clients based on either financial ability to pay or through the programming they desire. Most club owners limit their sales by offering too few choices that appeal to a limited number of people. For example, mainstream clubs only usually offer a monthly membership to the club, coupled with one-on-one training. In this case, there are only two offerings that miss other clients who might be interested in joining at other price points or who seek alternatives to the elite training model.

Traditional training gyms are even more limiting in that they only offer training for the elite client who wants one-on-one training. This is changing somewhat due to programming, such as boot camps, that attracts a wider variety of clients at a lower price point, but most of these training facilities still rely on sessions and packages to service the clients.

Apple is a perfect example of a company that understands using varying price points to attract the widest range of buyers to their family. As of this writing, you could buy an entry-level iPod® for just $49 and from there you could keep moving up the line and spend ever-increasing money for an almost endless array of products. In other words, it doesn't matter how much money you have or what your interests are because Apple has a product for you and will take your money at any level.

What are the goals for an effective pricing system?

- The system must have an entry point low enough to attract the widest range of qualified potential members.
- It must be able to generate a higher return per sale (higher average EFT) over time.

- It should be simple enough to be able to be explained by the dumbest person on the staff.
- It should make the first step to join the gym easy or an impulse to get started.
- Effective pricing systems should be based on five to seven different layers of pricing reflecting four to five different products. The more price points and products you offer, the wider range of members you will attract to that business.
- All memberships should be offered on a monthly and a weekly basis. Weekly payments lower loss rates and increase retention, especially with our younger clients. For example, a membership that is sold for $129 per month, such as team training, could also be offered for $29.79 per week. There is no downside to an owner who offers weekly payments and no risk in offering this option, but you will find that many of your members who are under 40 will stay in the system longer because their membership matches how they get paid in their lives.
- All training is offered on 12-month memberships and packages and sessions are eliminated.
- The more you pay, the more you have included. For example, if you become an unlimited small group training client, you can also drop into large group team training on your off days and you can also have full access to everything else in the gym. Put another way, you get everything offered under your level as part of your membership.

The most important thing we are trying to achieve is to show a low entry point that attracts the widest range of members but that also leads to a higher return per membership sold. For example, it doesn't matter if your price is $19 or $39 as an entry point as long as the average monthly payment generated comes in higher than those numbers. The only way to do this is by creating a layered pricing system featuring a number of price options appealing to a wider range of clients.

Let's look at this sales day in a typical box club. Disregard the membership fee here. We are only worried about the monthly fees and what they average. This club's simple access membership is $39 per month per member. In this example, the club is also offering group personal training, which is 12 to 20 people with a coach, meaning that clients are sharing the cost of a trainer and doing a workout in a structured group setting offered 8 to 12 times per week. In this case, group personal training people are paying $79 per month for 12 months to be able to attend—instead of (not in addition to) the club's base membership fee of $39 per month per member. In other words, the club's membership is included in the higher fee.

Group personal training, or team training, appeals to 24- to 44-year-olds who love group dynamics and who like a challenging workout. Team training is all about the experience and the group dynamic offered through challenging training. As weird as it is to contemplate, this experience of 20 people sharing the cost of a trainer and sweating as a group is missing in almost all mainstream fitness businesses. Even the businesses that offer boot camp products usually kill the program due to turning it over to the group exercise people instead of letting the coaches do their job. The group dynamic in training has been part of almost every client's life at some time or another. It is the rare member who hasn't been part of some type of team at some time in his life, such as organized sports, bands, scouting, or some other group experience. Being part of a group has been part of his life forever, but most gyms eliminate this social vehicle and force all the clients into a one-on-one situation.

Team training is about the energy, music, and experience. The workout should be the same from Monday to Sunday so clients can gain a sense of progressions in their workouts. The program designer should also keep most complicated movement patterns, such as Turkish getups or power cleans, out of this group and save those movements for small group training where the coach/client ratio stays at around one to four.

This club is also offering a semiprivate group option based on a coach with a group of two to four clients who attend according to a schedule offered each day by the club and pay $129 for a limited small group experience, meaning they can attend five times per month, or $169 for unlimited small group training, which is usually defined as a maximum of 12 workouts in small group and then guided workouts for that client on off days. Guided workouts mean that the lead trainer will write workouts the client can do on days he is not attending small group training that match the client's personal goals or physical condition.

This small group training model contrasts with the large group in dynamics and materials and the age of clients it attracts. For example, the larger group team experience might change only once a week, is heavily music driven, and is limited to clients who can keep moving and who understand the basic components of fitness. Team training usually attracts the 24- to 40-year-old client who likes the challenge and the energy.

On the other hand, the small group is more intimate and usually based on the workout of the day, attracting clients in the 35- to 55-year-old range. These groups are usually a little older and are the ones who might like much more coaching in their workouts instead of the challenge of keeping up with a larger—and usually younger—group who is pushing the limits. The key to small group training is intensive coaching. This is where you can add movements not suitable for one coach, with many clients knowing that the more complex the movement, the more coaching should be involved.

It is important to note that the entire group does the workout of the day in small group training and the clients do not have individual workouts. If a client has a unique need (such as medical) or he is training for a sports-specific event (such as a race of some type), then he should be in one-on-one training. If clients have unique issues—and there won't be many older than age 50 who don't have some type of wobble on their wagon—the exercise in the workout that day should be modified for that participant.

For example, if a client has a shoulder impingement and the workout that day calls for a pressing movement, the rest of the group should do the press while that client should do a modified movement suitable for him. In other words, modify the movement for one rather than try to individualize the entire process for all of them. Remember, we are seeking general athletic conditioning here, and if the client needs work, such as specific rolling and stretching, he should do that prior to the group workout.

Traditional one-on-one training also has a role in the business and there will always be clients who will pay for this service. Your goal as an owner is to dilute the penetration rate in your membership over time. For example, if you have 1,000 clients and you have a 5 percent penetration rate using the one-on-one tool, this means you have 50 clients who regularly support this offering.

This one-on-one group doesn't disappear and this group will not usually want to take part in the group offerings either, but you can add another 35 percent of your membership—in this example, another 350 clients—to your training revenue through the addition of types of training that appeal to different types of clients that your businesses has attracted previously.

The average return per sale is everything in today's business model.

Today, this club sold seven memberships using $39 as the entry point but achieved a much higher return per sale by using a layered price structure featuring a wider range of offerings and price points:
- $39
- $39
- $39
- $39
- $79 (large group team training)
- $39
- $129 (small group personal training)

The total of all these memberships is $403. If you divide $403 by seven memberships sold, the average is $57.57. This club shows an entry point of $39 but in reality generates an average of $57 per membership sold, giving it an enormous advantage over a competitor who shows $39 but then discounts for virtually every membership it sells.

For example, look at this traditional mainstream fitness center and what it would generate for its memberships sold on the same day:
- $39
- $34 (senior discount)
- $24 (second member of the family)
- $29 (student)
- $39
- $39
- $29 (corporate)

The total of all these memberships is $233. If you divide $233 by seven memberships sold that day, the average is $32.29 per client. In other words, this gym has an entry-level price of $39 but only averages $32 per client sold. Contrast this with the previous gym: Both show a reasonable price to join but one—by using a layered pricing structure—generates an almost double return per client served.

We should also look at a small training gym for a contrast. This gym is 3,000 square feet and is in a suburb in an Eastern city. The gym uses a layered pricing system that will be more fully shown a little later in this chapter. The following is one month's memberships for this gym:

- $99 (team training)
- $129 (small group limited to five sessions per month)
- $99
- $169 (small group unlimited)
- $299 (one-on-one training limited to five sessions per month)
- $99
- $99
- $169
- $499 (one-on-one training unlimited based on a maximum of 12 per month)

This training gym sold nine new training memberships that month and is generating $1,661 in new monthly member payments. You can join this training gym for as low as $99 per month for team training, but in reality, it is averaging $184.55 per member served.

In these examples, we can see a wide range of effectiveness. The traditional gym is chasing volume by showing $39 per month per member but in fact is discounting everyone and is only creating $32 per member. The hybrid mainstream player, who has added layered pricing to his regular memberships, is showing $39 per month but in reality is getting about $57 per client in his business. The training gym—in the same market but chasing a different clientele—shows an entry price of $99 but generates nearly $185 per client.

The Rule of 8

If a member walked into the club with a red shirt that said "I am quitting today—this is my last workout," would you stop the guy and talk to him for a minute trying to save the client from leaving? Of course you would. You would be worse than a horrible businessperson if a client takes the time to give you a hint he is unhappy and intends to leave and you do nothing about it.

In reality, the clients do give this warning. The International Health, Racquet & Sportsclub Association published a paper a number of years ago titled "Why People Quit." One of the many key points in this piece was that of the people surveyed on why they quit: The common denominator was that all of them were working out less than eight times per month at the time they left their perspective gyms. If someone drops below eight workouts a month—and now this person is likely to leave you during the next few months—would you not take action? The number eight might be the most important number in the fitness business because the future of every member in your gym is tied to reaching that monthly total of workouts. We call this the Rule of 8.

The problem with most club operators is that they wait too late to engage. Talking to the client now and solving a service issue now might save a few clients who are headed out the door, but the bigger issue is that something happened earlier in their experience that led to a client dropping below the magic eight workouts per month.

Assuming that client usage of the gym is a major issue in retention, one of the things we can do is design all pricing systems to help overcome this problem. Most current systems take a contrary stance and work against the member staying. For example, training clients currently buy sessions, and if they want to train more, they must pay more. This approach makes sense financially, but this also leads to clients cutting back on their workouts a little if their sessions run low.

We also limit other aspects of attendance. For example, most programming is limit to small offerings and the ability for the client to get help is also restricted. Clients start with personal fitness goals, but these people do not qualify as personal training clients they are often lost in the process. The ones who don't go to group exercise and who can't or won't pay for one-on-one training are set up on a simple circuit, and once that circuit fails, the client he has nowhere to go within the system and then must rely on friends, books, or online videos. Not knowing what you are doing in a gym is a limiter and an eventual membership killer. Why go to the club if you don't have a set plan of attack to reach those goals and, most importantly, why keep financially supporting a gym that won't help you get anywhere unless you pay a lot more money?

Keeping the Rule of 8 in mind, most of your offerings should be sold as unlimited and priced accordingly. Using the word _unlimited_ encourages the client to attend more often. For example, most of your training programs should be priced as unlimited versions. Remember that if the client appears more than eight times per month, he will stay longer and pay longer than members who disappear before reaching eight visits.

The following is the base membership model for a mainstream box club using the key points discussed in earlier paragraphs. Prices will be added after we explore the working model itself. Keep in mind that clients also get everything listed below their level and the prices listed later include the club's basic monthly membership fee:

- _Unlimited one-on-one pampering membership:_ This would include clients training for special events, those with medical issues, and those who simply refuse to play with others and who want their own coach and are willing to pay for this more expensive service. Also remember that the word _unlimited_ does in fact limit the client to 12 times per month with a coach. The goal is to get the client into enough training sessions to meet his needs but without overtraining the client and hurting him. This client would have a guided workout, designed by the lead trainer, that allows the client to come to the gym more often and do other workouts that enhance his goals, not overtrain and hurt him.

- *Limited one-on-one training membership (five sessions per month, but these sessions do not roll over):* This option includes five training sessions a month that can be used all in one week or once per week at the client's discretion. These sessions do not accumulate for additional months.
- *Unlimited small group semiprivate training model (two to four clients per session with a coach):* This all about intensive coaching in small groups.
- *Limited small group semiprivate training model (two to four clients per session with a coach):* This option includes five small group sessions a month and then unlimited use of the rest of the gym, as do all the programs beyond simple membership.
- *Unlimited large group team training model (12 to 20 clients per session with a coach):* This is also the premium programming level, which would include advanced cycle, yoga, boxing, and other programming offered regularly and that is priced beyond a simple access membership. The goal at this level is to give the clients options at an additional price that keeps them moving and from getting bored from doing the same program over and over each month.
- *Group exercise as a slightly more expensive option (would include regular group exercise and basic group exercise style cycling).*
- *Simple access to the gym, which includes the equipment and cardio only.*

One of the keys here is that if you buy a membership higher up, such as limited one-on-one training, that membership includes everything beneath it. Again, you would not pay a membership to the club and the training membership. When you go above the simple access membership line, which is between the group option and the guided workout, your membership to the club is included. Don't waste time trying to back that membership number out of training memberships. Attaining that number tells you nothing and has no use in your business planning. It's either pay for simple access or pay for a more inclusive membership and tracking the membership has no bearing because all we are chasing is a higher return per client.

It is smart to track the memberships above the group exercise option line as a separate file within your system. For example, look back at this annual revenue from a typical box club mentioned in an earlier chapter:

Membership Revenue	Training Revenue
$960,000 a year in net membership income	$84,000 a year in training income
($80,000 x 12)	($7,000 x 12)

In this club model, the membership income is strong, but how much better can this club do in the long run to increase it? Competition, the maturity of the club in the market, the number of people who live within the club's market sphere, and drive time to the club all create natural limits as to how far the club can push the net membership number.

On the other hand, this club has barely touched the training revenue and could conceivably within 12 months have the training revenue in the club equal or surpass the net membership income. However, this is not possible unless the club changes away from using sessions and packages targeted as a small percentage of its memberships and shifts to a layered pricing structure that allows the club to drive up the average return per member.

This potential number sounds high, but look at this simple example: Let's say a new generation training club that is 6,000 square feet has gross annual revenues of $1,000,000 and only 312 members, which is a return per client that is becoming quite common in the training industry. Is this really hard to achieve? Take $1,000,000 and divide it by 312 and you arrive at $3,205 per year per member. If you then divide $3,205 by 12 months, you arrive at $267. In other words, this club only needs to average $267 per member per month to hit a million dollars.

Owners trapped by the volume approach in the fitness business struggle with this, but in reality, you only need 300 members to make this model work rather than 3,000 in a typical box club and the training members have proven to stay longer and pay longer over time. Why can't a traditional mainstream player who has 3,000 clients in the system just get 300 or so of his current members to embrace the training model and the new product offerings? In other words, why can't the box players create a training gym within their gym?

Your goal then should be to build a membership model that maximizes the memberships available to you in the market, but also allows you to exploit return per member through training, which should be the largest income stream in the club if we apply a new generation business model to the problem.

The following is the sample membership model for a mainstream fitness facility that is adding layered pricing:
- Unlimited one-on-one pampering membership = $599
- Limited one-on-one training membership (five sessions per month/do not rollover) = $299
- Unlimited small group semiprivate training model (two to four clients per session with a coach) = $169
- Limited small group semiprivate training model (two to four clients per session with a coach/five session per month) = $129
- Unlimited large group team training model (12 to 20 clients per session with a coach) = $99, which includes the premium level for offerings, such as boxing, advanced cycle, floor Pilates, yoga, or other specialty programming
- Group exercise (would include regular group exercise and basic cycle) = $49
- Simple access to the gym, which includes the equipment and cardio = $39

All memberships would be based on 12 months. Members would be locked into each level for three months, but the members can rewrite their memberships at a lower or higher level by signing a new 12-month agreement if they desire to change levels.

In this model, you could enter the club for as little as $39 per month, but you could pay as much as $599 per month for an unlimited one-on-one training membership. In this case, the pampering membership means that the client would not only get unlimited access to training, but they would also have their supplements, protein powders, munchies bars, and other support items or amenities (such as spa services) included, which the club would offer to add value to this membership. If you add extra services at the higher level, make sure you are profitable when you do and adjust the prices accordingly.

Group exercise is broken out in this model, called destructuring a membership, but group could also be included in the base level simple access membership. Clubs around the country have varying degrees of success with group exercise, and many are finding that the stronger the training program, the weaker the group exercise program becomes over time, as many of the group participants seek better results with a trainer/coach and with the newness of the program itself. In this example, group might be strong in this club—defined as at least 20 percent of the gym's membership using it on a daily basis—but the owner needs to show a lower price to be competitive, so he retains group at a higher rate, showing just $39 as a simple access membership.

It is important to note that cycle is also broken out of the group exercise/ aerobics domain and is placed in the training department as a premium group training option. Cycle works well in this environment and can even rise to a higher perception of status if it is charged for separately, as was done when it was first introduced into clubs in the 1990s. Other premium group offerings, such as yoga or boxing, could also be offered at the higher price level.

Training clubs would use fundamentally the same model but would eliminate the bottom two options on the list. One of the mistakes that many training clubs make is that they are too limited in options by generally restricting their memberships to just one-on-one elite and also using archaic rules, such if you are not working with a trainer, you can't come to the club.

Even training clients like to sometimes just do their own thing and the traditional training club model actually forces clients to get memberships at other clubs because they can't ever solo in the training club. New generation training clubs are solving this problem by offering hybrid memberships, meaning that every client is a training client but that all the clients can have access to open times in the club. If you are still operating a training gym that is less than 3,000 square feet, you most likely won't be able to offer this option, but your goal at some point should be to give the client total access to your gym as part of his training program.

Another mistake training clubs have made is that the point of entry financially is too high, eliminating a number of clients who would pay for and appreciate their services but who don't want to be a one-on-one client. The alternative to this is to offer at least one membership below $100 in most markets and to offer layers where the group dynamic comes into play. The assumption that one-on-one training is the only tool dates to the bodybuilding era from the 1970s, although throughout the history of fitness—going back to the early 1800s in this country—fitness has always been done in group formats.

Many training club operators have assumed for years that there is only one client and that this client only wants to train in a one-on-one setting. The reality is that there is another client out there who loves the dynamics of the group or who might not have the money for traditional training. This client can be served by the group offerings because in this model, he can get the group dynamic and a cheaper price by sharing the cost of the trainer.

Other Membership Options

The overall goal as you build a new price structure is to eliminate as many short-term, or garbage, memberships as possible. Most gyms, meaning mainstream and training gyms, can eliminate the need for shorter options by offering 12-month memberships as the base tool and then allowing the client to take any program he wants for an extra 20 to 25 percent per month, with the ability to go month to month with no obligation. In other words, this gym owner is offering the client a chance to save money by supporting the gym on a long-term basis or if the client wants the freedom to come and go as he please, he can pay a little extra each month. This avoids the need to offer three-month and six-month options and other versions gym owners use to fill in the gaps or usually as tools to try to please every client every time.

The daily option

Every club should offer a daily drop-in option, but many clubs make a mistake by pricing the daily fee too low. A drop-in single workout should be a minimum of $15 to $20 depending on the region—whether the club is in a resort area with high peaks of usage through the year or whether it is in a highly transient area, such as a club near hotels. Even the fitness facilities in smaller communities should establish at least $12 to $15 per visit fee for guests.

One option for resort clubs is to offer a punch pass rather than a one-week or a one-month membership. A punch pass usually generates much more revenue for the club than a short-term membership.

For example, a club with a $20 drop-in fee might sell a 10-workout punch pass for $169. The club still gets $17 per workout, the member thinks he is getting a deal because he saved $31 off the regular drop-in fee, and the club is not giving up unlimited usage for a fixed fee.

Everything in the sample structure is designed to minimize the loss rate and to increase the yield. Other options, such as family and corporate memberships, will be discussed later in this chapter.

Club cancellations and the effect on yield

Loss rates can cost a club about 1 to 4 percent of its membership each month depending on the tool used. A scary concept is that many clubs give away another 1 to 4 percent on top of the loss rates because they don't have a strong, consistent policy in place to handle cancellations. Cancellations affect your total outstanding receivables base, such as loss rates, but are categorized differently. Loss rates are usually the member's decision not to pay. There is an obligation, but the member breaks it by ignoring the contract. Cancellations are decisions made by the club to let a member out of a contract.

Some are valid, such as moving more than 25 miles away from the club. Most are not valid and could be saved, except that the club chooses to let the member out of the valid contract anyway. For example, a member tells the manager that she is losing her job and doesn't want to pay anymore. The manager believes her story and cancels the contracts. Legally, the club has no obligation to cancel this agreement. This is lost money that the club should have collected but didn't because of no set policy to handle these situations.

Most states have specific laws that dictate how clubs are supposed to deal with members who sign contracts and then try to get out of them. How clubs choose to vary from these laws in favor of the members is where the problem occurs. For example, the law that states the club has to cancel a member that moves more than 25 miles from the club is pretty standard around the country. This is a fair law for the member and the club. But how this law is enforced in the club is the issue.

If a member walks in and says she has accepted a job in the next town and wants to cancel, the manager who knows the member and likes her as a friend simply believes the story. The contract, which the club acquired through marketing, sales, and administrative costs, is cancelled and becomes a loss for the club. Should the manager cancel in this case? Yes, if the member verifies the move. The mistake the manager made is not having a strict and verifiable policy in place. The manager should have said: "Yes, we'll cancel, but please send us a copy of a utility bill with your name and new address on it first. When we receive that, we'll be happy to cancel you immediately."

Cancellation losses usually mean that the club simply lets business it paid for disappear either because the manager is too nice, there is no formal club policy, or the management doesn't want to be the bad guys because they unreasonably fear bad word of mouth in its community. No matter the reason, the club is losing money that it should have collected.

To prevent unnecessary losses, set up a strict policy, follow the rules dictated by the state you do business in, and be reluctant to give up business you already paid for.

A good goal for club cancellations, which reflects the normal moving and medical action most clubs encounter, is to try to keep cancellation rates the same as the loss rates for 12-month contracts. Again, this rate is about 10 to 12 percent annually or about 1 percent a month.

This additional loss drives the yield down even further. A 12 percent loss rate, coupled with a 12 percent cancellation rate, means that the club loses 24 percent on every membership dollar it generates and these numbers are at the end of the scales compared with the large majority of clubs around the country. The wrong tool and a manager who can't say "No" can easily get the club to the 50 cents on the dollar loss mark.

Remember that the owner has the discretion to break the rules. An owner can believe a hard-luck story if he desires because the loss is ultimately his money. But the rest of the team should have a formalized policy to follow and the owners or senior manager should handle the exceptions.

Cost of collection

There is always going to be a cost of collection. It doesn't matter if you're a control freak and try to collect your own memberships or if you use a third-party service company. There is going to be some amount of collection cost for every dollar of membership revenue.

The real issue is how much you get in return for that dollar. This is where many owners get confused. These owners only look at what collecting the memberships costs and not what is generated in return for that cost. Your sales team can write all the memberships in the world, but if you use the wrong tool and have an inefficient collection system, you will eventually fail.

A few basic collection rules

You can't be the good person and the bad person at the same time.

In the fitness business, we are in the business of relationships. The members begin to trust us and feel that the club is a mix of their home and their favorite bar or other social hangout.

Once the clients become regulars and often friends, they become hard to collect from each month. Some of the members have real financial difficulties we just can't become involved in if we want to continue to run a financially successful business because personal involvement with too many members with problems—and most everyone will have a problem at some point in his life—ends up costing us money. Other members on the more aggressive side try to work us over for a lower rate because they don't want to pay that month and are often just cheap people pounding a young staff for a lower rate. We really don't want our staff in the middle of that story either because believing one leads to believing others and those also ends up costing us money.

Members associate attendance with payment.

Where you collect member payments is almost as important as how you collect. When members pay at the club each month, they start to associate attendance with payment. Associating attendance with payment means if the member works out that month, he feels an obligation to pay. However, if he stays away from the club, he doesn't feel he has to pay, even if he has a contract and a financial obligation to the business.

More money will be collected in the long run if the member's regular payments are handled outside the club. The only payments that should be collected in the gym are the ones from problem members. Most club owners would collect more money if they would stay out of the collection process and let their third-party company handle the regular payment. The club should only be involved in the collection process if the member is severely past due—usually in the 75- to 90-day range.

Three methods for collecting your membership money

Do it yourself.

Most owners try collecting membership money themselves at one time or another, but this method of collection has many problems that make it a poor option for most clubs.

First of all, you can manage more than you can do yourself. Control freaks love to collect their own memberships because they have a stronger illusion of control. But one person can only do and control so much. As with accounting and legal issues, you're better off to farm out these processes and then manage them instead of trying to create all these systems in house.

Collecting your own memberships also eliminates the power of a third party and members do associate attendance with payment. Even if you set up your own image of third-party collection, you're still collecting your own paper and the members do figure out that it's still you.

There is also no cost-effectiveness when it comes to collecting your own memberships. The club incurs costs whether the membership is collected or not. You can pay a lot to set up your own collection system and still not really collect that large a percentage of the outstanding receivables base.

This system is also very vulnerable to employee instability. If your entire receivables base is entrusted to one or two employees and something happens to those employees, the club is at risk because the receivables base is the most valuable asset the club owns.

Use an outside processor.

Processors are companies that specialize in the simple processing of EFT accounts. If the accounts are clean, meaning everyone pays and no one moves or closes an account, then these companies can do a fair job. If the member accounts have any problems, these accounts are sent back to the clubs to be handled. Processors mean just that: They process accounts but provide no collection effort whatsoever.

There are several problems with this system that affect the receivables base and, ultimately, the yield. First of all, losses are too big too soon. This means that many of these accounts that are kicked out of a processor's system and returned to the club could have been saved, but these clubs are usually not set up to handle member account problems. The club tries a few simple phone calls, saves an account or two, and then sends the rest to a full-blown collection company that charges 33 to 50 percent of what it collects.

If there had been a real collection effort earlier in the process, many of these accounts could have been saved at a more reasonable cost. Keep in mind that we are selling future service paper and not tangible assets. It takes a more sophisticated and strategic collection effort to handle future service contracts. Processors provide no collection effort at all and the club usually does not have anyone trained in the consistent collection of memberships on their staff.

Another problem with using processors is that collection problems are not handled quickly enough by either the processor when the problems first occur or by the club when the contract is returned. Speed is of the essence when it comes to solving collection problems and this system doesn't allow this.

There are also many false and unnecessary costs when it comes to using a processor. The processing companies charge when they collect, as they should, and also when they don't collect, which they shouldn't. They get paid whether they get your money or not, which reduces the overall yield from the receivables base.

Involve third-party financial service companies.

While there are only a few really legitimate third-party financial service companies in the industry, this is the best option for the majority of the clubs and gyms to use.

Using a third-party company means you pay someone else to service and collect your membership contracts. It also means you don't incur any cost unless the member's money is collected.

Many of our members in the fitness business are in their 20s and 30s. It's not unusual for these folks to spend just as much as they make each month—if not more—by using credit cards and short-term debt. A strong third-party financial company brings the illusion of power to the game and trains many of our younger and more leveraged clients to become good, regular payers.

Using a third-party company also separates the good guys, which are us, from the "bad guys," which are those people who actually collect bills in our name. This allows the club to maintain its relationship with its members who were so hard to build in the first place.

This doesn't mean that the club has to abuse and ignore members who don't pay. A combined effort by the third-party company and by the club, which only happens when chasing those severely past due members, should produce a higher return per member when it comes to the yield.

A final point about the use of third-party financial service companies is that it allows for verification of a club's receivables base. If an owner wants to borrow money from a bank or sell or buy a club, the most important asset to be considered is the existing receivables base. Used equipment is only worth so much and claiming to have a certain number of members means nothing unless they are individually represented by a part of the receivables base.

If the club is collecting its own paper, it's almost impossible to verify the authenticity of the numbers. The obvious method would be to tie the receivables base to bank deposits, but a few unethical owners in the past have been known to pad deposits prior to the sale to drive up the price. Without a complete member-by-member audit, you could never completely verify a receivables base collected at the club. There are simply too many ways to fake the numbers. If a legitimate third-party company holds the receivables, the verification of the asset is much easier and much more reliable.

A working average for collection cost should be about 7 percent of what's collected. Keep in mind that you might find a way to do collections for less, but what do you get for that cost? Again, it's not the cost but what you can get in return.

Where is the yield at this point?

In our examples so far, the yield from a member payment has been reduced by a loss rate, a cancellation rate, and by the cost of collection. For example:

Member payment	$40.00
10 percent loss rate	−$4.00
	$36.00
10 percent cancellation rate	−$3.60
	$32.40
7 percent cost of collection	−$2.26
Final yield	$30.14

The final factor: Giving away everything in the name of member service

Member service is not usually defined as giving away a lot of stuff for free. But many owners confuse the giving away of services with providing member service. Coffee is a good example. Many clubs have gotten into the habit over the years of giving away free coffee to the morning members.

Is member service giving away free coffee? Or is having two kinds of a high-quality, fresh coffee for sale in oversized cups with sippy lids member service? Is it the cheap but free coffee or the availability of a high-quality, fresh product that sets the club apart from the competition and provides what the members really want? Yes, there is that one member moron who'll leave because he didn't get that free cup of cheap, tasteless coffee. So, send him to the competition and let him drink its free swill and reduce its yield.

Another example is child care. The average 15,000-square-foot fitness facility with 2,000 members will lose about $1,200 to $1,500 a month on child care. Why? Because the common belief in the industry is that you have to have child care and it has to be cheap. And because the club down the street gives it away for free, we think we have to do the same. It loses money because it has a bad business plan. Therefore, we lose money because we copy the same bad plan.

Is member service child care in a small, cramped room for free? Or is it a larger, better-decorated room with a better-trained child care provider that's offered at a reasonable price? Would parents prefer free but low-quality child care, or good, high-quality child care at a reasonable price?

Member service doesn't have to always be free or cheap and we definitely don't have to lose money just because the competition is stupid enough to lose money chasing the image that free is cool.

The problem with the coffee, child care, group exercise, and other free services, such as towels, is that it lowers the yield. For example, if your free child care program costs $2,000 per month to run and if your club has 2,000 members making payments each month, you've lowered the yield by a dollar per member. Throw in two or three other free services and the yield drops even more substantially.

Starting with the yield example we illustrated earlier, we're working with $30.14 out of a payment of $40 before subtracting free stuff. The adjusted example is:

Yield after loss rate, cancellation rate, and cost of collection	$30.14
Cost of child care, towel service, and free coffee	−$2.00
Adjusted yield	$28.14

The yield—or the money the club really has to work with out of the member's $40 payment—is only $28.14 per member each month.

In other words, owners need to learn to charge for or eliminate these services and amenities. With the increased cost of doing business in today's market, we can't afford to give these things away free. Even free coffee, which used to be so cheap, now can cost a club with 1,500 members $700 to $800 per month. Another way to look at this is that $800 equals 20 $40 member payments before yield adjustments and 28 member payments after the yield adjustments are applied. This also doesn't count the sales and advertising costs to sell these memberships.

Other Factors That Affect the Yield

Corporate rates, family discounts, student rates, and other specials that lower the membership payment—and therefore the yield—are beginning to fade from the industry.

Where in the real world do you get half off for a second member of the family? "Hello. Dinner for two please. And can I get my significant other for half off please?" Most restaurants worth eating at would laugh in your face and then toss you on the street just for asking. Corporate memberships are also starting to lose popularity.

Except for a few notable exceptions, most clubs don't do well selling corporate memberships. The clubs have to dedicate too much money and too many of its resources to reach companies that want discounts that are far too great. Some clubs still do well with corporate memberships, but would they get the same members anyway at full price if the club was the convenient option in the neighborhood?

So, what's the trend? It's away from offering so many discounts and specialized memberships that lower the return per member. A few pioneering clubs are actually giving no discounts to second members of the family and no corporate rates. Everyone pays full price for their membership—the same that the other members in the club paid. These club owners are feeling that it's better to make more money from fewer members than it is to discount everything for the sake of having a larger membership number. However, there is a compromise position for those owners who can't break away from the discounting tradition. For example:

> The club has a $65 membership fee and $39
> per month payments for 12 months.

If you feel the need to discount for options, such as second person at the same address, then limit that discount to no more than 20 percent off the basic simple access for one member. If you want to go after corporates, try taking a different path and offer additional time per person rather than offering a lower rate. For example, the gym that is charging $39 per person might offer 15 months for the price of 12, therefore effectively lowering the effective rate but still keeping the price at $39.

However, some gyms in rural markets may want to offer a flat family membership. A family membership should have a membership fee of no more than $90 and the monthly payment—no matter how many kids in the family—should stay under $100. If a family had four kids, those parents have probably already suffered enough financially. Don't add to their financial misery by charging more than $100 per month in payments.

Summary

Profitability is the desired goal in business. In the fitness business, the ability to make a profit is often determined by the choices the owner makes when it comes to putting together the club's financial foundation.

The profit goal for most fitness businesses is to net 20 percent pre-tax. Most clubs can never achieve this because the tools the owner chooses for charging and collecting from the members prevents this net from happening. If the owner picks the wrong tool—for example, 24-month contracts—then the receivables base is weakened, which affects the final yield the club can expect from a member payment.

The yield is what the club has left over from a member payment. The club may sign up members for a $40 payment, but that doesn't mean the club has $40 to work with when the member pays. The actual yield may be less than $30 in many cases.

The yield from a payment is affected by loss rates, cancellation rates, cost of collection, and the club's adherence to 30-year-old outdated practices, such as offering losing programs because the competition does. All these lower the yield in some manner.

Therefore, the owner's goal should be to make choices in the business that strengthen the receivables base and increase the yield. A simple choice, such as using a strong third-party collector rather than collecting your own memberships, can affect the yield from a payment by as much as $5 or more monthly or $60 or more per member on an annual basis.

The choices an owner makes when it comes to charging members also affects the entire way the club will be operated. For example, an owner who uses a complicated, low-yield system will normally end up with a sales-driven club that spends most of its time and resources chasing endless new sales. Clubs that use efficient and simple systems can have a lower cost per sale and put more money into the service end of the business. This allows the owner to concentrate on renewals, which decreases the dependence on new sales.

The yield is the return we get from a single payment. Our overall goal in mainstream fitness facilities is to chase the highest return per client we can get while still showing a moderate entry price. We do this by moving away from the volume approach and toward a layered pricing strategy that offers the widest range of products with the widest range of price points. Different products combined with different price points attract a different client than most gyms usually get. Achieving this means we move toward creating a system that generates the highest return per client and gets the most results for the most members over time.

January 2, 2014
Three questions you have to answer now

- What is the single most important thing you want to accomplish in your career this year (open a gym/new job/move to a new town/financial)?
- What is the single most important thing you want to accomplish in personal development this year (bad habits/workshops/new skills)?
- What is the single most important thing you want to get done personally this year (family/spiritual/personal adventure)?

Put each answer on a card and carry them with you until they are done. Write a backup to each card because you will most likely get the first one done and then need to add another replacement. If you don't know where you are going, then you are just wasting your life and time. Don't be afraid to think big. If your goals aren't big enough to scare you, then they aren't big enough to change your life.

January 13, 2014
Something to work on with your clients

Avoid telling people what you do, meaning how you train, your style, or your beliefs, and spend a week telling your clients what the expected outcomes will be if those clients work with you. We get caught up on what we do, which to the client doesn't really matter as much as "What happens to me if I work with you?" It's not the tool. It's the carpenter and the clients will respond much more strongly to someone who projects them into the future. In other words, just focus on the outcomes the client can expect if he works with you and much less on the tools you will use to get it done.

6

Everything About Staffing

Staffing a fitness business is more complicated than seeing how many hours a week your relatives can work. Staffing any type of fitness business is almost more of an art form than a science for most owners. Learning to staff by creating the key positions, learning to use a staffing budget plan, and learning to hire by levels are all part of an advanced approach to running your business.

Of course, you could still use the system many owners use when they first get started. Figure out how many hours you're going to be open, total up all relatives, and then divide. This is okay when you first start and it would be really scary to imagine how many gyms there are out there staffed with two or three family members working for desperation wages, but eventually, you're going to need something more comprehensive to make your business grow.

Before we discuss staffing basics, first look at how staffing budgets affect the overall business. For many years, most owners in the business looked at what staffing costs as a percentage of sales—or in other words, a percentage of the total money or revenue the business brought in that month.

The problem with this system is that the staff always expanded as revenues increased. This continually drove up expenses as the revenues grew and also left the business severely overstaffed when revenues dropped. If you anticipated endless increases in volume, then this might have worked and the system itself dates back to an era where you might have shown continued growth for years in markets with little or no competition.

The more advanced way to look at your staffing budget is to compare cost of staff in relationship to the monthly base operating expense (BOE). This percentage ratio has also changed over the years. During the 1980s and early 1990s, a financially sound fitness business would have its BOE divided into these percentages:

Rent/mortgage and any additional landlord add-on charge
(triple net) = 33 percent of the BOE

Payroll and payroll taxes and any commissions
or bonuses = 33 percent of the BOE

General operating expense, such as supplies, repairs and
maintenance, or utilities = 33 percent of the BOE

The club's monthly expenses were divided into three distinct areas, each of which equaled a third of the club's operating expense. These numbers were a good starting place for analyzing a business as a beginning to the problem-solving process for gyms that were for some reason not functioning according to plan. For example, it's common for gyms that overstaff by carrying too many managers or make other staffing mistakes to have a staff percentage that's way over an acceptable percentage.

However, the percentages in the sample have changed dramatically during the last several decades, starting in the mid-1990s. The cost of payroll and related payroll expense, such as commissions, bonuses, and other basic business expenses, has risen faster in comparison to increases in rent or the cost of owning a building. Today, a properly balanced club financially now looks like this:

Rent/mortgage and any additional landlord add-on charge
(triple net) = 20 percent of the BOE (This number can go to
25 percent in gyms that have rents of $25,000 or higher.)

Payroll and payroll taxes and any commissions
or bonuses = 37 to 45 percent of the BOE

General operating expenses, such as supplies, repairs and
maintenance, or utilities = 40 percent of the BOE

Payroll and other payroll costs are now 37 to 45 percent of most fitness facilities' operating budgets and can be substantially higher in gyms using traditional one-on-one training as their primary profit center. This type of gym might have a payroll percentage that runs as high as 50 percent or more but without a supporting profit margin. In other words, the revenue and expenses are high in the old one-on-one model, but the true profit is often low in the under-30 percent range.

Again, looking at overall percentages of money spent in a business is a good place to start analyzing a business and the problems it might be having. If payroll costs are higher than the suggested 37 to 45 percent range, the club might be wasting payroll dollars, keeping too much staff around too long, overpaying for classes or training, or incurring any other number of ways an owner can waste payroll when he isn't paying close attention. Keep in mind this 37 to 45 percent of the BOE target as you try to improve an existing facility or start a new one.

If payroll expense is more than 37 to 45 percent, then most club owners are wasting money—usually by making some basic staffing mistakes. Some of the common mistakes include trying to give everyone 40 hours a week, having a sales system that is too complicated and forces up the cost per sale, simple overstaffing, giving everyone titles and the associated costs that go with them, and rewarding longevity instead of performance.

There is also a lot of waste on the training side of the business. Owners stuck in the era of traditional one-on-one training usually pay too much per hour for a trainer and could save a great deal of money by simply moving most trainers to a flat wage. For example, in most markets, trainers make about $35,000 per year. If you live in a major metro area, such as New York City or San Francisco, you can adjust this for your area after you are done laughing at this admittedly low wage in comparison to those areas.

What owners don't realize or acknowledge is how hard a trainer has to work just to make that limited amount of money. You're there early in the morning, off for a few hours midday, and then back again for a long evening session. If you're any good as a trainer or if the owner is trying to get the most out of you before you die, you are also there Saturdays until late afternoon. All this work might get you about $17 per hour average for hours actually worked and about $4 per hour for all the real hours you are there waiting to work.

Converting the trainer to a flat wage—let's say $20 per hour, which is a little more than $40,000 per year—would give you a stable employee who is there for full blocks of time and who can handle all your training needs including one-on-one training, small group, team training, fundamentals for the new clients, and whatever else you need. He has a steady job, real time away, and perhaps insurance and benefits. Everyone wins in this case and the owner can now achieve about a 40 percent margin in the training department because all sessions of any type are now flat wage instead of the owner having to pay large amounts of extra money for the number of people in the session or if it is a one-on-one training. Just because we have been paying ineffectively for six decades doesn't mean we can't stop and figure out a better way for all involved, especially the owners who can cut payroll expense drastically.

Save Money by Redefining Full-Time Work and Allowing Flextime

Two basic concepts that are somewhat new to most operators could save you a very large percentage of your payroll. The first is reconsidering what's considered full-time employment and the second is the use of what's called flextime hiring.

Three o'clock in the afternoon is the kiss of death for owners trying to keep the payroll under control. There, standing at the front counter, is a small herd of staff all bored to tears and waiting for the evening rush to flow through the door.

Most of these folks are there because we're still trying to apply 1950s work theory to next generation workers. No one works like our fathers used to back in the day. Gone are the days of straight 8-to-5, 40-hour workweeks, working for the same company your entire career, and endless overtime in the name of the company. Also included here is the end of the authoritarian period of management discussed in other sections.

Employees in the gyms now (and they all don't have to be in their 20s to feel this way) want more free time, participation in their jobs and the decision-making process, opportunities to grow through education and advanced training, and work schedules that fit their lifestyles.

At the base of many of these problems is the full-time issue. Except for several key people on the management staff, who will be discussed later in this section, full time should be defined as 32 hours of work (or more) per week. By setting full time at 32 hours, you'll eliminate a lot of wasted payroll by trying to find busy work to fill 40 hours for all your full-timers.

Being full time should have a great deal of status in the gym. Full-timers should receive the most education and training, get the most perks, and be treated like the serious investment they are in your business. Most clubs need that central core of full-timers who carry the load for the business and who are supported by a cast of part-timers that changes depending on the age of the club, time of year, and needs of the club's target population.

Full-timers are the kings and queens of the business and the part-timers are the scourge of the earth barely fit for the consumption of good food. Full-timers should have a status in the club that makes becoming one desirable, especially if you're a low-life part-timer. For example, full-timers might have a free membership for their spouse or significant other, 30 percent off all clothing, supplements, and special programming (such as yoga), and vacation time and other perks that separate them from part-time people.

Hand in hand with declaring full time at 32 hours is the use of flextime for scheduling. For example, a full-time salesperson might only work Monday through Thursday from 1 p.m. to 9 p.m. and still receive all the benefits and perks of being full time at 32 hours.

This person might be the lead salesperson and still have the chance to achieve all the bonuses and commissions a salesperson would get but would only work four days a week instead of five. This would be a very desirable job for someone who might be into sports and needs an extra day of training per week or who has kids and just needs the extra time. This also saves you the additional eight hours on Friday when sales are traditionally slow anyway and still provides the person a decent living because he has a 32-hour base and commissions from the prime sales times.

Flextime simply means not every full-time person has to work five-day weeks. Another example might be a weekend person who also supervises the club on Saturday and Sunday. That person might work Saturday, Sunday, and Monday and still get in 32 hours. The same person could also work four days of 10 hours each and still be full time.

The consideration here is overtime. If an employee is working a 40-hour week and he voluntarily decides to accept four 10-hour days, then that person needs to sign a simple form giving up the right for overtime for those additional two hours a day over eight depending on your state laws. You don't want someone coming back years after the employee has left, looking for overtime pay for something he wanted to do at the time.

What Are the Key Jobs and Responsibilities in the Fitness Business?

When you're restructuring an existing club or starting a new one, always go back to the key positions in the club and what they should be doing. It's easy to overstaff when we hire two or three people to do parts of what one person should be in charge of in the business. Unclear expectations by senior management also drive up the cost of staffing because we have no clear concept of what one person could or should do as part of his job.

The following sections discuss the key jobs in a typical training-centric business, the hours needed to get that job accomplished, and what these people should be doing. There are variations, of course, but this should give you a good starting point. Salaries for these people will be discussed in the next section.

The manager

The manager is the one ultimately responsible for the club's financial position. If the owner is on-site and filling the manager's position, then he is the manager and you should have an assistant manager to help. Avoid the confusion for the lower staff of having the owner on-site and someone else using the manager's title. It's hard to work for more than one boss at a time. Having an owner and a manager on-site makes it more difficult than it needs to be for your staff.

The manager should be the chief watcher of the business. Whoever has the manager's job—whether it is a separate person who works for an off-site owner or the owner on-site acting as manager—should be responsible for most of the following tasks:

- Establishes the base operating expense for the business and is responsible for bringing the gym in under budget, along with meeting or exceeding revenue projections. The manager has to be sophisticated enough to manage both sides of the business, meaning sales and training. The manager should be a certified personal trainer, although it is not mandatory that he ever trains anyone, attend annual training conferences to stay current in the field, or be a regular training client in his own gym. Expect that revenue from the training side of the business should exceed revenue from the membership side in training-centric mainstream gyms and it is key that the manager understands and can manage that product. In training gyms, the owner is usually the manager and will have an assessor and a lead salesperson on his senior team.
- Writes all checks—either manually or electronically—generates reports based on the gym's computerized check writing system, and takes care of all deposits and banking concerns
- Is in charge of daily production reports and the tracking of all the key indicators and numbers in the business

- Works with the third-party financial company on problems and reporting
- Leads sales by example. The manager should do at least 10 to 20 percent of all sales to set the pace and stay in touch with the problems encountered by the salespeople. In a smaller club (meaning fewer than 600 members), the manager may do more of the sales load. In clubs with more than 2,000 members, managers may not get to do many sales but should still turn in a few per month to keep their finger on the club's sales pulse.
- Responsible for the monthly tracking of the multiple profit centers, including a profit and loss sheet on each profit center in the club
- Staff training is a major part of the manager's job. The manager should coordinate all training in conjunction with the assistant manager, including weekly group training sessions, weekly one-on-one training with each full-time staffer, and other special training, such as bringing in outside speakers.
- Responsible for any other numbers reporting and financial analysis, such as tracking sales per square foot, cost per sale, cost per lead, or renewal percentages.
- All marketing is handled by the manager, including working with the ad people, supervising distribution, and managing ad budgets. The manager should also supervise all electronic marketing for the gym but doesn't necessarily have to be doing all of it himself on a daily basis.
- The condition of the club is also the responsibility of the manager, including scheduling a cleaning service, repairs, and maintenance of the gym's atmosphere during working hours, which includes music, staff uniforms, and club cleanliness for the sales effort.
- Daily promotions of the profit centers are split between the manager and the number two person in the club.
- Interpretation of the club's policies, including disciplinary action against the staff, handling of all cancellations of memberships, and the final action in all member service problems that may arise
- The manager also supervises all other management staff, including the lead salesperson, the assessor, the lead trainer, and the lead nutrition professional if your gym has one. The assistant manager would co-manage these people in reference to expected production and goal setting.
- When all else is accomplished, the manager should be on the floor most evenings helping generate business. Production is still part of the manager's job, along with the watching function, but the manager is not the prime producer during these hours, but he is there on the job to make sure production is happening and clients are getting serviced professionally.

Of course, these aren't all the possible duties for the manager. However, if you have a significant amount of other duties, consider that the manager is usually the watcher of the business and manages the back end of the business while the assistant manager is considered the doer or the person who is in charge of generating the business for the club. One creates the business while the other watches the back shop to keep expenses under control and guide the business for long-term growth.

The hours a manager should work have always been somewhat controversial. Some old-style owners believe nothing short of seven days a week will do. Some managers think they're in power positions, and as soon as they get the job, they start leaving the club at 5 p.m.—just when the real work begins.

Done properly in a mainstream fitness facility, the manager's job is 45 to 50 hours a week. The manager should be in the club Monday through Thursday to do whatever it takes to get the job done. Paperwork is usually done during daytime hours. Once primetime begins, the manager should be out on the floor. After about 4:30 p.m., we don't make money in the office in any type of gym business. The action is at the counter and on the floor and that's where the manager should be, acting as traffic cop to keep everyone focused on the moneymaking aspects of the business.

On Fridays, the manager should be in the club from about 9 a.m. to 3 p.m. to finish paperwork for the week and then be gone. The assistant manager can finish the day and the weekend supervisor can handle the weekend. Managers who are good are very valuable assets and shouldn't be worked until severe burnout sets in and kills their productivity.

Training gyms have several advantages when it comes to hours worked. First of all, training gyms seldom have a need for Friday hours later than 6 p.m., Saturday hours after 2 p.m., and most gyms of this type don't offer any Sunday hours at all. The basic idea, though, is still the same for this type of gym. You still need someone to drive sales (acquisition of new clients) and someone to place the person into the system where he belongs, called the assessor. Put simply, training gyms still have to have someone run the back shop and manage the money and processes and several people up front who do nothing but create revenue for the gym.

The lead salesperson

The lead salesperson should be the one who generates the most sales in the club. This person works the best selling hours, which are usually Monday through Thursday nights, and is the one who tracks and controls all prospective members. Larger clubs with high volume would need more than one during the heavy hours and everyone on the team needs to be cross-trained to do sales.

It is important to note that this role changes greatly in a training-centric business model. In the old days, the salesperson was often the most important person in the gym because he was the one who generated the highest amount of revenue and, in the traditional club business model from the 1950s, usually the only revenue for the gym. If you're moving toward a training-centric business model, you now have two teams concentrating on driving revenue from two separate revenue streams.

The lead salesperson is now your first line of offense in the gym. His role is to handle all trial members or any other leads from initial marketing, enroll referral sales (buddy sales), handle walk-in traffic if the gym generates that type of leads, and, most importantly, works directly with the assessor and the training team to get all new clients or potential clients using the gym on trial memberships into an appointment with that department. His goal is not to sell training but to get the person into a session with a fitness professional whose only job is to assess the client and get him into the right training program in the gym. The assessor is explained in the following section.

In large volume clubs with a membership of about 1,000 members or more, the club might need a sales manager. This person would also be the lead salesperson whenever he is on the job and would also be responsible for sales training the rest of the staff.

The lead salesperson is part of your management team because training-centric businesses have to have that constant interaction between the sales department and the assessor. In a smaller training gym—defined as about 12,000 square feet or less—the lead salesperson can also assume other management jobs and can help with marketing and retention.

It is important to keep in mind that if you own a training gym, many of the systems important to running a financially successful mainstream business directly also apply to your gym. You still need sales—defined as the acquisition of new clients—and you still need an assessor, whose primarily job is to patiently and professionally bring the new client into the system and place him exactly where he belongs. In the past, individual trainers handled this job, but the revenue potential is so large in this style of gym today that you should only let trained professionals handle your most valuable asset, which is the new or potential client.

The following are a few responsibilities the lead salesperson might have as part of his daily job:

- Responsible for 30 to 40 percent of the sales goal depending on the size of the club. In the training gyms, he would be responsible for controlling and tracking all leads for the month.
- In charge of training every member of the staff in basic sales. Every full-time employee should have continuous sales training for two reasons: one is to serve as backups on the off hours and the other is that every staff person will do a better job supporting the other members of the team if he understands the other person's job.
- Responsible for follow-up training and review of the sales staff on a monthly basis
- Responsible for keeping all sales supplies stocked
- Expected to assist in any stressed area in the club at any time if there are no sales tours going on at the moment

The hours for this job would vary according to the club size. A lead salesperson in a smaller club would probably have a larger variety of duties and would most likely work more than 40 hours a week. In the 600- to 1,800-member clubs, the lead salesperson could work 32 to 35 hours per week over four days.

The assessor

The single most important job in the gym business is one that most of you have never heard of in your careers and probably would have never read about in the magazines or heard about at the trade shows.

This new job is the assessor, who has the sole function of being the first workout/gym experience for as many of your new clients as possible and who then places the new client where he belongs in the system. This person should be a trainer with experience who isn't afraid of asking for money. Any trainer who has been training for a long period of time often gets bored and wants more from the job than just another day of sweating with the regular clients and the assessor job is a great way to move up and beyond the tedium of just doing the same thing over and over again every day. The goal for the assessor—through this first training experience for the new or potentially new client—is to place new these clients somewhere in the training membership system based on a first assessment and a review of goals, time frame, and commitment.

There are currently two systems in use in most fitness facilities. The first is based on the salesperson trying to sell a basic training package along with a membership. This package is usually just a small traditional one-on-one experience that does nothing more than get the client in front of a trainer, who then tries to sell the client more training in the future. The salesperson is always restricted to just a small package because he has neither the training nor the skill set to sell long-term training packages. It is hard for a typical salesperson to explain and sell long-term training if he is not a trainer and can't set goals, analyze the client's true needs, discuss prior injuries, or lay out a long-term plan that would meet the client's immediate needs now yet still cover long-term goals, such as weight loss.

The second method of selling training in the industry is more common. This model is where the gym's salesperson sells the client a basic membership to the gym and then turns the new member over to a trainer. This trainer then gives the potential client a workout or two, attempting to sell him an extended training package almost always based on a series of options based on one-on-one training done with that trainer.

The key question here—and why this method is horribly ineffective—is how much sales training did that trainer ever have? Most trainers receive zero sales coaching, but they are often responsible for the gym's potentially biggest source of revenue and are simply not qualified to do the job. The sad part of our business is that most of these trainers really do nothing but check out the potential client to see if he has money, and if the person doesn't "qualify" as a one-on-one training client, he is blown off, given a giant workout card dating from the Nautilus days of 1970, and sent to the circuit from hell room, doomed to go in a circle until he gives it up and quits—on average, about seven months later.

Both of these systems are utter failures and are doomed from the first hello. People visiting a gym don't want to talk to salespeople. They want to talk to someone who knows something about working out. The failure is that the potential member goes to a gym thinking he is buying fitness and a solution to his ever-present fat ass. This means he expects to talk to someone who might really know something about fitness and getting into shape. He doesn't want or need to talk to a salesperson. He wants to talk to a fitness expert who can provide a solution to his problem.

Remember, the potential client did not come into the gym to buy a membership. He came in to buy a solution to a problem. The old analogy is that no one buys a drill because he needs a drill. He buys a drill because he needs a hole somewhere. The same is true with a fitness membership. You don't buy a membership to own a membership. You buy a membership to solve a problem, which in this case is the fat ass syndrome. The salespeople just can't get past selling the drill and all the cool stuff it does, while the people who can tell you how to use the drill to get the best hole are the trainers.

Gym salespeople usually work out and many look fit, but they are not qualified to talk to a person about fitness and a solution to the fat ass problem. They are trained in sales, not physical training, and if they do sell anyone anything in training, it is too often just a small hundred-dollar or so package based on about three workouts.

On the other hand, there is also absolutely no one more stereotypically worse at sales than a trainer. Trainers are by vocation passionate and by birth usually intrinsic people who love to help people and who in most cases would give training away just to be of service to humanity. Stated more clearly, trainers can't sell, most weren't born to sell, and few were ever trained to sell and the majority of all trainers hate selling anyway because they feel they are above the process, so they suck at it anyway.

The system also works against selling training in most gyms, especially the chains. The vast majority of gyms worldwide only have two products to sell: You either buy a membership or you buy one-on-one training. This basic two-prong system effectively eliminates the younger clients who love the group dynamic (and we wonder how CrossFit got to be around 7,000 units), anyone who is on a budget, and anyone who finds that traditional one-on-one training often becomes more boring than watching old people walk slowly through a supermarket. In other words, the pricing system and training model itself is eliminating much of the profit potential for the business.

The solution is to use a two-team sales attack. You would still have a traditional salesperson handling basic memberships, such as referral sales, walk-in traffic, and potential clients who come through the door for the gym's trial membership, and an assessor, who creates the first training experience for the new client and then places her into the system. The assessor's job is to primarily create revenue for the training department and to feed the rest of the trainers.

It is important to note that no trainer should ever have his own stable of clients in your business and that everyone is team trained. You have to control the quality of the product and the membership structure and you can't do this by allowing trainers to run their own businesses within your business using their own training philosophies and their own pay structures. Remember that this is your business—representing your training philosophy—with the house owning the clients, not the individual trainers.

The assessment itself takes about an hour. You have to slow the first experience down for all new clients. It is also important that you never test body composition or do a full screen at this point. The guy knows he is fat and he is in your gym because he understands this point. His friends are making fun of him, his wife is threatening to leave him, and his girlfriend doesn't want anything to do with him and that fat belly. Pulling up his shirt and testing body fat is not necessary to prove that his life sucks. The goal of the assessment is to build confidence in the client and then find the right program for him. There is still a need for a full functional movement screen and body composition but only as baseline tools after he becomes a client.

This business system is based on the concept that you would have a five- to seven-layer price structure, including large group team training, small group intensive coaching, and traditional one-on-one training. The assessor would at some point place the client into the group where she has the most interest and also where she fits financially.

For example, the team training often has up to 20 people in it and is perfect for the person who is 24 to 40 years old and who likes music, energy, and the group experience. The people who do team training are not too poor for one-on-one training, as the chains believe. They just want a more exciting and challenging product than the traditional boring-ass training.

This system is especially important for training gyms where the owner gets trapped doing most of the workouts. The old adage is true: You have to stop working in your business and start working on it. You should be your own assessor, feeding your training team until you master the job and can then teach it to others, but you should also control the workouts and product too. Stop training clients and start selling clients into your system.

The lead trainer

There have been a number of issues through the years that have finally forced almost all fitness businesses to step away from using outside, or contract, trainers. Legally, it is hard to defend independent contractors the way we normally do it in the business. For example, if you collect the money, set the time of training, require the trainer to wear a uniform, or require him to do other work in the gym, then most likely you are breaking the rules that govern the difference between employees and real independents. The risk is too high for most owners to try to beat the taxman, and as of now, most mainstream gyms have eliminated almost all independents and replaced them with in-house trainers.

Because it is really an issue of control, most clubs have eliminated all outside trainers and have gone with all in-house staffs. In the past, when trainers were hard to come by, many clubs let the trainers pay rent to use their facilities. The problem with the control issue was not only the issue of taxes but also more importantly with the more current issue of quality and consistency of training in the gym. You could have seven trainers in your gym who practice seven different training methodologies and advocate seven different nutritional approaches.

You have to remember that training is our main product, not just selling access to the equipment in the gym, and that we have to be able to deliver a consistent product based on a consistent methodology over time. The equivalent of this breakdown in the product in the real world would be going to a national high-end steakhouse and having three chefs in the back just doing their own thing and ignoring the menu the house publishes. Each chef has his own agenda and wants to do it his way and to hell with what the restaurant owner believes is right for the customer. It is your house and your clients and every trainer has to deliver a consistent product based on your belief system and method of training.

Another problem was that the independent trainers also sold their own clothing and supplements, did their own diets, offered boot camps in the park and kept the money, and worked when and if they chose, therefore bypassing the gym's other programming and profit centers. What we created was a entire crew of trainers who literally ran their own businesses within a business with no controls and who as a team reflected the true image of the gym to the clients, which was at best mediocre.

Many owners are also finally grasping the fact that it is senseless to give up so much of the profits to the trainers while the gym gets so little in return. The premise of this book is that we are moving away from the traditional high-volume membership model that has sustained this industry for so many years toward a training-centric business model where getting the maximum results for the maximum number of clients in the shortest period of time is the goal. This simply means that creating a steady receivable base of training revenue, with the goal of exceeding the monthly revenue from membership, is now too important to treat the training department as a second-tier product with little revenue—and even less profit—potential.

The key to the training-centric model is to create a system that generates a higher return per client served. This can only be done by getting a significantly higher percentage of your memberships involved in a training program based on a 12-month membership and not using short-term tools, such as sessions or packages. Remember that the national average of penetration into a mainstream gym's membership with training is about 3 to 6 percent—all of which is usually done in traditional one-on-one settings.

Based on all this, the lead trainer now has a much more important role in the gym than in the past due to the impetus of chasing a much larger revenue stream in the business. In the past, the lead trainer was hired mostly due to being there the longest or perhaps having slightly better credentials than the other staff trainers and the size of his personal stable of clients was always a factor. Today, the skills we need most in a lead trainer are the ability to train a team, the ability to generate revenue, and the ability to control the quality of the total training product. It is no longer about the lead trainer training any clients as long as he can train a team that can handle a much larger and diverse training clientele.

The lead trainer can also be your assessor, but once you move beyond about 150 clients, you will most likely find that you have to separate these positions. However, it is important that the lead trainer and assessor are always cross-trained so each one can always back up the other in case of an emergency.

You should get to the point that your lead trainer trains no one but other trainers. The exception to this is that it is good to let this person take a team training or do a special workshop just to keep fresh and be seen by the clients, but if you are trying to develop a team that can generate high revenue, then your lead trainer should not ever be allowed to do one-on-one training because that is the least effective method of creating revenue in the training department.

The lead trainer needs to be in the gym about 45 hours per week over five days. The trainer also needs to make sure everyone on the staff is cross-trained enough to at least master the gym's basic workout methodology, handle the diverse product line (such as team training and small group intensive coaching), be able to begin to spot dysfunction in training clients, and to stay current on any new tools that are added to the department. By training every trainer this way, there will always be someone on duty who can at least answer a member's basic questions.

The lead counter person

Who runs the counter in the primetime hours in most mainstream fitness businesses? It is usually a very young and very inexperienced person working a position that has the highest turnover in the club. Most gym owners consider front counter people as strictly entry-level folks who are expendable—just bodies to be replaced as the next one leaves us for a better job. The reality is that during primetime, which is usually around 4 p.m. to 9 p.m. from Monday through Thursday and Saturday morning until 1 p.m., you will see most of your members and generate most of your revenue. Training gyms have two primetimes because this type of business usually has that strong morning crowd from opening until about 10 p.m. from Monday through Friday. In the mainstream fitness businesses, we often have our worst employees running the front counter area during our busiest times. We don't need inexperience and inability during the rush hour. We need the best we can put into the game.

The lead front counter person, who is the person who works from about 4 p.m. to 9 p.m. from Monday through Friday, is one of the most important people on your staff. Your lead counter person is the first and last person every member sees coming and going from the club. The lead counter person is the standard for the gym's member service image. The lead counter person is the one who can make or break your profit centers because of her presence at the counter during primetime. In other words, this shouldn't be the weakest and youngest person in the club. It should be the best communicator and one of the most mature people you have who can deliver client service consistently day after day to everyone who visits your business.

Over the years, we have practiced a reverse discrimination in most successful fitness businesses by hiring women employees for all the key jobs in the gym, including manager. Women in our businesses have demonstrated better communication skills across a wider range of people and better member service skills in the form of an empathetic attitude and they have been more dependable and stable over time and respond more sincerely to recognition for the work they do.

Women have often been given a bad reputation in the business world that is simply not true in the reality of the workplace. Women are not the hormonal ones. It is the young male in his 20s that is usually the disaster employee and it's always the young males who come running into the office shouting: "I quit. I met a new girl! We're moving to Miami tomorrow. Gotta go." When you're hiring key people, you are looking for stability and the ability to multitask—something that women seem to bring to their jobs at a much earlier age. This does not mean you should never hire a young male, but it does mean that any young male you hire should exhibit a maturity level beyond his years.

Anyone could be a front counter leader, as long as he is mature, can communicate, is an outgoing and empathetic person, loves to be in the center of action, can manage other front counter people, and loves to help people figure out solutions to their problems. You might notice by reading this list of traits that we're not talking about the typical 22-year-old male here. We're probably talking about a female in her late 20s with great communication skills and practical customer service experience gained in fast food or retail.

In smaller clubs, this person might take on a bigger role and do sales or even help train. However, once the club gets more than 600 to 700 members, the club needs a dedicated counter person at primetime hours who can set a standard for member service. The hours for this person are about 32 to 35 hours per week. This would be a great job for a housewife returning to the workforce or a person who wants free time during the day.

Training gyms can't ignore this position by thinking you are too small or it doesn't apply to you. By the nature of your clientele, meaning training gyms that usually attract people willing to spend more money and who are looking for a higher level of service, you have to add this position as soon as you can. Once you reach about 125 clients or so, you most likely need someone there during your evening rush hours at least from Monday through Thursday. This is assuming your gym is at least 3,000 square feet and that you have added a recovery shake bar, a front counter, and a logo wall, which is nothing more than a wall with the counter in front of it that separates the front door from the training floor. No scared potential client wants to walk into a gym and find himself immediately standing on the training floor. Every gym needs that safety zone up front where the client can meet your counter person and then peek around the wall to see what is happening in the gym.

The weekend supervisor

This would be somewhat of an old school job that has been lost in the mainstream gyms during the years. Most fitness facilities operate with an eclectic group of weekenders—usually chosen by their low status on the totem pole or by their inability to find other work. Young? Not too bright? No friends? Nothing to do on weekends? Then, welcome to the gym, you new weekend guy.

However, this position is also a key job in the gym. Most gyms simply give away potential weekend business with their unwillingness to staff properly. Saturdays have always been strong in every fitness business, but the inexperience of the weekend crew usually restricts the revenue potential. In the smaller gyms, most owners are so burnt by Saturday that going back to the gym is the last place they want to be, but the reality of the business is that weekend mornings have the potential to generate a lot of additional revenue for the business.

Sundays have always been declared dead, but is that because Sundays are really dead or is it because we create a self-fulfilling prophecy and put the weakest staff on the weekends and kill it anyway? With a little work and creativity, such as opening Sunday up to any member guest without needing a guest pass or without paying any additional fee, Sundays can be developed into a fair sales day and a strong profit center day.

If Sundays are slow in your business, you don't really have any reason not to go creative and try to fill up the gym with at least warm bodies that might spread good word of mouth and maybe buy a smoothie. For example, if you're in a competitive area, try opening Sunday up to members from any club in the area if they can present a current membership card. These gym tourists get to see your club and they also get a chance to spend money in your profit centers.

Your new weekend supervisor is the person to start making these things happen. This person is part of the management team and is usually sort of a trainee manager who gains experience by taking over the club on the weekends.

This person should be in the same training program as the rest of the management team. Think of the weekend manager as part of your farm team or as a future manager in training. Give him the same sales, numbers, and production training you would give your manager and other lead positions.

This person could get all his hours done in three or four workdays. It might be better to have the person work Saturday, Sunday, and Monday (instead of Fridays). No one will really give up those three days on a consistent basis if he has any life at all.

If the person is there on Monday—traditionally one of the busiest days—he could handle some of the floor action and also be part of the backup sales team. In smaller clubs, the person might have to work four days to make enough hours. Hours for this job would be 32 to 35, although a smaller club might need a 40-hour person over a four-day period.

Training gyms don't normally have to worry about this position until the gym's membership crosses 300 clients and then you have to have someone in charge on Saturday mornings—assuming you are closed on Sundays—who can handle membership problems, process guests and new trials, and make appointments for your assessor.

The morning person

This is not a management person, but it is a key position. Good morning people—those who show up 30 minutes before the gym is to open, have everything ready before the members arrive, never miss a day, and even get a few sales now and then—are not just good employees. They are the acts and proof of a divine being.

The morning crowds in most fitness facilities are usually a hardcore group of regulars who get to know each other as friends over time, have insanely regular routines (which they hate to have disrupted by even as much as moving the equipment six inches to the right), and expect to get through their workouts with minimal fuss. The morning person is the one who supplies the glue that holds the whole morning ritual together. You normally don't get a lot of sales in the morning, but you can certainly lose a lot of memberships and revenues over time with a chronically bad morning person.

Hiring for the morning position is always erratic. We normally look for students or someone else young and cheap who has little experience in the fitness business but who is willing to work hours that for most people are not very desirable. Maybe we're looking in the wrong place.

Your mother would be a great morning employee. Let's say she's retired as a real estate broker, thinks getting up at 4 a.m. is fun and does it anyway every morning, is a great people person who would know everyone and his dog in a week, and would be extremely consistent. She would also work for $8 to $10 per hour just to keep busy.

Instead of someone like her and her demographic, we historically look for someone who by his choice of lifestyle is just getting in at 4 a.m.—instead of just getting up. After a while, these folks leave us for other less disrupting jobs for their way of life. Replace these folks with an older, more dependable person and your morning business should increase.

The morning job is in the 32- to 35-hour range over five days. It's good to have the same person during every weekday to build consistency with morning members. Morning people usually receive a shift deferential, which is usually $1 to $2 per hour, that is added to their base pay.

These are the core jobs for almost any gym of any size. If you're restructuring an existing gym or building a new one, start with these positions and the responsibilities and then expand as needed. Most facilities farm out their membership payment collections, thus eliminating an office staff of any kind, although large clubs still need a liaison between the financial company and the club who can also function as a general-purpose paperwork person.

Using a Staff Budgeting Sheet

All staffing should work off a budget. A common mistake for many owners is staffing by personality instead of what is actually needed in the club. For example, your loyal employee Joe has worked 20 hours a week to put himself through school. Joe is now getting married in a few months and wants to go to 25 hours. Normally, most owners would simply expand his hours to meet his request because most owners find it hard to say no to someone who wants to work, and more importantly, most owners would be afraid of saying no and pissing off a decent employee for fear of losing him altogether.

Another hazard in putting together a staff budget is staffing by employee quirks. Mary can open on Monday and Tuesday, but she volunteers at her son's school on Wednesday and she can't come in on Thursday until 9 p.m. Add four or five other employees to a schedule with their individual quirks and you have a complicated piece of work that forces you to redo the entire schedule every time someone leaves or wants to change hours.

The way to avoid this is to staff by using a block system. A block system is creating a set job on a set schedule and then hiring for that specific block. Managers should also do a staff budget once a month based on the block system and expected needs for the time of year. A budget sheet could look like this:

Day: Today's date

Club: The Gym (more for multiple clubs)

Total hourly expense: $139

Total salary expense: $320

Bonuses and commissions: Four sales at $25 each = $100
(There would be other bonuses.)

Payroll taxes: $139 + $320 + $100 = $559 x .13 (worst-case tax scenario) = $72.67

Total payroll for the day = $631.67

This illustration is a one-day sample and doesn't have an entire staff listed. To use these effectively, do one for each day of a typical month. Some days may be redundant, but it's still a good learning tool to do an entire month the first time. Redo the budget sheets each time you lose an employee or there are other major staff changes.

Thoughts on Paying Your People

How we pay has changed dramatically through the years in this industry. In the old days, people were hired for very low salaries but were paid high commissions. This created a culture of people who were willing to tell any lie or break any rule in order to get the sale that day. Because salespeople were the stars of the show, no one else was paid much and it was assumed that anyone who couldn't sell every day was expendable and those people came and went as the market dictated.

If you tried that in today's market, you wouldn't have much of a chance to survive over time. Competition is tougher and as much as 10 times or more dense in many markets. Even the best salespeople from back in the day would struggle today in a business where the average consumer is tired of the old sales pressure and tricks and is far too sophisticated to be fooled by the "You must buy it now or lose it" sales theory that worked so well when the clients were less sophisticated and less experienced with sales techniques.

How people buy and why they choose to stay with a business have changed and that means the employees we hire have to be better, more mature, better able to service, better trainer, and more patient than the accepted standard from the old days. Business is harder, competition is tougher, and you and your team have to be better.

The new generation employee now wants stability, benefits, recognition, and the feeling of belonging to a team. There is also a lot of current research that illustrates that heavy commissions simply don't motivate today's employees and the type of person who wants commission-only work most likely isn't going to work in an industry where the financial ceiling is so low. This type of person also wouldn't most likely fit into a modern culture where the customer and his goals are far more important than slamming the guy in an office and then ignoring him until he gets frustrated and leaves.

Paying higher bases has been mentioned throughout this book. Higher base pay attracts a higher-quality employee in this market. People want the stability from receiving a living wage and that type of person will usually do the work for that pay without the need to attempt to drive work through commissions.

Perhaps the biggest change you will have to understand is that commissions and bonuses should be rewards for good work and not whips used to drive the work. In other words, if you hire right and attract good people through a decent base pay, the commissions we used in the past to drive productivity are no longer important. If you produce, you should get some rewards for your success, but these rewards just don't work to drive more production out of any employee in today's business environment.

As mentioned elsewhere in this book, the difference between hiring a minimum employee and someone who can produce is usually about a $2 to $3 difference per hour in most markets. For example, you might be able to hire someone for $8 an hour in your market to work at your front desk, but for $10 an hour, you might be able to hire someone with the talent, enthusiasm, and life experience that enable him to actually do the job well. It has been said before, but it's worth repeating: if you pay peanuts, you get monkeys, but if you pay real money, you attract talent capable of helping you grow your business.

The following sections offer some thoughts on pay for each position. Keep in mind that what is good in one state or country might be truly horrible somewhere else. Read this not as an exact guide to what to pay but as a model as to how to pay. You will have to adjust these numbers for your market and your business, but if you understand the basic concept, you will be able to build a sustainable structure that will allow you to attract and keep people who will make a difference in your business.

Front desk people

These people are your front-line troops who become your service image over time. You have to stop hiring the cheapest and least qualified people you can find and start hiring adults with communication skills who can solve problems and provide customer service to each and every client in your business. You will most likely need a manager for the front desk. Managers' salaries can be easily calculated if you set your front counter position rates first. For example, if you pay your front counter people $10 an hour and attract adults who can talk and deliver service, a front counter manager can usually be found for about $3 to $5 more per hour depending on age, work experience, and real-life experience the person brings to the job. Creating your own managers from within is desirable, but go outside if you don't have the right person when you need to hire.

It is important not to be cheap here. If you have a budget set for this position for $13 per hour and an experienced person from the real world who has solid retail experience is willing to work for you and wants $14 to $15 per hour, then hire her. If you are wrong, then correct this within the first 90 days to keep your potential loss down. Good people are hired by the hourly wage but in reality produce income that negates the extra dollar or two per hour. If you're wrong and the person can't add to your team, then try again, but remember that it probably isn't the system—it's the person you hired. Sometimes, you're wrong, and when you're wrong, move on.

Salespeople

There are really two ways to sell. Old school is pressure and tricks and is part of our history. Modern sales technique is based upon communication skills and the ability to solve problems and build relationships. Again, if you set the front counter rate for an employee for your market, then you can hire a sales person based against that rate. For example, if you pay $10 per hour for the counter person in the illustration above, then your sales person is probably going to cost you about $15 per hour to get someone who has sales experience and who is a real adult with strong communication skills. You will also pay commissions, but keep them smaller than you would think and remember these commissions represent rewards for getting the job done and not incentives to drive the work. In this example, you most likely would pay about $10 per sale in addition to the base, but keep in mind this is just a starting point and you might pay a lesser base rate and smaller commission in smaller towns and in the southern portion of the country or you might pay a higher base and stronger commissions in metro areas where the cost of living is so much higher.

Trainers

Paying trainers might be where we make the biggest pay mistakes in the business. The tradition has been to pay them a split or percentage of their hour rate, but because they work limited hours, the pay per hour has always been high.

The assumption has always been that the trainer is the one who brings in the business and then resells that business each day. There is also the assumption that the trainer is writing long, complicated programs for the clients and that justifies the additional pay per hour. The question is, what if none of this is true anymore? If it isn't true, which it isn't in the business system advocated in this book, then we are overpaying for someone who is merely carrying out the mission with a client who was sold by someone else, who will be doing a workout designed by someone else, and who will be re-signed yearly by a professional sales team and not that trainer.

At the time this book was written, the average trainer in this country was making about $37,000 per year and working his butt off to reach that number. Yes, there are super trainers in the big metro areas who would laugh at that low pay, but keep in mind that those trainers and those markets are few and are the exception to the rule that represents the top end of the average pay.

Trainers are also suffering from an illusion that they really make more money than they actually do. For example, a trainer might do a split, which means he is splitting an hourly fee charge to the client with the gym where he works, and his share of this split might be $40. In this trainer's head, he is a $40-per-hour trainer and he only works for that rate. But does he really make $40 per hour and is he really a $40-per-hour guy?

Let's say the trainer works the following schedule for a typical week:
• He gets to work at 5 a.m., Monday through Thursday morning, and works until about 11 a.m. In that time period, he trains three clients.
• He comes back at 4 p.m. (working a split shift that allows him to see more clients) and stays until 9 p.m. During that time period, he trains another two clients.
• He trains three sessions on Friday and two on Saturday morning.

All this work adds up to 25 sessions per week, and remember, he has to do splits and weekends to get that done. Doing 25 sessions is good for an average trainer, and if you get up above 30, you are working your ass off and are in the gym even longer than the example here. Our hero in this story was in the gym for 52 hours that week to train clients for 25 sessions. The rest of the time in the gym was spent on the Internet, working out, or keeping busy.

25 sessions per week x $40 each = $1,000 per week

$1,000 x 4.2 average weeks per month = $4,200 per month

$4,200 x 12 months = $50,400 per year

$1,000/52 hours per week = $19.23 per hour actual wage

There are a lot of questions here that need to be answered. First of all, how long will this guy last in this job? Research shows that the average trainer lasts about eight years and is then gone, but it takes about four years or more to become a trainer who is capable of training and coaching at a higher level of pay. In other words, just when this guy starts getting good, he gets gone.

Secondly, how effective will this trainer be over time? This is a tough schedule and the longer you try to do this, the more your effectiveness suffers. It is tough for any employee to work so long to get so little over time.

Because this system is so ineffective to begin with, we fail as owners by trying to throw more hourly pay at the trainer to keep him, but in reality, you can't really pay this person enough per hour to keep him in the system. The system itself is flawed, and even if you gave the guy all the money from the client, he is still going to fade over time. There are simply too many hours needed to collect too little money.

The solution is to switch to flat rate pay for trainers, which provides stability, structure, and a life for the trainer and also allows a gym owner to increase his profits through the training department. For example, let's take the trainer from the previous example and convert him to a flat rate:

- If we offer him $23 per hour, he will make $1,035 per week (based on a workweek of about 45 hours). Paying him $1,035 per week gives him an annual salary of $52,164 ($1,035 x 4.2 x 12). The advantage to the trainer is that he can now work from 5 a.m. to approximately 2 p.m., Monday through Friday, and have a set pay he can count on, he can have hours off that are regular, and he doesn't have to sell in this system. In other words, the guy has a life and a steady job for the first time in his training career.
- The owner also wins in that he now has an employee he can load up with team training, small group training, one-on-one training, and other needs, such as orientations and fundamentals training, every day at a fixed, known rate. The owner also has another great benefit in that he needs fewer trainers in this system. Instead of having a squad of trainers he needs to feed at a high hourly rate, he now can pay fewer people a decent living wage and get more work and a higher return per client served, giving him an overall higher profit margin from this segment of his business.

The assessor

The assessor should be the highest producer on your team and, therefore, will most likely be the highest-paid person you employee. The assessor is usually given a higher base and is usually a salaried person because he will most likely be managing others on the team. In this example and in relation to the other jobs discussed in this section, the assessor might get a base of $2,500 to $4,000 depending on experience and the market. The assessor would also usually get a commission base representing 20 to 40 percent of the payment amount he sold. For example, if the assessor sold a new client a $129-per-month membership for 12 months, he would get 20 to 40 percent of the $129 once as a commission ($129 x 20 percent equals $25.80). This is a production-based job that takes a trainer who wants to move beyond simply handling clients every day. Offering a strong base and solid bonuses in the form of commissions will usually attract someone who can produce a lot of revenue for the business.

The manager

In the past, a manager used to be the highest-paid person in the gym, but that doesn't have to be the case these days if you have a strong assessor. The mistake we make is to create managers who are not tied to production.

The ultimate role of that manager in every type of fitness facility is to create monthly revenue. Fitness businesses are production-based businesses and the manager is the person who has to keep the production happening each month through the supervision of the staff.

Manager pay is also such a broad topic that it is hard to really give direct numbers. In this ongoing example, the manager would receive a base similar to the assessor, which would be in the $2,500 to $4,000 per month range. But keep in mind that this is too high for rural markets and far too low for major metro areas. The manager should also have bonuses/incentives in place each month for hitting the key indicators of the business. For example:

- You might pay $500 if the manager hits the targeted total sales number for the month.
- You might pay $500 if the manager grows the net receivable base by $1,500 for the month.
- You might pay $500 if the manager hits the total targeted deposit for the business for the month.

The key is to pay a decent-enough base to get a manager capable of leading staff, creating revenue each month, hiring and firing, and handling service problems. If you do all this as the owner, then you are the manager. If you don't do much of this and hire someone who does, then you need to pay the person more as a base for the additional responsibility he assumes for your business.

Summary

Mistakes in staffing can increase a typical gym's payroll by at least 10 percent over what it should be under normal conditions. The rules in staffing have also changed over years and could add even more waste to the club's budget. For example, keeping staff costs as a percentage of total revenues (sales) continually adds to the expense side of the club without necessarily adding to the net.

Payroll and related payroll expenses should be about 37 to 45 percent of the gym's monthly base operating costs. If the gym's percentage climbs above this number, the gym needs to analyze the waste and start cost-saving controls to bring that percentage down.

Gyms can save payroll expense by redefining today's worker and what he wants from his job. Flextime, full-time status at 32 hours, and staff budgeting can all help reduce the cost of employees in your business.

When starting a new business or restructuring an existing one for more profits, start with the actual staff structure. If jobs aren't narrowly defined and you can't produce an exact job description for each job you are trying to create, then the gym ends up with more employees than it needs because the owner ends up hiring people for specific tasks that arise instead of redefining who should really be doing that work. Create the structure first and the responsibilities for each position before adding random jobs that could be done by someone else already on your payroll and in your system.

Another starting point when you are restructuring a business is the use of staff budgets. By setting staffing budgets and by working off a budget sheet, you can get away from staffing by personality or availability and shift toward a block system. A block system allows the club to create a set period of time over set days for the job. The employee either accepts the block offered or not. If an employee wants to add hours, it is done so only if there is a block of time open on the budget sheet.

December 5, 2013
Integrity

Integrity might be the most difficult word for a fitness professional to internalize, but integrity is what really sets the true professional apart from the pretender. Integrity means you live with an internal code that constantly guides you to always do the right and ethical thing. Is that workout the best for the client or is it really all about your own ego and needs? Do you become close friends with your clients and even date them, crashing through that professional plane that should never be violated? Do you stay true to your promises, keep your word, and live up to your obligations or do you find excuses to avoid your responsibility? Are you endorsing a product because it is truly good or are you doing it just for the money? Integrity is a shield that will protect you for life if you master it but giving up your integrity drops you from the ranks of the truly great and the true professionals who fight so hard to make the fitness industry an ethical and wonderful world to work in.

December 16, 2013
Intensity

Your word for this year is "intensity." We usually define this word as a fitness term, but it should also define your approach to life. In fitness, there is no gain in cardio or strength without the application of intensity. In your life, intensity is represented by the depth of the commitment you are willing to give something. The most successful people in their fields are the ones totally, deeply committed to their life's work. Life without intensity is a life not worth living and is something you lose one day at a time until you wasted the most precious gift in the universe. Question the depth of your commitment, and if you are in, then never waste a second doing anything without total focus and without your total commitment. If someone says "She is one intense bitch when it comes to fitness (guys, do your own word here)," you have now mastered the word and are now fit to lead others down the path.

7

Changing the Culture in Your Gym

Here are two things you can start thinking about now to change the culture in your club from that of failure and the feel of do-it-yourself fitness to one of success for every member. Change is coming and you will either be part of the next generation of fitness professionals or the very power of the change itself will bury you and your business where you stand.

During the next six months, turn your business into a training gym: No matter how big you are—and that goes for the 100,000-square-foot giants who have always relied on their physical plants as their main retention tool. How would you like to put $25 million into a club and find out that the 3,000-square-foot guy down the street has a higher retention rate than you do because he gets results for his members and you don't?

It is that simple and you have to put all your efforts into becoming a training-centric business if you want to create a sustainable business model for the coming years in fitness. We simply don't touch enough people or make enough change with the present business system and our current training model that only reaches about 5 percent of the gym's membership in a mainstream gym has failed in most commercial facilities.

The training guy down the street is right. He tells his clients what to do, tells them what to eat, and tells them what supplements to take. He then takes them through an amazing workout based on upright, functional training and changes their lives. Most importantly, he is charging about 5 to 15 times more a month for the privilege of working out in this small and often underfinished gym.

The fitness business should be a business of trust. We take money in exchange for the client's trust and his belief that we can help him change his life through our leadership and guidance. The reality in most mainstream clubs—unless this person can ante up the necessary money to declare himself elite and, therefore, buy leadership through personal training—is that the member is left to seek fitness on his own through magazines or help from other lost members. He signed up to get in shape, but to us, he is nothing more than a replaceable score on that day's sales sheet.

Break down a typical commercial center and you can easily see that we fail more than three-quarters of the people who trusted us to help them. Assuming the club has group exercise, you would find that about 3 to 6 percent of the members are in one-on-one training and about 20 percent take part in the club's group programs. Rounding off, only about 25 percent of the club's membership has any type of ongoing relationship with the business, such as the instructor/client in the group setting, or is getting any type of help and guidance through the trainer/client arrangement.

Put another way, 75 percent of the members in this club don't receive any help or have any relationship other than that warm and fuzzy feeling they might get from their favorite treadmill. This is the first owner who will complain loudly that the low-price guy is killing him or that the nonprofit is taking all his business. What he doesn't realize is that he has no relationship with his members and they will quickly leave him for the cheapest club in the neighborhood because fitness to him is all about the treadmill and he will go to whoever can rent it at the lowest price.

The members enter the business believing we will help them, but we set them up with antiquated circuit training, including the giant workout card, that fails clients after a few weeks and then ignore them until we need them again at the end of their membership. If a member wants to get in shape in these clubs, he has to work hard on his own because the club simply won't or can't provide the leadership and help he needs to be successful over time.

If you have relationships with your members, they will stay longer and pay longer. Without this relationship, you are nothing more than another club that rents equipment by the month and the lowest-priced competitor in the market will own that niche.

Leadership sells and people who get results will never leave your business, but most mainstream fitness businesses aren't designed to achieve that level of penetration or success.

Even how we lay out and design clubs will change in the coming years. Cardio will get even more important, functional equipment (such as the new generation multiplane cable equipment) will rise to another level, and you will drain the fitness tool warehouses to fill your gym with kettles, ropes, medicine balls, and other tools that professional sports people have been embracing for years. As a side note, when was the last time you watched a professional athlete on any of the sports shows on TV go around a circuit as his strength component?

You will still always have a core line of single-joint stuff, but your functional cable equipment and workout tools will take a higher-volume position and you will also reintroduce lifting platforms and other tools that challenge and delight the members. Free weight areas will no longer be designed for bodybuilders but for functional people and the tools we select will change dramatically.

This type of training has to be infused throughout your business, not just set aside in one room. Your culture has to change from that of failure to one of success for the most members you can touch. Training is what we do in this business and we have to return to our roots because people who get results are the ones who never leave, which is what retention is all about.

The second thing you can do is to begin to teach the fundamentals of fitness during your trial periods or during the first 30 days a person is a member. Somewhere in the past, we made a decision that all new members will be set up on a circuit, given a stupid card that we keep in a huge box on the edge of the floor, and are left to their own devices. We don't teach them how to work out. We teach them a simplistic workout that everyone knows will fail the client in about six weeks.

Couple fundamental classes with your trial memberships and teach people how to work out based on mastering the fundamental movement patterns of fitness, such as the goblet squat, hinge, lunge, press, pull, and carry.

Add about six to eight fundamental classes on your schedule and teach the basics of getting a good workout. For example, a fundamentals class might be based on the basics of a dynamic warm-up, strength moves (such as a kettlebell swing), a lunge, a body weight squat, some type of pressing movement, a row, and a dead lift movement—all considered the essentials of any fitness routine. Without these movements, the person is doomed to machines and the circuit will fail them—and if they fail, they leave. If you are more progressive and have functional movement equipment, then teach that too. Using a little parody here, if you give a man a workout, he comes to you for a day, but teach a man how to work out and he is your member for life.

Also teach the person cardio. We all know that those members walking endlessly on a tread reading while watching the current daytime talk show queen are failing and we should know that they will all leave us because they are not getting results after it dawns on them that walking slowly for an hour brings them to a plateau that can be broken by simply adding more days of working out or taking longer walks each day. Teach effective cardio and teach it early. If members get results, they will stay longer and pay longer.

The guests in the trial might be in the fundamental group all month, which is fine, or if they master the basics, they should be sent to other group experiences, which allows you to service the most guest and members at the lowest cost. Do everything in groups if you can and stop isolating the members. Most of us have grown up doing every social activity or athletic endeavor in group settings. Boy Scouts, Girl Scouts, sports teams, band, church groups, or anything else you might belong to are all examples of group dynamics, but when you come to the clubs, we do everything we can to isolate the person.

For example, look at the trend in cardio. When we added the TVs to the machines, we essentially locked the person out of the group dynamics in the club. The members don't talk to each other, don't look around, and don't get involved. You would be better to not buy the TVs and just order more cardio in your club.

Everything we do in the real world is about social groups, but everything we do in the gym world is about isolating the member from all the others in the club. Again, if my only relationship in the club were with a small TV and treadmill, why would I not simply go to the lowest bidder in the market?

Your club has to become the epitome of a large training facility. We forget that people come to us to change their lives, but because our businesses were designed for nothing but the acquisition of new members, we fail more than 75 percent of our members. Get results from the most people possible and you will have the highest retention rate you have ever achieved.

There are two parts it takes to build a successful training-centric business that almost every owner misses. These two pieces give your program that finished feel and are two keys that separate you from your competitors. Remember that it isn't the big things that usually kill your business. It is the combination of a hundred small things done badly that will ultimately take you down.

The first missing piece of building a financially successful training-centered business is creating a culture—in writing and one that can be taught to everyone on the staff—that becomes the central focus of who you are and what you are trying to accomplish. Culture is a nebulous word that is hard to grasp, and in this case, it means you create a belief system based on your philosophy as to how the client is trained and serviced during each visit.

The second missing key is the introduction of consistent coaching cues. For example, a trainer/coach who has a small group in progress but who spends time talking to other coaches on the floor has obviously never been taught that this behavior is bad service and bad coaching.

The example we will use here is from a women-only, 14,000-square-foot training gym that currently has 1,400 clients. The gym has no fixed equipment, a full line of cardio with an emphasis on treads, a full line of multiplane cable equipment, a large cycle room, a large group exercise room, and several big rooms with turf, slam walls, a row of heavy bags, a rack system, and basically enough open space to train groups of up to 30 easily using several coaches.

The key to success for this business is the stress on culture. As mentioned, there are currently about 1,400 women in the gym and about 40 percent of them are currently involved in training. This gym was once sold and the owners had to take it back as a damaged business. The first thing you have to do when you get control of a business or try to grow an existing one is establish why you are there and what you are trying to accomplish as a team.

If you want to make changes in your business, your team has to know what you are trying to accomplish each day. Why are we doing this? What do you want from us? What kind of business is this and who is it for in the community? All these are legitimate questions that have to be answered if you want to build a cohesive team that can affect the largest number of clients in the shortest period of time.

The question is: How can you train staff, especially the training staff, if you don't have a clearly written statement of what you believe and how you want your clients treated and trained? If it isn't in writing, then it isn't real and whatever you say merely reflects your thought of the day and not a long-term guideline that can be used to train and motivate all staff and clients.

The management team in the gym used the culture guide shown in Figure 7-1 as the basis for training of all coaches and group exercise instructors. Of course, you will need to modify it as needed for your gym, but once you create your own version, use it as a review to start every staff meeting you have with your trainers and also share it with every new training client.

Many of you may disagree with some of the actual methods, but for the sake of applying this to your gym, look at the creation of culture as your main goal and not whether you agree with the particulars of training as mentioned here. Also keep in mind that this makes a great handout for potential clients because it positions you well against competition.

Remember, most of your competitors are selling memberships and you are selling maximum results for the maximum number of members in the shortest period of time. You have to differentiate yourself from everyone else in the market down to the smallest details. The potential members don't just want a gym. They want to give their money to people with strong beliefs and a strong message as to how things should be done.

Once you establish culture, you can work on coaching cues. The following section provides an elementary list. Pros could do full-day workshops on just this topic alone, but these are the things that most trainers ignore—and that irritate the paying clients the most. If you want to keep people paying longer and staying longer, start with these rules.

The Basic Rules of Coaching

Start and end on time as advertised and as promised. Our clients have lives and we are grateful for their time and money. Your job is to respect both these things. Focus on those assigned to you for that time slot. Put away your phone (except to use it as a timer if needed), keep your conversations limited to those who are paying to see you that day (except to help another client who might be doing something that will result in injury), and always know the names of those in your group.

Every client is thanked every time he works out with you. You get paid because they paid the gym and you should be grateful for their support of our business.

Practice the acts of involvement. We are not rep counters. We are professional coaches. Place your clients where you can touch and coach them easily. Never, ever lead a session with a coffee cup in your hand. Never stand with your arms crossed, acting as if bored. Never sit on the floor cross-legged counting reps. Never lean on equipment while coaching. Never do the full workout with the clients as if it is your own personal workout. Pay attention to your client, coach closely, touch as needed to correct, offer guidance, and stay involved.

Why Does This Gym Exist?

This business was created to shelter and nurture women who are seeking a more fit life but who can't find the help and support they need to be successful in traditional, mainstream membership clubs. We are here to supply leadership to the women in our area who struggle with their health and fitness and who cannot find the answers they need to be successful in typical fitness facilities.

Why We Feel Training Is the Key to Success

Fitness is motion and motion is life!

If a woman wants to maintain the highest standard of living throughout her life, then she needs to participate in a challenging fitness program at a minimum of eight times per month. The core to achieving long-term success in fitness is strength training, which is the heart of our training program and is the key to sustainable health and fitness over time.

Our Motto of Success

Strong women are beautiful women. (Strong women are beautiful.)

Our Mission Statement

We change lives.

This gym exists for one reason and that is to constantly challenge and lead our members to achieve the highest level of sustainable fitness they can reach. We have an obligation to our members to provide a safe environment and to help as many as we can reach their goals and beyond. We are here to change lives and we have the opportunity to do that every single time a client walks through the door. Our staff ask themselves at the end of the workday: "Did I make a difference today? Did I change someone's life today?"

The Philosophy of Success in This Gym

- We provide leadership and guidance in fitness through training.
- Everyone is trained as an athlete no matter the age or current conditioning.
- All clients are treated as equals. We never prejudge potential by the current condition of the client, by her age, by her color, or by her orientation. Everyone sweats together in this gym.
- Strength rules. Strength training is the foundation for success in this gym, and if a woman has only one workout a week, it should be strength.
- Upright, holistic, full body is our constant approach.
- You can't out-train a bad diet. We teach nutrition by the art of reduction. We do not believe in diets. We believe in seeking a healthier life through better food choices.
- Cardio only works if intensity is present.
- Never to failure—but always to challenge.
- Lift heavy, lift often, and lift like you mean it.
- We do not say "No, you can't." We do say "Not yet—later"; "Let's work on it"; and "Yes, it can be done, but you have to do the work." "No" is not an option in this gym for our clients. We believe that the only limits clients have exist in our heads, not theirs.

cont.

Figure 7-1. Sample culture handout for a women-only training gym with a combination of 22 full- and part-time trainers

- We see every client as someone who has an issue that needs to be solved. We believe there is no such thing as a perfect client. There are only real people who have physical issues and who need our help.

We never forget that time is the enemy of fitness. Our clients have busy lives and need to get in here, get it done, and get on to other things in their lives.

Our core workout format (maximum of 50 minutes per workout) is designed so every client can get in and out of the gym in less than one hour total. This format is what we use in all physical training sessions, including team, small group, and one-on-one training:

- The one-minute meet and greet. Every client needs an opportunity to meet the other members and to build relationships. We do foam rolling and other corrective work prior to workouts in one-on-one and small group settings.
- Twelve minutes of graduated, dynamic warm-ups. We warm up for the exercises we will be doing that day.
- Core exercises. The core has to be strong and built to last. Core building is part of every routine and every session (one to two minutes).
- Strength (20 minutes based on two minutes on and one minute off or one minute on and one minute off)
- Dan John heavy carry—carry heavy, carry long, and carry big (one to two minutes)
- The big burn to put the finishing touches on a good workout (three to five minutes)

The group hug and thank-yous to our clients. Our clients have other choices in this market. It is mandatory that every client is thanked for being part of this business every time she is in the gym. There is no exception to this rule.

The Stages of a New Client

- During the client's first 30 days in our gym, we establish movement patterns using a higher 15 to 20 rep count. We engrain the patterns and basic movements of the key exercises our clients will be doing in all their workouts in the future. Correct movement first prevents injuries later. We keep the clients safe and teach them how to move correctly prior to putting any loads on them later.
- Over the next 30 days (or for most of our clients over time), we seek advanced conditioning based on 8 to 15 reps. They can now move, so we load and train for overall conditioning.
- The third stage used in building a long-term client fitness foundation is based on seeking strength. This is usually done for one week per month for our long-term clients who have established decent bases. This is based on lifts of three to five reps. Everyone in the gym is trained as an athlete. We believe most of the barriers our clients face are in our heads, not theirs. Once the client has the proper base of conditioning, we can do a week a month where we push the client a little and build strength. Remember, strong women are beautiful women.

Figure 7-1. Sample culture handout for a women-only training gym with a combination of 22 full- and part-time trainers (cont.)

Dress as if you respect the client. They are paying you to be there. Be clean and professionally dressed and remember that you are not there as a role model. You are a professional coach who is there to provide leadership, offer guidance, keep the client safe, and make sure each workout is the best you can deliver.

Conclusion

When you start your shift from a membership gym toward a training-centric business model, start with building a culture of success for every member, delivered through every trainer and group exercise person, and see if this works for you. If you haven't ever written out your personal or gym philosophy, then how do your coaches know how to act and perform? Culture is not a verbal five-minute lecture at a meeting but is a systematic approach to creating an environment that separates you from every other gym in town.

January 15, 2014
Just because you don't agree with me on an issue …

Hey, just because you don't agree with me on an issue or a way to do things doesn't automatically make me a bad person. One of the strongest indications of personal maturity is when you can separate the person's position on an issue from the person. It is far too easy for someone to dislike another because that person doesn't happen to agree with his own ideas. You have to remember that just because he has a different idea or belief doesn't mean you have permission to dislike the person. The mature thing is to discuss and debate the position, but then afterward, spend time getting to know the person behind the position. This comes up a lot in the professional fitness world, where beliefs are entrenched and debates rage over how to train or get results and there are people in the industry who haven't spoken for years to someone who disagreed with them in a workshop or on a post. Do a personal inventory and ask yourself if you are capable of looking past the person's position into who the person really is and if this mistake is getting in the way of your personal and professional relationships. It is okay to disagree on positions. It is not okay to be angry at someone who merely disagrees with you.

December 10, 2013
The lying clients

I love when clients look you straight in the eye and lie their ass off as to why they aren't getting it done. The following are my three favorite "you lying bastard" stories:

- *"There is so much conflicting information in the news that I simply don't know what to eat."* Nowhere on any known nutrition plan is that big-ass donut you just ate controversial. Nor is that entire pizza and those two pitchers of beer. We know—and he knows—he just lied to himself and us.

- *"I did everything exactly as you told me and it still isn't working."* Your trainer did not tell you to watch nine hours of TV a day. Your trainer did not tell you that fat free means eat the whole damn bag. Your trainer did not tell you that when you work out, you shouldn't sweat. And, yes, you lied when you said you only eat salads.

- *"I don't have the time."* It actually takes more time to get fat than it does to stay thin. If you eat better, you eat less often. If you work out, you have more energy and get more done. If you turn off the TV and get off your ass and move for several hours, your kids, spouse, and pets will also get in better shape. You managed to find the time to get fat and you have even more time to get into shape … if you stop lying to yourself and make that goal important in your life. Some days, you just want to beat them with an old jump rope.

Section 2

MONEY
AND
CLIENT
RETENTION

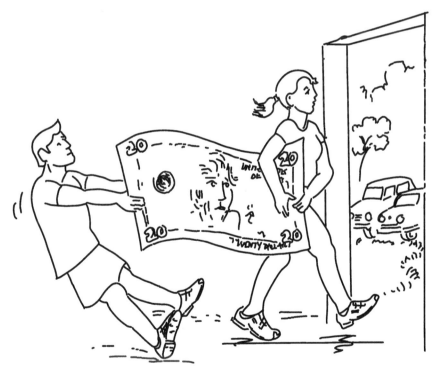

8

Competing in the Era of Low-Priced Competitors

There has been a strong surge of low-priced competitors entering the market during recent years and you will see more players attempting this business model in the coming years in every market in the country. Competing in the $19 to $39 market requires an entirely new business model few owners understand or are able to get to work effectively without getting new information. Most importantly, is this lower-priced model something you should be considering for your business?

The surge has been mostly in the very low-end range of the price market, especially in the $9 to $19 territory. Much of this growth has been totally reactionary to a few chain clubs that showed success with the $9 to $10 model in the early 2000s. These models stripped down the clubs, removing group exercise, child care, salespeople, and trainers, along with eliminating most free weight equipment, such as limiting the size of the dumbbells to 50 pounds or so. The primary tool in this model is the ad price, although some of the more sophisticated players, such as Planet Fitness, buried price in a marketing campaign aimed at contrasting their clubs against the old-style clubs in the market from the 1990s that were more fashion show and bodybuilder oriented.

The major problem is that when all you have to sell is price and someone takes that away from you by going even lower, you have nothing left to compete with in the market. Price is the hardest thing to defend over time and is what makes the low-priced model—defined here as going low and then going strictly for sheer volume with no or very limited other sources of income—so hard to sustain over time.

For example, if you set your price at $10 and the guy down the street hears you sold 300 memberships that week, then all he has to do in his mind is post his prices at $9 and now he has basically dismantled your primary means of attracting new members. It is like being in a fight with five guys and the first pulls out a ball bat, the next a knife, the next a pistol, the next a shotgun, and then the last guy runs over to get his tank. The only limit in the low-priced fight is $0, which is as low as you can go without paying someone to join your business.

Some owners have tried to creatively get around the low monthly fee by charging a little more up front. For example, there was a club owner on the eastern seaboard that ran a price special of $79 down and just $3 a month on EFT. His theory was that all he needed was about $100 per member per year to keep the doors open and this system allowed him to show $3 in his ads.

His system was a direct response to a competitor who was at first running $20 and $19 a month but then dropped his price to $10 down and $9 per month. It is interesting to note that both these clubs failed, which highlights another problem with basing your plan on just price alone: The cannibals eat the cannibals.

Every market has natural limiters built in. For example, it might be parking, drive time from the club, a river that needs to be crossed, or a bad section of town or simply that there are only so many people who live near enough to your business to support it. When other players dilute your market by copying your business plan, something has to give—or in this case, someone has to fail—because there are only so many potential members in the market to support the clubs.

For example, imagine a town of 30,000 people. Once a year, the Girl Scouts in that town sell cookies. What if there was only one Girl Scout? She would own the market and be able to sell cookies to everyone in town who wanted cookies. Her personal limit would be her ability to reach all 30,000 people. Now what happens when you have five Girl Scouts? The return per Girl Scout would drop since all five are trying to sell to the same limited marketplace. Now imagine you have a troop of 30 Girl Scouts selling in that town. The return per girl is now dropping significantly since there are so many young women trying to sell the same product in a limited market. In other words, each additional Girl Scout added to the mix reduces the return per girl in the market.

Many mainstream owners, especially those who have been using a higher-priced model for years, are now considering exploring low-priced options for their own businesses. What we have done as an industry in the past—based on the 1995 big box model that relied on the ability to sell an almost unlimited amount of volume—does not work anymore.

It is not the economy that is making the club business tough. It is not the competitors who are hurting most businesses. It is the business model itself used by most owners and that has been copied for years from generation to generation based on what worked 20 years ago that simply does not hold up in competitive markets, but most owners either refuse to modernize their business practices or don't know what to do and merely keep trying to use tools and techniques that failed a generation ago.

This business model fails because almost every single mainstream box-style club in the industry uses the same tools: high volume, limited income from key areas (such as training), dated marketing based on price specials, and virtually zero attention to retention, which in competitive markets should be the thing you master and fight for the hardest. You may not get as many new members as you did in the past, but you can still learn to fight for the ones you have and to make a lot more money from the members we still get.

The next generation business plan in the industry—a direct result of the advent of the low-priced surge—is toward showing the lowest entry point you need to attract the widest range of clients and then adding a layered pricing model that allows you to reap the highest return per member possible in your club.

The new generation training clubs in this country have proven that layered pricing works and many of the more successful dedicated training facilities are doing gross revenues only dreamed of by many mainstream clubs. It is common now for 6,000-square-foot training clubs to gross more than a million a year—something that is still considered a hard goal to reach for many of the box-style operators.

This training-centric business model will work for all fitness facilities and can be installed into any club no matter what size you own. Training does work and it does generate revenue, but the training business model most clubs and most training facilities use is based on a failed model that never created the income we need from the members we get.

Setting the price too low is not the problem by itself. The issue is that we set our prices too low and then rely on volume alone to drive the revenue for the gym. It seems like the biggest and most oft-repeated mistake in the industry would be something that is talked about more by potential owners. Failure is not about opening with the wrong partners. It's not about being totally undercapitalized. It's not about dumping your spouse and running away with one of your good-looking personal-training clients. The biggest mistake we make is simply pricing the gym too low for the market and then building the business plan on the concept that there will always be an endless supply of new memberships to replace the ones we attract but burn up through our inefficient systems.

Microtrends

Going for the low price is nothing new in the industry and pricing is really nothing more than a good example of a microtrend. Microtrends are short-term cycles—usually about 10 to 12 years in length—that reappear in the industry over time.

Microtrends have four distinct stages:
- The long, slow buildup phase
- The "hot" stage where you can't live without the product
- The quick fade
- Oblivion

Aerobics in the late 1980s might be the perfect example of a microtrend. There was a long, slow building period in the industry after aerobics (before being renamed group exercise) during the 1980s between the Jazzercise era and the full introduction into the industry as a staple of programming. At the peak of aerobics, there were national competitions, packed workshops around the country, cult instructors on TV (such as Joanie Greggains), and the introduction of step aerobics, which represented the peak of group exercise in the industry.

Then, in the late 1980s and early 1990s, it quickly faded. The instructors were desperate for their own identities, resulting in newer and more extreme products and programming, the members had a bad case of "been there, done that," and owners were beginning to tire of paying instructors ever-increasing pay versus the sudden lack of new clients entering the clubs.

Around 1993, aerobics was relegated to a few diehards, the rooms were mostly empty, and the members had moved on to the newer equipment in the club, such as the first plate-loaded products. For all practical business purposes, the sport was dead and remained that way until approximately 1999, when a dynamic instructor in California named Billy Blanks marketed Tae Bo® and new generation group exercise was born, replacing the dead concept of aerobics. Every sign of a microtrend was present here, including the long, slow build, the burst of energy and excitement at the top, the quick fade, and the period of oblivion lasting until someone dusted off the basic concept of group exercise again and reinvented it.

Pricing is also a microtrend. Low-price memberships featured as the key feature of a club's business plan is not new and cycles through the industry just like aerobics did. For example, in the late 1960s, Lucille Roberts started a chain of clubs in the New York region that featured a price under $10 per month and innovative marketing, growing the business into a national player at the time of her death. Looking back, you can find at least one attempt every decade of a new player going low and making an attempt to capture the market by offering the lowest price.

Price wars and going low hit the market hard, have a long, slow building period as other players copy the first players in the game, hit a hot spot where price dominates the national discussion, and then fade quickly. The attraction for owners to go low is almost irresistible. Drop the price, write a big number of memberships, destroy the market, and make millions is the lure that can't be denied in this model.

The problem with the low-price models is not the price itself but the return per member that is generated in the business. If you just base your membership on price, you need virtually unlimited volume to make the plan work over time. In this model, the price—and therefore the resulting membership numbers—is the only source of revenue in the business. For example, if you charge $10 for a membership but have no other income-producing segments of the club, then your return per member is $10 or less depending on discounts, such as buddy deals or families.

The low-priced model is not a sustainable business plan over time because you will get copied and the imitators just don't match your price but usually go lower. For example, if you base your entire business plan on doing heavy volume at $10 per member, why would you think as an owner that the guy down the street won't go to $9 or that his competitor won't go even lower. If price is all you have in your arsenal of business tools, then you in essence have nothing that can't be taken away from you over time.

The reason the low-price model gets attention is that it does have factors that make it successful. For example, if you are the only club in the market chasing a low price, it will work, but if you get another low-price player in the game, both these units end up chasing the same target market, therefore diluting their ability to do the volume they need to survive.

The following sections detail some of the reasons the low-priced model does work, along with a few of the myths associated with going low as the primary component of your business plan.

The Low-Priced Model Does Appeal to a Broader Base of Potential Members

The lower the price, the more the potential buyers is a self-evident truth. If someone can't afford something today and it becomes cheaper tomorrow, then you theoretically should attract more buyers at the lower price.

But this concept does have a bottom level that is mostly ignored by many practitioners of the low-priced business model. In other words, you can go too low and end up working against yourself by alienating the members you did attract. The old rule that likes attract likes does apply here, and in many markets, if you go too low, you attract an element that disrupts this rule.

For example, if you develop a low-priced model based on a homogeneous population in a small isolated town where most everyone is employed, there are no bad parts of town, and the bottom of the affluence level is fairly close to the top of the pyramid, then no matter who signs up for $10, in that market will most likely be a friend, neighbor, or someone similar in look and interest. Likes attract likes, and even if you make $75,000 a year and are standing on a treadmill next to a younger person who makes $20,000, in this environment, you most likely know common people, ski the same areas, go to the same church, or perhaps eat at the same restaurant, although the $20,000 person might be the waiter and the other guy is the customer.

However, the model breaks down when you go too low in some markets. The reality in life is that there are bad parts of towns and there are people who bring negativity to a club and can destroy the business, and if the club's price is too low, you can attract a clientele that drives out the other members who you would most likely like to keep.

So, what is too low? In many markets, anything less than $19 might be too low and a club owner using $10 in this market might destroy the club by chasing members who will eventually run out the other members. In most markets, the low price that works to attract a wider range of potential members yet won't destroy the club is either $19 or $39 depending on the club and the other competition in the area.

Low-Priced Memberships
Keep People Paying Longer

There is a theory that if the price is low enough, the person just keeps paying the small fee, thinking that even though he isn't using the club, he will go back at a later date. In other words, he will cancel a bigger payment if he doesn't use the club for a month or so but won't cancel the $9 payment because it is so small and he thinks that life will straighten out and that he will get back to the gym next month.

This theory has been kicked around for years, but it seems to fall in the urban myth category, along with the alligators in the sewers and Bigfoot. Money is relative to the owner. If you make $100,000 a year, then the $39 payment a month most likely shouldn't affect you and why would this guy cancel because in his world, the $39 is probably the equivalent of $10 to the guy making $30,000 a year? If it applies to one population, then it should apply to both because the relative amount of money is the same.

There just isn't any firm evidence anywhere that this is true. In fact, one of the largest chains in the industry used a $5 per month renewal option for its membership for a number of years believing the same thing. The theory was that the client would pay a regular membership for a year or two more consistently because he knew there was a big reward at the end, which was a replacement of his regular monthly dues by a $60-a-year renewal fee. The belief was also that many clients would automatically pay the $60 just to protect it even though they might not be currently involved at the club. The $60 was supposed to just be too good to let go.

Again, there is no hard evidence that this worked, but anecdotally, the chain suffered a number of bankruptcies, so while the system was copied by many other chains, there is no proof that the idea of a low price or a low renewal fee keeps people paying substantially longer if they are not using the club. The other side of this, of course, is that money is money and very few people will continue to pay for a long period of time for something they aren't using no matter if the fee is $10 or $50.

The Third Year Is the Pivotal Year
in a Low-Price Business Model

The basic concept of a low-priced business model is very simple. Hold a long pre-sale and sign up 3,000 members or more, sign up 250 to 400 a month for your first two years (steadily growing your receivable base), and then in year three, you arrive at a replacement mode stage where you sign up 250 new members but you now lose 250, which is acceptable because you had two years and a strong pre-sale to grow that receivable base into a substantial number.

This idea is also theoretically sound until it meets the realities of the market. If you return to the model mentioned earlier where you develop your business plan in an almost vacuum environment with no competitors in the same class, this should work, but the reality is that there are simply too many other factors in a market for this idea to work over time.

The following sections detail a number of factors that would prevent you from either accomplishing your first goals or from moving into a replacement mode going into your third year if you own and operate a low-price model. Keep in mind that about 85 percent of your market comes from a 12-minute drive time from your facility during primetime for most mainstream box facilities and about 20 minutes if you are a specialty training club, sports performance center, or another niche player, such as a women-only club.

This drive time penetration determines your market segment or market share due to the limiters that exist in this ring around your business. For most clubs, this drive time represents a ring of about three to five miles, which might be extended to five to seven in more rural markets or just a matter of blocks in a major metro area.

The total density in your ring

There are only so many people who live within that drive time, represented by the three- to five-mile ring. Many rookies first look at their town, explore the total population, and then adjust their plan to include potential members who simply live too far away from the club. Your market is whoever lives within 12 to 20 minutes from your club on a Monday night at 6 p.m. (primetime for most clubs) and there are very few people who will drive further than that or past too many other competitors to get to you.

The other competitors in your ring

Mainstream box clubs and low-price players have a disadvantage in that their business plan is generalist in nature. This means that most of them attempt to service everyone in the market and the closest one to the potential member's house will usually win.

Next generation clubs, such as sports performance centers or upscale hybrid training centers that offer all levels of group and personal training as well as limited membership options, are more specialist in nature and the consumer will drive past a generalist to get to a specialist who he believes can answer his need. For example, if you are older than 50 and looking for a training center, would you go to a facility that advertises as a generalist who can service everyone or would you go to a specialist that advertises "We specialize in fitness after 50"?

The low-price clubs can exist in this market as long as there is only one of them fighting for that particular market segment. In other words, training clubs will survive, women-only clubs will survive, upscale full service clubs will thrive, and a low-price player can also coexist because everyone on the market is chasing his own market segment. Where this fails is when competition shifts away from the specialists to too many generalists all seeking the same segment. In this case, if the first low-price $10 guy is followed by several more all in the same price range, then there will not be enough people in that market segment to feed all the players who need heavy volume to succeed.

Awareness

There are only so many people in any given market who want to join a fitness facility. This varies from region to region of the country, with a heavier user base in markets such as California and a much lighter base in the southern states. According to recent IHRSA numbers, there are still only about 16 percent of the total people living in this country that belong to a fitness facility, meaning there are 84 percent who have no interest or haven't yet joined. One reason many markets become overly saturated is that there simply aren't enough people in the market to support the number of clubs that open. Once you reach this point, someone has to fail unless there is a sudden influx of interested potential members who arrive in the market.

As a side note, a sophisticated owner will spend most of his marketing investment developing interest in the market rather than just constantly trying to exploit the small percentage of people already interested in joining a club.

Influx/outflow

This is the one point that does work heavily in the favor of a low-priced club owner. In markets such as Orlando, where there is a constant flow of new people arriving in town seeking work that balanced the constant outflow of folks moving on to other opportunities, there is almost unlimited potential for the low-price players as long as you can tie up the market by being the only chain. If you lose control of the market, meaning that other copycat competitors get a base foothold in the market, you at that point have the same issue of just being in an overly saturated market, which is simply too many clubs fighting for the same market segment.

Perhaps the biggest issue that always seems to end the cycle for low-price players is that at some point, the cannibals always end up eating the other cannibals. "Imitation is the most sincere form of flattery" goes the old saying, but in the business world, if your only product to sell is price, then you can't protect your business. Image is everything in the fitness business, and if the illusion exists that you are making a lot of money doing almost anything—from pricing to equipment to some type of new programming—you will be copied quickly and widely.

When this happens, the low-price clubs that need so much volume to survive begin to fail because there is not enough potential members in that market area to support a number of players all using the same price model as their primary marketing angle and product. When the cannibals start devouring the market share of the other cannibals, someone will fail and the survivors— or those who ran businesses based on something other than price—start to slowly raise the prices again and normalize the market. Oblivion sets in for a few years, low pricing goes away and stays dormant until the next player a few years later comes out with a new angle, and then the microtrend begins again.

Another problem with the price being too low is that it affects virtually every other part of the business. If the price is too low, the club is forced to sustain an unrealistic number of sales. If the price is too low, the collectability of the memberships may decrease. And most importantly, if the price is too low, the multiple profit centers in the club may not work because the club is filled with price-driven members—the cheapest human beings on the planet. Keep in mind that it's hard to sell multiple profit centers to guys who bring empty milk jugs full of cheap sports drinks they purchased at Walmart. And senior citizens who are in on the lowest membership possible aren't likely to kick in for that expensive nutrition program or support a higher-priced training membership.

Pricing has grown to be the biggest mistake because it's so misunderstood. It's often left to last when it comes to developing a business plan because it seems so simple: Look at what the competitor charges, set our prices a few dollars lower, and then claim that our club is better than anyone else's. Therefore, the member is getting a better buy from us. Again, does the member really logically believe that your business can be the best and the cheapest at the same time? Or does it seem logical to the consumer that he will really have a good experience and get enough help and service in a business that prices itself at $9 to $19 per month?

Setting a price has almost taken on magical proportions to some owners in the industry: "Find that one magic price and every potential member will buy." The myths associated with pricing have evolved to become some of the biggest sacred cows in the business. "Sacred cows" are beliefs that are repeated so often that they become the unquestionable truth.

For example, one very entrenched cow in the industry might be "You have to have a child care room in the club. Most members won't use it, but they want to see it when they join." Another cow might be "Without group exercise (aerobics), you'll never get any women into the club." And don't forget an all-time favorite: "Cash is king. You have to go for all the cash you can get when you open your club."

All these premises were thought to be the absolute law at one time or another in the industry. And all were eventually proven to be untrue. Clubs don't have to have child care to be profitable and cardio and other styles of group workouts, such as group personal training and cycle, have already started to diminish traditional group exercise and paid-in-full memberships lower the return per member so substantially that most owners, especially those who run multiple units, are much better off without the cash.

But the pre-eminent sacred cow of all time in the fitness industry is setting the price low so the club will attract more members. The rule was that the lower the price was set, the more members, or higher volume, the club would attract. For example, why set your monthly price at $40 and limit your membership? Why not set it at $20 and attract a lot more members?

Hey, why not set it at $2 per month per member and hope every living human being—and maybe a few dogs too—who live in a 15-mile radius around the club joins. These are also the same theoreticians who suggest building endlessly bigger clubs without regard to the market or club's focus. "Hey, John opened a 20,000-square-foot club and has 2,000 members already. I'll open a 30,000-square-foot facility and kick his butt because I'll have 3,000 members."

The assumption is that the bigger your facility, the more members you will attract. This follows the previous assumption that the lower the price you set, the more members you will attract. If this flawed logic were true, all you would have to do to be successful in the club business would be to build a 200,000-square-foot facility and offer $10-a-month memberships.

And yes, this does work exactly that way. The lower the price, the more members you get, but two things happen that counter this. First of all, the core model itself is so far outdated that it is not sustainable.

The first wave of low-price clubs that emerged in the last microcycle evolved as very stripped-down versions of mainstream box facilities. Child care, group exercise, and even salespeople were eliminated from the business plan, supposedly leading to reduced expenses. However, many of these owners found that a lot of this eliminated expense came back as additional maintenance on the club due to the high volume and increased equipment costs to stay competitive and quite a few found they still needed more staff than first thought to just keep the place under control.

Secondly and more importantly, fitness has evolved past the low-priced guys. Many of these players built their units with the fewest moving parts, such as eliminating dumbbells over 50 pounds, most of the traditional free weight stuff, and any esoteric equipment, such as medicine balls or suspension trainers, relying instead on just a lot of cardio and circuit equipment. The market and consumer have evolved around the low-priced guys. However, the consumer has tired of circuit training and other limited fitness options that were the centerpieces of these clubs.

Another factor was the explosion of functional training, driven from the bottom up by trainers and sports performance guys, at the end of the first decade of this century. Kettlebells, suspension tools, giant ropes, balance equipment, and boot camps flooded TV, were the themes of bestselling fitness books, and all the magazines carried articles about actors and sports celebrities training with functional tools. All of a sudden, the low-priced guys started becoming the guys from the early 1990s who owned shops selling pagers and wondered why all the customers were leaving for those new portable phones.

Some low-priced operators have created a more hybrid model that uses a lower price, such as $19 per month, but then still offers group exercise and training. This model only works in very unique markets and you have the combination of high density relating to the number of potential members available in the market, along with a more sophisticated consumer who seeks training, and other auxiliary revenue sources in greater numbers. However, most of these have failed because low price in these models often means low quality and reduced options.

Return per Member Is Everything

Volume has been the key in all fitness businesses since the start of the modern fitness era in 1945. Open the door, sell as many memberships as you can, and then replace those that fail and leave.

As we discussed in the last chapter, volume is being replaced as an operational philosophy by return per member and this has been a difficult adjustment for owners schooled in the traditional volume approach. For example, a traditional 20,000-square-foot Gold's Gym from the mid 1990s with 2,000 members might do $1.2 million a year in gross deposits with a pre-tax net of maybe 15 percent. Today, training clubs that are only 6,000 square feet are doing $1.3 million a year with only 300 or so members and are doing a pre-tax of 20 percent or more. The interesting thing to note is that the Gold's Gym from that era might have charged $39 to $49 for a single membership per month, but today, that same club might charge only $9 per month as compared to the training clubs that get an average of $149 per month per member or higher.

The issue here is that mainstream fitness has evolved as a commodity viewed as generic and where it is all pretty much the same, while the training clubs have evolved as true service businesses where the consumer buys expertise. The real-life comparison is that mainstream fitness has become Walmart and the training clubs have a financial service company selling investment information and advanced financial services. One is a product with no difference between offerings, while the other is a specialization that has a higher perception of value.

Commodities, such as the cheapest toilet paper, are based on selling very large numbers of the product to as many people as possible (volume) and are hard to rebrand as top-line products. On the other hand, training clubs have done this well, concentrating more on the return per client rather than sheer volume. In the coming years, the smaller training facilities will have a huge advantage in the market because they can survive and thrive on so many fewer clients, which also leave at a lesser rate due to the high quality of results the typical training client achieves compared to a simple membership at a box club.

Again, we aren't selling a commodity. We're selling a service. And in most service-based businesses, the consumer thinks that the highest-priced service is the best. For example, if you're suffering from some terrible illness, do you want the cheapest doctor you can find treating you? If you are in serious legal trouble, do you want the cheapest lawyer you can find defending you?

Did O.J. Simpson have his nephew right out of law school defending him? Did Casey Anthony get a schmuck from behind the convenience store? Or did our notorious defendants have the best and most expensive lawyers they could find? With services, the cheapest is usually the worst.

Most of the time, the consumer equates price with quality. The higher the price the club charges, the higher the quality of service the member will receive. The cheaper the price, the lower the quality of service the person will receive. Price is part of the club's image.

Most owners believe they have the best club around, but if the price is the same as the competitor's price, then the club is exactly the same in the consumer's mind. Price is part of our image and many sales are lost or won before the potential member ever gets into the club.

Another major problem with low pricing for most owners is that this business model pre-determines the club's operational philosophy. Low prices usually force a club into a sales-driven style of operation. In other words, low pricing determines how you have to run your club.

Sales-driven means the club has to focus on sheer sales numbers. The lower the price, the more members the club is forced to sign up. Once the club becomes sales-driven, it can no longer be service-driven. The two types of operational approaches are mutually exclusive. You can't run a sales-driven club seeking high volume and also offer individualized customer service. These two business concepts just can't exist at the same time in the same gym.

When a club is sales-driven, all the club's resources have to be spent in the generation of new sales. For example, it's usually pretty easy to spot a sales-driven club. Once you're in the club, you notice the five or six sales offices by the front door. All the senior or high-level staff are salespeople who hover around the front, waiting for the next "up," or are in their offices working closeouts (you didn't sign up while you were in the club, but we going to give you one more chance at the end of the month) or making cold calls to people's homes.

In this type of club, it's pretty unusual to find anyone out on the floor helping members or providing any type of service because all the club's payroll dollars are spent on the sales force and the commissions it takes to keep them volume-running. The counter people in this type of club are also an indication of the type of operational philosophy the owners are following. Instead of a mature, service-oriented front counter force, you'll find a very young, undertrained, and underpaid counter person who probably hasn't been on the job very long.

The club simply can't provide service because the owners don't have the additional revenue and probably don't believe in it anyhow. Each day, the club is judged successful or not by the number of sales generated that day. Note here that there is little other revenue in these clubs from multiple profit centers because this style of club can't control these various parts of the operations. Why? Because all the real people are in sales and the rest are warm bodies passing through on their way to other jobs.

The owners and management have a hard time controlling these profit centers because they don't have the more experienced and mature person to supervise them. Again, the club doesn't have these people because all the best people are in sales, and because of their quotas, these people can't do anything but sell. Once you lower the price, you set all these other factors into motion that force you into this type of operational method.

These same club owners have also had little incentive to offer service in past years due to their ability to replace members lost in the process. The majority of this type of club signs up a new member and gives him three workouts with a trainer that is only interested in getting one-on-one clients, and if the client isn't qualified to spend more money, he ends up with a circuit workout and is left to fend for himself. He might pay to term or might be self-motivated enough to keep learning on his own, but he is usually gone in about five to seven months. These owners don't really care because there had always been enough new blood to replace these lost members.

However, things change dramatically when the low-priced craze hits the quick fade period. Once the market becomes saturated with a number of clubs all using low price as their main marketing tool, replacing that lost member becomes much more difficult, which is the point of no return for many of these operators, especially going into that crucial third year where you need to replace as many as you lose to stay in business over time.

There Are Really Only Three Things You Can Affect in Small Business

Small business is actually relatively simple. Once you establish your concept, there are only three things you can do to affect the outcome:

- Change the price up to increase return or down to increase volume.
- Decrease the expenses.
- Generate a higher return or additional sales from the people you already have as clients.

Small businesses that are successful over time reach a balance of the three. It is interesting to note that many "shooting star" businesses, which burst on the scene and become wildly successful in a short period of time, usually exploit number one but later fade over time as others copy their plan. This is the point when that temporarily superstar fades because he never had a grasp of the other two points, leaving him vulnerable in the market. Illustrations of this have been hot tech companies or even restaurants that are hot one minute and then gone a minute after that.

Constantly seeking high volume generally means that the club runs price-driven ads, meaning some type of sale of the week, as its primary marketing tool. Price ads eventually ruin your market because they only appeal to the 16 percent of the population that is already aware of fitness and who are probably working out somewhere now. In other words, the longer you run price-driven ads, the smaller the market gets because you've burned up everyone in your ring that is motivated by a cheap price and who is interested in fitness.

Ads based on low price, such as "Join now for $10 down and $10 per month," assume that the potential member already has some type of experience with a fitness facility, knows what he is looking for in a club, and believes that price is the deciding factor. These ads do nothing to attract someone who has no experience with a fitness club because he doesn't understand if the price is a good value or not without having some type of base of experience.

Low prices featured in ads also do nothing to attract those people who want to buy quality and are willing to pay for it. There are certain folks who want cheap and will take everything that goes along with a cheaply priced membership, such as lines, no help, and a worn or outdated physical plant. There are also folks who appreciate quality and who will pay more for more personal attention, the privilege of not having to stand in line, and for more services and amenities than the typical club can provide. Traditionally, most ads in the fitness market target the lower-price-driven potential member and even the ads that supposedly target the more sophisticated clients are still usually based on some type of price special.

Interestingly, the fitness clubs that are breaking this mold are the training clubs that are using more sophisticated marketing techniques aimed at a higher demographic simply due to the fact that this is their target audience. Paid trial memberships, such as 30 days for $69, work quite well for the more educated buyer whose main goal is to experience the product and service before committing—something seldom available in mainstream fitness.

The alternative to the sales-driven operational plan, especially in competitive markets, is the return per member philosophy. The return per member system strives for a higher return per member or learning to make more money from fewer members.

In this operational method, which will be the next level of owner growth in the industry, the emphasis shifts away from sales-driven toward a more service-driven environment that works off a low-pressure sales system, multiple profit centers, and an increased emphasis on renewals.

The owner learns to work off a lower number of new sales, make more money from the ones already in the system, and keep those members longer, driving down the continued need for high volume and driving down the cost of doing business. For example, if there were only 100 potential members in a market, the club would be better off with 60 of them paying $40 per month than having all 100 paying $25 per month. The club would make $100 less each month in this example, but the cost of the sales would be cheaper in lower commissions, ad costs would probably be lower, wear and tear on the club would be less with fewer members, and staffing costs would be lower with fewer members to take care of over the same period of time.

The club in this example with the higher price would also most likely make more money in the long run from its profit centers, such as personal training. Its members are already used to paying a higher price and were probably not attracted just by price. They would be much more likely to spend money on a club's profit centers because they didn't join because of a cheap price. They are used to spending money and will continue doing so.

These members will also be stronger candidates for renewal. Because the club has fewer members and is charging a higher rate for the members it does have, it should be able to provide more personal attention and member service—something the other club can't because of its lower return per member.

Another key point to consider in the volume versus return per member debate is the degree of vulnerability a business has. No business is ever 100 percent risk free. As an owner, you have to come up with a business plan that decreases your vulnerability yet gives you the best chance to make money.

The problem with a low-price/sales-driven business plan is that it's almost impossible to defend. A business based on selling the lowest price to the greatest number of members has nowhere to retreat in time of war, meaning competitors are trying to put you out of business.

Because a low-price/sales-driven club is based on volume, any decrease in the new member stream can drastically affect the club's bottom line in a very short period of time, especially if the club has no other source of income except new sales.

If a competitor came in and offered a higher price membership, such as a 7,500-square-foot, upscale training club, it wouldn't take away a huge number of members from the low-price operator. It doesn't have to take many to do damage. It only has to take away the best members, meaning those who will pay more for a club that doesn't have the implied problems the low-price operator does. A good competitor only has to take a small percentage of members (which is probably the low-priced guy's best members because they are willing to leave for a higher-priced but better quality gym) to hurt a volume-driven business plan.

For most low-priced operators, a 10 percent reduction in monthly business would severely hurt them because their profit margins are usually pretty tight. There are, of course, exceptions to every rule, but defending a high-volume, low-priced facility against aggressive competitors is not something most owners would wish to attempt.

Another point of vulnerability is that the club totally depends on just one source of income. In competitive markets, it's wise to spread the risk among several different areas. If a high-volume club totally depends on sales and has no other source of income, such as multiple profit centers, the club is at risk. For example, if just one or two people generate the majority of those sales and those people leave, the club's business will immediately suffer. In a return per member business plan, revenue should be spread over several different areas. In this case, if the club loses a key salesperson, it still has time to react and probably won't suffer too much because there is still revenue from the multiple profit centers.

Summary

The emphasis in the coming years will be away from sales-driven operational methods and toward trying to drive up the return per member. Sales-driven/low-price operations have been part of the industry since it began and continue to cycle through every 12 years or so in the form of microcycles, but with the increased cost of doing business, increased competition all chasing the same market segment, a more sophisticated member base, and more business-aware owners, this system is no longer the way to operate.

Owners also have more to risk now than ever before because the cost of starting up fitness facilities has dramatically increased over the years. With this increased risk comes the need to decrease the business's vulnerability. Running a business plan that's not defensible is not a method of decreasing risk.

Decreasing risk and vulnerability only comes from seeking a higher return per member or, in other words, learning to make more money from the members we already have. Because of their low-price/sales-driven system, most clubs in the industry simply spend all their time and money replacing the members they once had. To be successful in the future, we need to keep the members longer and make more money from those members already in the club.

The mistake that underlies the sales-driven operational style is setting the club's membership price too low. Once the club establishes a low price, the owner is forced to run the club in a specific method, meaning everything has to be geared toward developing volume.

We have to keep in mind that price is part of the club's image. To be the best, the club has to price itself accordingly. The consumer associates price with quality. If the price is too good to be true, then it probably is. Finally, keep in mind that we are selling a service, not a commodity. The better the service, the more the member would have to pay for it in the real world and the more the member should be paying for it in the fitness world.

Some key reminders to consider when you are trying to compete on price include the following:

- Setting the price too low is the biggest mistake we make in the club industry. Using price as the key component of your business plan is not sustainable over time because anyone can copy your price.
- When in competition with like businesses or with businesses in the same category, consider setting your price a few dollars higher. For example, if most of the market is $10 and no service, can you offer $19 and do a version of a full-service club with a layered pricing system on top?
- Price determines how you run your business. If all your time and energy are spent on just sales and replacing members you have had and then lost, slowly switch to a return per member system.
- To switch to a return per member system, do it over a year's time. Raise the monthly price slowly, and if you're discounting for cash, also slowly raise that price over the next year. If your business depends on cash, you don't want to hurt yourself by cutting the cash off too quickly. It's better to slowly wean yourself away from your current system.
- Add a little older and more mature counter people and then introduce one profit center at a time. As the profit centers start to work, your need for a high number of new sales should start to decrease. Your biggest profit center in mainstream fitness facilities should and always will be training revenue.

- Keep in mind that it's okay to lose a few people each month because your price is too high. Almost all your staff and most owners too panic if someone walks out because of price. A good rule of thumb is that if 20 percent of your potential members left because of a price objection, you are probably priced right for the market.
- The most objections on pricing you get will come from your young staff. To them, $39 or more a month is high and they judge all potential members according to their personal situation. Train hard and heavy on the true worth of your business and why you price accordingly.
- Change your marketing away from price-driven ads and replace them with exposure types of ads. Exposure means try before you buy. This type of ad attracts people price ads never will and brings in people more interested in service instead of price.

January 14, 2014
Many people aren't readers anymore.

In the age of information delivered in a few lines of badly written text, many people have drifted away from the power of reading, which means the power of learning. Many of you admire the gurus in the industry, and if you sit and talk with Gray Cook, Greg Rose, Alwyn Cosgrove, Mike Boyle, or Todd Durkin, you find that they are all intense readers who cover a variety of subjects way beyond just fitness. I asked Dan John for his top 10 book list and there wasn't a fitness book on it. If you want to grow and become that legendary person in whatever you do, most of what you need is in books. Read at least two books a week. Read every day. Read things outside of what you do for a living. Read about people who are successful in their own lives and find out why. You all work on your bodies, but not enough of you work on your minds.

December 11, 2013
Moderation sucks.

Anything good in life happens out on the edges, where the extreme happens, not in that safe middle. The day your child was born was not a moderate day. Your best day of vacation adventure ever was not a moderate day. If you are going to do something, go all in. If you want to be a trainer, then commit to being the best ever. Pick your friends carefully, but then commit and be the best friend ever. If you say you're going to change lives, then refuse to fail. Moderation is for old people who eat dry toast and wear diapers. For the rest of you, go extreme or get back on the porch and get the hell out of the way.

9

There Is No Business Plan in the World That Can Overcome Poor Renewals

Renewals—or keeping the business you've already purchased—is one of the most important issues, along with staffing and the ability to generate sufficient new leads, that owners will face in the coming years. As markets mature—defined as more and more competition in your competitive ring—and as more members continue to seek a fitness lifestyle that leads to a more frequent attendance year after year, it becomes more important for your business plan to learn how to keep the members you've already obtained, thereby reducing operating costs in the form of lower advertising costs, lower sales expenses, and less wear and tear on the club.

For years, the large majority of the fitness business has been geared toward creating business plans strictly focusing on bringing in new members. The base assumption for most of the history of the fitness business has been that you sell, ignore, and then replace a member because he is replaceable in the market with another person within the same demographics. For example, it's not unusual to see a rookie owner present a 150-page business plan containing 50 pages of marketing, demographic information, and sales training with only a paragraph or two toward the back on what he is going to do to keep those members over time once they are signed up.

It's even more sad to have a future owner point to a specific month in the future in this same plan and show the break-even point based on having a certain number of members. The pain arises because this owner never shows any members dropping out or ever leaving the club. The plan says he enrolls 1,500 new members during his first two years and then keeps all 1,500, and at this point, the club will break even. It's hard to look at their faces when you show them that even a good club loses about 50 percent of its members on a year-to-year basis adjusted for losses.

For example, the following is how the losses might arrive for a decently run club:

New members who enroll in January	100
Percentage (1 percent per month) who will move more than 25 miles from the club and will have to be cancelled, as per most state laws governing fitness businesses	−12
	88
Percentage who will not pay based on using a 12-month membership tool, which has the highest collectability of all possible membership options	−12
Members left at the end of year one	76

These numbers are hard to change in a fitness business. There isn't much you can do about members who move outside of 25 miles, as dictated by the state. The other 12 percent losses are a reflection of the tool you use to let members pay. Month-to-month memberships have a loss rate of 48 to 60 percent annually (4 to 5 percent per month) and longer-term memberships, such as 24-month memberships that were once thought to be the solution to losses, have loss rates of 5 to 7 percent per month in most markets, with very few exceptions. The 12 percent loss rate in this example is actually good when compared to other options the club might be using to enroll new members.

It is what happens going into the second year that club owners and their teams can most influence. These are the members who have paid you for an entire year and now have the option of going again for another year.

For example:

76 members left at the end of the first year (adjusted for losses)
x .40 percent (realistic national average on retention) = 30

In other words, this club owner started with 100 new members, and going into the second year, he is down to just 30 left that decided to renew. This loss is where the club owner and his team can have the greatest impact in the business because while losses as dictated by moves or divorce are hard to affect, losses that stem from internal sources, such as cleanliness, are much easier to change over time.

In the past, club operators have resorted to fairly sleazy tactics to keep these people going, such as letting the member slip from a contractual obligation at the end of the first year into a month-to-month option with the hopes that he won't notice and will just keep making those payments or just let the club keep drafting his credit card or checking account.

It is hard to imagine a club owner who invests everything he has into opening a new facility and then basing his business plan on the hope that his clients are too dumb to look at their bank or credit card statements after the 12th month of a membership. In reality, this owner is ignoring the business potential of retention, concentrating instead all his resources on just driving new memberships as illustrated by his plan to ignore the member for his year in the club and then keep drafting his accounts until he squeals.

Besides business plans, almost all the industry's literature about how to do business, most of our staff training, and most of the owner's thinking is devoted to sales, marketing, and doing whatever it takes to keep up the constant flow of new members through the front door. Volume has been everything in the fitness business for decades and almost every tool an owner can wield is centered on just the acquisition of new members that are replacing the ones who are leaving at the end of their first year.

As owners, we've never really maximized the potential of our businesses because we've never really maximized the vast untapped income available through renewals. And this significant source of potential revenue will become more important in the future for two important reasons: increased competition and the increasing cost of capitalization.

In theory, we all know that renewals gain importance as competition increases. Everyone sits around the bars at the trade shows, talking about how little worried they are that this month's going-public, mega-chain, discount fitness business is coming to their town. Why don't these owners act worried? Because they know all the right things to say to each other to cover their fear. "Our members love us because we have the best member service anywhere. These new guys may be successful in California, but their stuff won't work here. No one is going to leave my club." When all else fails in business, denial works.

Intellectually, these owners can say the right things, but then most turn around and do the opposite, especially when pressure is applied. For example, as competition increases and their sales decline, these owners then spend more money on new sales, therefore forcing them to decrease the money they spend on keeping the members they already own. Why? Because they secretly know their members don't really love the club because they secretly know they haven't spent nearly enough money to renew their physical plants in years. And because they lived in denial, they never really thought competition would come to their town, so they never really had to learn to be good operators.

The owners in this example really have only one option and that's to start buying new sales because it's too late now to change the other factors that matter in retention in a short period of time. Renewals have to be part of your one-year, three-year, and five-year business plans because when a competitor opens next month, it's too late to make the foundational changes necessary to protect your membership.

It is also interesting to note that there is a major difference between being lucky and being a good owner. Owners that open clubs in markets with less competition can usually do almost anything to attract and maintain new business simply because the market there is underserved and there is little if any choice of places to go for the consumer.

In these markets, it is easy to feel like a genius as an owner because everything you do works to bring in new members. Run a stupid ad and people come through the door. Add some new equipment on the floor and the members think you are a rock god. Anything you do seems like the right thing because the member has nowhere else to go in the market.

However, reality intrudes in this fantasy when competition enters the market. When competitors arrive with a fresh physical plant, aggressive marketing, and an energetic staff, the existing first club in the market will often suffer for one simple reason: The owner of that club never learned how to run a good business. He was lucky in the fact that there wasn't anyone to take his members, but he was unlucky in that he never had a chance to learn how to run a good business. For example, this owner probably never learned how to run a tight budget, train staff, reinvest as part of a long-term business plan or, most importantly, he never learned what it takes to keep members in the system over time.

Competition makes you a better operator, especially if you survive and thrive on a crowded field. Many of these owners have left the industry during the last decade because most couldn't or wouldn't learn how to compete and many left angry because they felt that the new owners had no right to get into their market. It is good to remember that you have the right to try, invest money, and open a business, but you do not have the right to succeed. Financial success is only guaranteed by hard work, smart business moves, and a will to make what you do work over time.

Maturing markets also force you as an operator to find a cap in the market for the number of new sales you can add each month and year. One unique point about the business is that virtually every component can grow by 3 to 5 percent per year, except for new sales, which will top out in the market due to the density, affluence, and number of competitors in your immediate market.

For example, your training revenue can increase by at least 3 percent per year almost indefinitely due to the fact that you add more members from the existing rate, add more products and programming, raise the training rates every few years, or attempt other methods that increase your return per training client. Even your total deposit can increase yearly because you can raise prices, add new offerings, or learn to keep a higher percentage of the members you do get over time. In other words, just about everything in the business can increase yearly except the number of new sales you can generate each month, which is limited by the number of people in your market and by the number of competitors you have.

This also means that one of the secrets to the business in the coming years will be to move away from seeking endless new sales volume and move toward a business plan that seeks to make more money from fewer members or, in other words, you work to drive up the average return per member over time. Retention is one of the keys to this concept because it doesn't take a big increase to make a major difference. For example, look at the following to see how just one extra month of renewal income changes the business:

The club in this example has 1,500 members.

The club loses 40 percent of its members
per year to attrition.

The club charges $39 per month per member.

1,500 x .40 = 600

600 x $39 = $23,400

If this club could increase its retention by just keeping
these members one more month, it would add
$23,000 to its gross revenue that year.

The second reason renewals are gaining importance is the increased cost of capitalization. Increased capitalization (the money it takes to create a new fitness business), coupled with a steadily increasing cost of running a fitness business on a month-to-month basis, forces up the cost of buying new sales. Simply put, as gyms cost more to build, which adds to the ever-increasing cost of running a business on a monthly basis, capitalization forces the clubs to spend more to buy new sales.

The solution to this problem is where the biggest controversy in the industry is currently stemming from today. On one side, you have the new generation owners following much of the advice offered in this book and in others I've written about the business of fitness who seek a moderate entry point for a client, such as $19 or $39 per month per member, and then try to increase the return per member through a layered pricing system. For example, look at the following structure that might be used in a 25,000-square-foot full-service club. We will disregard the membership fee at this point to keep it simple. All the memberships would be offered for 12 months at a time on a contractual obligation:

- $39 per month for one member, allowing simple access to the club, including use of the cardio and equipment
- $49 per month for members who want simple access and who also want group exercise
- $59 per month for a guided membership that includes a monthly template workout suited for the client
- $69 per month for group personal training done with a coach and limited to 12 people. This would be offered about 8 to 12 times per week. This membership would also include full access to the equipment and group training.
- $99 per month for small group, semiprivate training limited to groups of two to four. This would be offered on a schedule based on the workout of the day and the members can attend as many times per week at they like.
- $299 a month for limited one-on-one training that includes five sessions per month, which can be used at any time that month but do not roll over into the next month if not used.
- $699 a month for unlimited one-on-one training, including full supplementation, protein powders, meal replacement bars, and other services the club could include to enhance the value of the membership

This type of structure offers a number of advantages for an owner. First of all, you are showing a lower entry fee to the marketplace, but your plan is to create a higher return per member. The lower price will appeal to a wider range of potential clients in the market, therefore attracting a broader range of potential clients.

The layers on top of the entry price also allows the club to get more people involved in training, along with appealing to different types of clients. There is always a certain segment of the club neglected by traditional one-on-one training that would be captured with this model. The group most often left out is the younger demographic, which seeks the group dynamic. These are the people who seek 10 or so people working out together with a coach, accompanied by good music and a very challenging workout. This group will not partake in traditional training because it is often simply not challenging enough or is too boring.

There is also a group of folks who have fitness experience of some type and who don't want to spend money on training. However, they *will* spend a little extra each month to have someone create a workout for them. These guided workouts are template driven, meaning the head trainer doesn't sit for an hour and a half individualizing the process but will create a sequence of workouts in a template format that matches the age and goals of general groups of clients.

The goal, of course, is to drive up the average return per member. The following are sample numbers from a typical membership day in this club. The club does seven memberships for the day based on the prices outlined previously. The numbers shown here are the monthly payments the member would make for the category of membership he chose. Another version of this example was used in another chapter, but for the sake of making this point simple, let's look at it again:

- $39
- $39
- $49
- $39
- $299
- $99
- $69

The total of the monthly payments for the day is $633. Stated clearly, this sales team sold seven memberships that day and generated a return per client of $90 ($633/7).

This club shows an entry-level price, which is competitive in the market, of $39 but in reality averages $90 per monthly sale in its average return per member per membership. This would be a hard club to hurt in the marketplace because it is making a lot of its money internally from members already in the system.

Perhaps the most important point is that this club will also have a higher retention rate over time with this model. By segmenting the price structure, you allow many more members to get help and guidance, therefore more will get results and the foundational thought is that people who change their bodies will stay longer and pay longer than people who simply do a circuit a few times a week and ultimately fail because their bodies adapt and then stop responding to that limiting method of training.

This system solves two major problems well. First of all, you can show a lower price in a competitive market if needed and this club could use $19 as its base if needed. Remember, it isn't the price that matters but the return per member that is the key. If you just show $19 but don't have a layered pricing system on top of the low price, your actual return will most likely be less than $19 due to discounts, such as seniors or second members at the same address.

Secondly, you turn the short-term nature of training revenue, which has always been based on sessions and packages, into a recurring income stream based on members already in the system. In other words, you are making more money from fewer people and you already have the people you need in your business.

The other side of seeking a solution for the increased capitalization issue is the complete opposite of the approach just discussed. This side of the argument stresses the volume approach and is based on showing a low price, such as $9 per month, and then going for as many members as you can attract for the business. This method was popular starting in the early 2000s but was already showing fatigue just a decade later.

The problem with the low-price/heavy-volume approach is that is not sustainable over time. This is true for two reasons. First of all, no matter what price you set, others in your market can and will go lower, taking away whatever marketing advantage that this system might have initially enjoyed.

Secondly, there is only so much volume in any give market that will respond to price. There is a term quoted often by businesspeople called the *law of diminishing returns*. This originated as an agricultural term from England from the late 1800s. The law states that an action repeated often will have a less and less return each time. The original concept was based on planting corn and stated that if you plant corn in the same field year after year, each harvested crop will be less than the year prior.

This can also be directly applied to the low-price players. Each time you run a price ad in a limited market, you will get less and less response over time. Remember that your market is limited to about a 12- to 15-minute drive time from your club during primetime, which is usually early evening in most markets. A significant number of people won't drive more than that time to join a club. It is simply too far and not convenient to get there easily as part of their life.

Where low price does work for a more extended period of time is in markets that have high turnover. The influx of new people into the area gives you a new market each mailing but is still not enough to overcome the law over time.

Perhaps the biggest negative in this system is in retention. Going into year three in the low-price model, you enter into what is called the *replacement mode*. The low-price business model is based on a steady growth in new members and the resulting receivable base. During the first two years and then going into the third year, you enter into the replacement mode, where you might lose 250 members per month but you theoretically replace them with a fresh 250.

Increased competition and the law of diminishing returns kill this concept quite quickly in many markets, but in reality, it might take several years for a club that has had a solid first two years to fade, and if you have strong turnover in the market, it might even extend the decline further into the future, but it will come eventually.

Perhaps the most dramatic change in the club business in recent years has been the increased cost of buying a new member, which is another reason club owners are finally being faced with the reality that retention is important if you want to stay in business over time:

- Cost per marketing lead (what it cost in marketing dollars to bring someone through the door divided by the club spending $6,000 per month for marketing and averages 70 new sales): $85
- Cost of commission (what the club pays a salesperson to write the sale, keeping in mind the more complicated the system, the higher cost per sale): $30
- Hard costs to start the member, including paperwork and staff needs (there is a hard cost to start every new member, which includes labor for the first month of group workouts, paperwork and administrative costs, and any other auxiliary costs, such as first-visit incentives): $35

In this example, the club would spend about $150 to buy a new sale. The formula gets more complicated when the cost of doing business for the gym increases, as it does every year due to such items as increased utilities, taxes, marketing costs, and labor. The higher cost of doing business, coupled with a low renewal rate for a typical club, means a greater demand for new sales to feed the business.

This dependency on new sales, called *front loading*—or running the business by the front door—has a history in the industry that dates back to the 1940s. High-pressure sales, tied to extremely low-priced renewals, such as $60 a year offered by the chain clubs in the 1980s, created a system where no one really cared if expired members came back or not. In a business sense, it was actually better for the club if the expired members didn't come back because the return per member from the discounted renewals was so low. At $60 per year, if the person takes a shower each time he's in the club, you would lose money. And it's a total loss if he uses any toilet paper.

What's actually good for a renewal rate? Keep in mind that a renewal rate means how many members stay with the club year after year. In the example at the beginning of this chapter, the club started with 100 new members, but a year later, after adjusting for losses outside the control of the club, the owner ended up with 76 members who might renew going into their second year. If the club owner renews 40 percent, he would end up with just 30 members at the beginning of year two for those members.

There are a lot of owners out there who would consider selling their spouses and throw in the children for free if they could hit and maintain a renewal rate of 40 percent over time, especially because the realistic average for a lot of club owners is a pathetic 20 percent or so.

The question, then, is not whether the club is doing well with 30 renewals. The real question is what happened to the other 60 percent who didn't renew? What are we doing wrong in the industry that drives more than 60 percent of our existing members away on a yearly basis and why are we so ready to continue to pay such a high cost to buy new sales? All most clubs really do is replace the lost members they lose each month rather than being able to use the retention of current members as a competitive edge in the market.

Most owners start at a disadvantage in the first place when it comes to retention. These owners assume, as have many of their predecessors, that the member will not renew anyway no matter what they do as owners. But is this really a self-fulfilling prophecy or the reality of the fitness business?

For example, it used to be common for an owner to sell 24-month contracts to members rather than the more efficient 12-month contract, so the client would not have to make a second buying decision at the end of the first year. But 24-month contracts are harder to sell due to their length of commitment and require more pressure at the point of sale. This requires a better salesperson, who requires more money, which decreases the money in the gym available for customer service and reinvestment in equipment, which ultimately leads to the member not renewing because he didn't get the help and service he wanted.

The assumption and the supporting management style was that the member would never renew if given a chance. In this example, the owner was correct because the member really never had a chance to renew. All the resources of the gym were dedicated to generating new members, leaving very little to service the members who have already bought.

There was one chain of clubs in the southern part of the country that refused to believe that the member would ever stay in the club past his initial membership. And the club did everything possible to make this come true. The sales team comprised the largest percentage of the staff, received most of the training, and by far took the largest percentage of the payroll, which was high anyway because of the emphasis on driving new sales.

Marketing expenses in this six-club chain were high because the clubs depended on new sales that they had to spend a great deal of money every month to buy new leads. The staff also turned over often due to the pressure of generating these new sales.

The front counter and other support people in these clubs were the youngest and cheapest employees the club could hire because all the money went to the salespeople. This meant that service in the club was very poor because the staff was undertrained and inexperienced in the positions they held. The only trainers in the club were outside trainers who were not interested in servicing or helping people—except for money.

The physical plants were also very rundown, including your basic white walls, no juice counters, and outdated or insufficient equipment. And the locker rooms would make your mother cry because they were so disgustingly dirty.

Would this type of club have very good renewals? Of course it wouldn't. It would have been easy to see just by standing at the front counter that the club and salespeople were only interested in the member before the sale, as indicated by the large number of staff hanging out at the counter or in the offices on the phone opposed to the one independent trainer on the floor. There was absolutely no interest in the member after the sale and the club philosophy was that because every member wouldn't stay long anyway that concentrating on getting more new meat each month was a priority.

These clubs were eventually sold because this type of high-pressure front-loading system will only work for so long, especially outside of very heavily populated markets. After a while, you burn up the market because you can only feed so many members through this system before running out of potential people. Remember, more than 80 percent of our members come from within a 12- to 15-minute driving time from the club. Unless you change your marketing and attract a different type of member that is even more service driven, such as the deconditioned folks, you'll run out of sufficient new sales.

Without a strong renewal base, most clubs go this same route. The club may be hot for a year or two, but eventually, you run out of potential members because you burn up your marketplace. The renewals would eventually compound over the years, adding up to a steady and continually increasing source of revenue for the club that would eventually start to decrease the dependency on new sales.

One of the more important breakthroughs in recent years has been the realization that we can now help people get what they really came to us for in the first place. Advances in training style, philosophy, and equipment have made it easier to get sustainable results for a much larger percentage of the population.

In the past years, most owners wanted to do the right thing for the members but were limited by the technology they had at their disposal. Alwyn Cosgrove, a functional guru who has had a powerful influence on how trainers today think about how we train people, once said: "Just because I have changed my mind doesn't mean I was wrong then. It just means that I have learned so much new since then." In other words, we were right at the time, but we are wrong now.

The problem with technology from the last century is that it didn't get enough results over time for enough people. Therefore, retention was a difficult thing to just base on results received by the member. For example, expecting someone to do a circuit three days a week for a year is like asking someone to sit and watch a 90-year-old woman push a cart through Walmart. What we asked this guy to do is the same thing we asked the client of the last century:

Take the beating no matter how painful the journey. Circuits are boring and nonproductive after a few weeks and doing circuit training becomes like going to the dentist, where you know the pain is needed to get results, but it is also something that maybe you can put off until later.

In today's fitness world, we have the tools, education, and trainers to get results and we can do it with energy and fun, creating an experience where the client looks forward to coming. Results not only sell, but they keep people in the system longer. Even group exercise has broken through in recent years. In the past, everything was body weight and dance based. Today, many of the group exercises programs feature modified resistance training in some form or another and the participants in these programs are getting better results now from their workout than was possible with the first generation group in the 1980s.

The next logical step is to learn why people who have paid us for 12 months decide they no longer wish to be part of the club. When people join a club, they initiate a trust relationship. If they don't renew, that trust relationship was somehow broken along the way. People who have a strong relationship with the club will stay longer and pay longer than those who just have a relationship with a treadmill. Relationships are dynamic and are between people and the club that can tap this power will keep members longer than the ones that don't understand this concept.

Most people who join a club make a commitment to that club. They say: "Okay, I'm here and I trusted you with my money instead of those guys down the street. Now let's get this relationship started." However, as gym people, we usually say: "Yes, I know you're a new member, but could you please get the hell out of the way? I'm busy trying to sign up new people to replace you because I'm planning on giving you little or no service or help."

Nine Basic Renewal Mistakes

There are nine core mistakes most owners make when it comes to renewals. These are the basic mistakes that experienced owners can move beyond with time and a good business plan. If your renewals are mediocre or you're new in the business, start here and build.

Mistake #1: The club fails to bring each member into the club at least eight times a month.

The IHRSA fitness industry trade organization (International Health, Racquet & Sportsclub Association) published a report titled "Why People Quit." In this survey, 969 former members were interviewed as to why they quit their clubs. The most interesting part of the entire report was that every single member was working out less than eight times per month when he quit. Not just a few. Not just a certain percentage. All 969 former health club members dropped to less than eight times per month when they quit.

The report went on to discuss many of the reasons these people cited as to why they left. The point that might be the most relevant, though, was left out and the question that should have been asked was: "Were you working out enough in the club or on your own to meet and sustain your fitness goals?"

It is good to move and someone who is moving once or twice a week is probably going to be healthier and happier than one who doesn't, but most fitness professionals and organizations recommend that you move actively up to an hour a day and, in a perfect world, about five to six days per week.

In other words, if you aren't moving on a regular basis, meaning at least more than eight times per month, your body isn't going to change and you sure won't be renewing that membership to a gym where you seldom go anymore.

Keeping all this in mind, club owners should build the feeling of unlimited access into as many of their programs as possible. For example, group exercise should be sold as unlimited group exercise and training—as illustrated in the sample price structure detailed earlier.

You want people in the gym and you want them there more than eight times per month if you want to keep them staying longer and paying longer. Special events, special workouts, unique class offerings, or anything else you can do to get the person in the gym and sweating will add up to more retention over time.

Mistake #2: Management and staff do not foster relationships with and between members.

People with relationships stay longer and pay longer. And people don't have relationships with fitness equipment. They have them with other people.

People who work with a coach in any type of personal training, group exercise, weight loss program or boot camp or in any capacity that involves a leader and followers will have a higher retention rate than someone who just comes to the club and does nothing but walk on a treadmill. And the treadmill walker will also be the first to leave you for a cheaper club because his relationship in the club is with treadmill number four and not with any of your staff.

Cycle classes are a perfect example of the double whammy. The clients get to know other members in the class, but they also develop a friendship and loyalty to the instructors. These members are less likely to leave their friends for a cheaper club compared to the member that just slinks in the door, wanders around the back for a while, and then leaves.

In good clubs, members also have relationships with the staff. Managers who work the floor during primetime, strong counter employees who get to know names, and trainers who are willing to answer questions and guide folks on the floor all are part of the relationship-building process and all contribute to a stronger member retention over time.

Mistake #3: The club fails to understand the importance of a person's first 30 days as a new member.

When do members make the decision to renew? Most clubs weight the decision toward the end of the member's time. For example, a club may send out a 60-day notice of renewal and a 30-day notice and then call the member during the last two weeks of his membership.

This is okay for a small percentage of members, but it's way too late for most—about 11 months too late for most. Many members make a decision to renew during their first 30 days, not their last. It's a lot like golf. If you are well grounded in the basics early in your career, the game is more enjoyable and you might stick with it longer.

It's the same in a gym. If you get started right, are accepted into the club by the staff and other members, and start your fitness program with a good grounding in the basics, you will most likely stay longer and pay longer than a member who did not have a good start to his membership. Another analogy might be a meal in a restaurant. The meal is mediocre, the service fair, the atmosphere nothing special, but the waiter comes up and asks if everything is all right. You say yes, but in your mind, you know you'll never come back again. You just want to finish your meal and be gone.

It's somewhat the same in the gym. The service is average at best, the atmosphere is nothing outstanding, and the equipment is adequate but maybe a little outdated. But when anyone asks if you're happy—a special feat in itself— you say "Yes," knowing you made the wrong choice, but you'll live with it until your membership and then you can get on to the next club.

Many clubs actually create barriers to their members' happiness during the first 30 days. A limited number of start-up workouts, not enough support material as to the systems and happenings in the gym, limited opportunities to meet other members, and an uncaring and service-limited staff are all problems a member would have to overcome to remain a happy member for any length of time in that gym.

For example, let's take a new member who's deconditioned, in her late 30s, and hasn't been in a gym environment for a number of years. The club has a policy that it will work a member out three times and then she's on her own if she is unwilling or unable to pay for one-on-one training. Three times is probably not enough for a deconditioned person with little if any fitness experience.

She comes into the club after she is turned loose, tries to figure it out on her own by reading a book or magazine or perhaps goes online to look at a few video workouts, gets frustrated when nothing changes with her body, and she then leaves. The club writes her off as someone who wasn't really serious about fitness and would have quit anyway. The member writes the club off because of its lack of service. What's the chance she'll renew at the end of her year or if indeed she will ever try a fitness facility again because they are all probably like the one she did try?

One of the most important things you can do to get this member started correctly is to provide as much training as possible during her first 30 days, with an emphasis on teaching her how to work out rather than just starting her on a simple workout that no one will ever upgrade for her.

Most club owners are unwilling to provide much help due to the expense of providing every new member a one-on-one coach and this is a legitimate concern. The solution is to move all training for new members and guests that are in the system due to marketing, such as trial memberships, into a group scenario.

The most effective way to bring qualified leads into your business is through the use of trial memberships. Trial memberships are nothing more than a way to let the potential member try the club, meet other members and staff, and experience the club's service prior to buying a membership. Trial memberships kill risk, which is for many potential members the biggest barrier to inquiry. In their minds, why try this club at all when you know you have to make up your mind to commit to a membership after only one visit? Killing risk or at least minimizing it allows the club to attract a potential member who will not respond to traditional club marketing based on discounts, such as 50 percent off the membership fee or some unbelievable special, such as a two-for-one pricing deal.

People who join after a trial will stay longer than members who just get started because the trial member had a chance to experience the club and make a buying decision based on the experience and not through pressure applied by a salesperson, which almost always leads to buyer's regret for the new member. Buyer's regret is that "What the hell did I get myself talked into this time?" feeling you have after getting beaten up by a high-pressure dinosaur salesperson.

Perhaps the main reason trial memberships are so successful is that there are too many moving parts in fitness. For example, would you walk into a bar, find someone exciting you want to talk to, walk up, spill a drink on her shoe, knock her off the stool trying to wipe the drink up, bang her head on the bar on the way back up, and then ask her out at that point? Good intent but perhaps bad timing on your part.

The same is true in selling an emotional-based service such as fitness. Asking someone who hasn't been in the club for years, who is out of shape, who is miserable after his first light workout, and who needs food badly to become a new member on his first visit doesn't make any sense either.

The goal of exposure marketing is "To know me is to love me." This means that more people will trust you and then become members if they have a chance to get to know you with minimal risk. If people work out a few times, meet other members going through the same process, and slowly develop a feeling that they can indeed do this, you are more likely to get them as members over time as compared to a club operator who hammers guests on their first visit to the facility.

There are two common memberships that are used for paid trials: 30 days for $39 or a risk-free trial, such as 21 days free with no risk and no obligation. Both appeal to different groups of consumers and both can be modified for the specific task. For example, the 30-day trial can be done for as little as $9 in a competitive market or can be as much as $129 for 30 days for a training club.

The goal of any trial is to get a broad range of potential members into your business for an extended period of time so you have a chance for the guest to experience your expertise and professionalism, meet the other guests and your staff, and to get a chance to get involved in fitness using a risk-free or minimum risk opportunity.

Keep in mind that when this was written, there were still only about 16 percent of the people in this country who belonged to a health club or any type of fitness facility. The rest of the people hadn't yet decided that joining a club is the solution for them to meet their fitness needs. This other 84 percent of the population doesn't have enough experience to even understand how a fitness business works or if it indeed helps them with their personal goals. Remember that for many of the folks that have never been in a gym before, the fitness world is a scary place where everyone but them is in shape and that there is nothing they can do in the club without looking foolish.

Advertising price to this group—which hasn't even decided if it is ready to try fitness—is a senseless waste of marketing money. Your marketing here based on the concept that the reader can accomplish his goals with you and that you will let him try it first to prove it to him gives you a nice edge over the clubs that just hammer price constantly, which only appeals to a small group of people loose in the market that might have previous club experience.

Guests who use the trial need to be treated exactly as real members to make this work and most clubs can't afford to train every guest, along with every new member, using a one-on-one method. This is why it is important to offer group aspects of training to all new members and trial guests during their first 30 days or with the matching length of their trial. You want everyone you can drag into group training to get all the help and service they can take during their initial time at the club. For example, how hard would it be to convert a guest who has been in the club for a month and who has never had a workout with a coach?

The basic tool to use for new guests and members who are in their first 30 days is called fundamentals. Fundamentals is a simple way to provide low-cost consistency for new members and guests during their first 30 days in the facility. We also use the format of fundamentals as an assessment tool that will be discussed in depth later in this book.

The paradigm shift that has to occur here is that you have to move away from the mind-set that we have to give the new member or guest a simple workout, review it a couple of times, and then let the person go solo, never to be seen again, toward the idea that if we teach the person how to work out with a mastery of the basic movement patterns, such as a simple squat pattern that makes so much sense when someone good shows it to you and is so hard to do correctly out of a book, the person can then get quicker results over a shorter period of time.

The old adage that if you give a man a fish, you feed him for day but that if you teach him how to fish, you feed him for life can be applied here. Teach a new member—and this includes even the deconditioned person, who we automatically prejudge as inept and unable to learn or move—the basic moves of fitness, including the goblet squat (counter balanced), the dead lift (emphasis on where the hips are going), the kettlebell swing, a pressing movement done correctly (push), a pull movement (perhaps a kettlebell row) and a lunge.

Teaching these moves in a group setting for the entire month gives the member a base he can apply to a different workout each week or month that is supplied by the club. For example, the club could post three workouts every Monday on a big wall in the club that gives every member an idea of what to do that week. Remember that one of the biggest complaints a failing member has is that he just doesn't know what to do each workout, which is another way of saying he is okay doing it on his own if someone else would provide the program design for him.

This concept gets a lot of pushback from the old school players and trainers who feel that program design should be something that everyone pays extra for as a member and that a simple membership just gets you into the club. This might have been true 50 years ago when you had no competition, but in today's cutthroat world, where the loss of even one client is painful, keeping every member engaged and on track for success in the club has to be the new business plan.

The format for fundamentals would look something like this:
- The one-minute meet and greet
- The 12-minute dynamic warm-up
- The 20-minute strength segment
- The three- to five-minute big finish (metabolic burnout)

The strength section would include these movements—in this exact order:
- Kettlebell swing
- Push movement, preferably an overhead press
- Goblet squat, which teaches the client the proper stance and hip movement, with a counter weight
- Pull movement, preferably a kettlebell row
- The lunge
- The dead lift, with the emphasis on the hips and the difference between this movement and the squat

The emphasis here is on the "how," not the "what," and getting the client comfortable moving into new patterns. The goal is not to give him an archaic circuit workout that he will be bored with in six weeks and that won't get any results past that point. We want the person to be successful and to be able to move from different workout to different workout each month without a trainer in the process.

This will not negate your training department or revenue. The trainer in a newer business model should play the role of personal coach and group leader. In the pricing example listed earlier, the coach leads and motivates the group personal training, provides guidance and personal coaching to the small group, and does individual programming design, education, and motivation for the one-on-one client.

You should also at some point move away from letting all trainers on the staff do their own program design. The more efficient—and safer for the club—method is to have the head trainer or owner do all program design and review all the programs that are being applied to the one-on-one clients. Having one source protects the club in that all training in the club is done using the owner's philosophy and belief system and that the trainers in the club merely carry out the mission. This protects the club in that the information and education the client is receiving comes from the club itself and not from an individual trainer who often feels it is all about him and not about the business.

The guest or client will first encounter fundamentals in the form of the assessment/induction process during their first or second visit to the club. The standard in the industry for years was to have a guest start with a salesperson, who explained the basics of the club and did the initial tour, and then turned the guest over to a trainer, who was supposed to write a program for the person and get him set up on a circuit. In a more efficient world, the guest or new member will meet with a skilled trainer, who will do an assessment (the induction process into the club) and then place the person where he needs to be to meet his goals.

The traditional method has failure written all over it, but it has taken decades to replace such an inefficient habit. The first failure is that the guest is in the club to discuss fitness and his goals and to pursue some form of getting into shape. The person this guest would really like to talk to is a trainer, not a salesperson who only exists to sell a membership.

The second failure is the trainer. The trainer has no sales training, hates to talk about money, and is only interested in getting the guest into his one-on-one training stable. If the guest is not qualified (no money or not interested), the trainer sets the guest up on a circuit once and walks away. Even though the club says you get three workouts, we know the trainer is not likely to put much effort into a person who is not a potential client.

The salesperson who first started with the guest now has to overcome the weak training experience or if the guest became a member first and then did the training, we now have a new member who is starting unhappy and with a half-ass workout that is doomed to fail him in about six weeks as his body plateaus and he faces circuit boredom. The inefficiency is compounded by the fact that the trainer has probably had no sales training and does nothing to give the guest or new member a sense that this club is any different from any other club in the area that starts every new member with "three workouts and then you go solo" policy.

The assessment/induction tool, which is a modified fundamentals format, is designed to overcome these deficiencies be getting the guest or new member placed correctly during his first or second visit and then set on the road to success during his first 30 days as a new member. Doing this requires some new thinking that breaks away from the traditional sales approach found in most mainstream box clubs.

First of all, you will need to create two sales teams. Your first team is the traditional salesperson in the club whose job it is to get people started on the right track and to help them eventually become members. The second team should consist of a trainer/salesperson, defined as an experienced trainer who wants a leadership role in the club and who isn't afraid to ask for money. This person will do all the assessments on the new clients and guests and then place each person where the assessor feels he needs to be in the club to best meet his goals—physically and financially.

Potential members only arrive in a club in two forms. The person is either a guest of a member or just walked in through the club's marketing or location. The first person, which is the proverbial buddy sale, would start with the traditional salesperson, get signed up as a new member, and then be placed with a trainer/assessor. Your available pool that would actually end up doing the assessment would be based on the following numbers. (Obviously, these numbers are for a mainstream full-service club. Training clubs should have a full 100 percent show up for their assessments.)

New guests or members at the club that month	100
Number who are too stupid to change from their pre-existing bad habits*	−20
	80
Number who would take part in the club's group exercise program**	−20
Number who need help and guidance in the club	60

Out of this number, we can assume that about 3 to 6 percent would end up in traditional one-on-one training anyway, but in this example, those people would still need to be placed into the system at some point. The true potential that would show up for an assessment is 60 out of every 100 guests and new members. Guests and new members are lumped together here because we are trying to not only get the new person education but to also upsell the new person into a training level once he has experience with the products.

The problem with the buddy-sale person who signs up during his first day is that he probably does not have any experience with any of the offerings on the price sheet above simple access. Solving this problem is simple: Just give the person who signed up during his first visit a VIP full-access pass to training for a full 30 days. This new sale is still invited to do an assessment and the salesperson should walk the new person directly to the trainer/assessor, who will set up the new member with the access pass. The script to use to get someone to do an assessment would sound like the following:

---

*We have all seen this guy—the one who will do the lat pulls by throwing his body backward off the machine until the brim of his backward-facing hat hits the floor and who now can claim he "stacked the machine." He most likely has been doing this since high school and you aren't going to change him much.

**Your percentage of takers for an assessment is usually small from this category of potential members. Most of the people who do group just do group and aren't usually interested in doing the assessment, although it should be offered to them. This number is variable depending on the club's group penetration rate.

Paul, our training philosophy here is quite different from most clubs you might have seen. We would like to get you started with us by setting you up with Randy, who is our senior trainer on staff and who will spend an hour with you finding out where you are on your path to fitness and how we can help you get there. He will also do an assessment, which will take you through some of the training techniques we encourage here, such as using kettlebells—something you might not have much experience with yet. However, the primary goal of the assessment is to get you comfortable doing all the basic movements you would need to take part in any level of our training programs. Let's walk over to Randy so I can introduce you and so we can get you set for that assessment as soon as you can get into the club again.

If the guy is dressed and ready, do the assessment today while he is in the club. If he isn't dressed for fitness, walk him over to Randy and have Randy set a time or have the salesperson do it if Randy is currently on the floor. Keep in mind that a good assessment will take at least an hour, so we want the client to be dressed and at ease as we start the process and not feeling rushed.

The purpose is to slow down the first encounter between a guest and the club or to add value and anchor the new member during his first 30 days in the club. Most sales encounters are almost always too rushed—often lasting less than 20 minutes. Slow down the pace, spend some time with the new people, and make sure their first encounter with your business is life changing compared to the other clubs in the market.

It is important to note that the purpose of the assessment is to build confidence in the client and to demonstrate the expertise of your staff and the professionalism of the club. Do not do a body fat composition during the assessment or anything else that will discourage the client. Testing is good and has its place, but it should only be used as a baseline tool for new clients already in the system. You want the client to feel that he can do it and that you are the club that will patiently help him learn new approaches to fitness, and tearing him down during the first visit does not accomplish this.

Trial guests who show up in the club using either the 21-day risk free trial or a paid trial should have full access to training during their initial time period. The goal is to get them totally immersed into the club's training culture before we ask for money.

The only variation with the assessment during the first visit compared to the standard fundamentals is the first 10 minutes. During the first 10 minutes, the assessor should focus on three areas:

- What is your goal with us?
- What is your time frame?
- How much time can you commit each week to fitness?

If the assessor gathers this information, he moves to the dynamic warm-up, to the strength segment, and then into the big finish. If the guest is really deconditioned, the assessor would modify as needed, but unless there is a medical reason the client can't move, then the goal is to get the guest involved and sweaty no matter what age or condition.

At the end of the assessment, the assessor takes the guest back to the table, where he coaches cardio. Cardio is probably the single-biggest myth for beginners who are venturing back into fitness. Often, their fitness goal is to just come to the club and walk on the treadmill, going three miles per hour and watching their favorite TV show. We need to take this fallacy away from the person and rearm them with realistic information. This is also a chance to demonstrate expertise by coaching some form of gentle interval training that gets the client thinking about his personal fitness from a different viewpoint.

There is one important question the assessor must ask at the end of the assessment:

> *Paul, are you the type of person who prefers to work with a personal coach or are you the type of person who prefers doing things in a group setting and sharing the cost of the trainer?*

At this point, it is up to the assessor to place the person where he thinks he belongs in the system. It is important for the assessor, as a professional, to suggest an exact program and plan of attack for the client to use to reach his goals. The question asked helps the guest to place himself financially without having to admit he might not be able to afford a personal coaching program or indeed he might be someone who really just likes the group dynamic.

If the person is deconditioned or not athletic, he can repeat fundamentals several times a week, which is probably enough of a workout for him anyway at this stage. Again, fundamentals should be offered four to six times per week and in a group setting so the members can begin to develop his own relationships in the club.

If the person is athletic, he might drop by fundamentals once if needed or not at all and he can then join any of the other group offerings during his trial visit or during the first 30 days of his new membership. The goal is to get his armed with tools he can use elsewhere in the club and then move him on to where he can get the most benefit and have the best experience in the club.

This system can be summarized with a few key points:
- The goal of the first 30 days is to get the new client or guest to move beyond hopeless beginner and to get him grounded in the club by being able to have an elementary mastery of the basic movements of fitness.
- The goal of the assessment tool is to slow down the first contact between the club and the potential member or to replace the antiquated "three workouts with a bored trainer and you are on your own" scenario with a system that gets the member on a track to long-term success. Remember, this is ultimately about retention, and if you set the person up correctly the first 30 days, he will stay longer and pay longer.

• This is a sales tool, but you are now adding a trainer with experience to the sales mix. The trainer/assessor's goal is to place the client where he needs to be in the club to get the maximum success in the shortest period of time. His other role is to feed the other trainers on staff, who have proven to be inefficient salespeople anyway.

Other issues that kill retention during the first 30 days

We also start the member relationship off badly during the first 30 days by not reviewing our procedures. For example, look at a new member who survives the training process and starts to attend the gym on a regular basis. Toward the end of his first 30 days, he tries to write a check for $18 for a ball cap from the pro shop as a gift for his brother. The new front counter person, who is just following the gym's policy, IDs this member who wants to write a check.

She doesn't know or use his name and IDs a person who has a $40-a-month contract, and by doing so, she creates a situation of nontrust with a new member. The policy itself is nonsense. We already have enough information on a contract to go after the person if he writes a bad check. The policy should be for nonmembers only.

And because this club doesn't understand the importance of member service in relationship to long-term renewals, it doesn't understand the value of having a competent person at the front counter. This is usually the lowest-paying and most undertrained job in the system, but this person has direct access to every member of the club. How many people a day does a badly trained front counter person offend and can you afford to replace members who start their relationship with your business poorly?

Your counter person, especially during primetime, should be one of the strongest employees on the staff, not one of the weakest. By not learning a member's name and by not knowing when to stray or question a club policy, she just cost this club a member. The member may not quit yet, but can he expect the service to improve over the rest of his membership?

Question all procedures in the club. Most club procedures are created from years of accumulation and from creating a policy for a "one of a kind" occurrence. For example, a member constantly books space in your classes or other programming weeks in advance but then she doesn't show for most of them. You get mad and create a policy that takes care of this problem by putting that crazy woman in her place once and for all. This policy states that no one can now book over three spaces at a time, effectively punishing everyone who booked seats and showed up as promised.

The issue is that you now have another policy that was reactionary and based on just one or two offenders but effects all the members and staff. You would have been better off to deal with the abusers privately by probably just cancelling their memberships and avoid punishing everyone for the actions of such a small group. Review all your policies and keep in mind that less is more when it comes to delivering good service at the front counter. Your goal is to make sure it is easy to keep members, not to make it easy for them to get mad and leave.

Mistake #4: Member service is not consistent.

Paying a membership payment every month to a business that doesn't know your name, waiting for equipment, and not even being able to buy a cold drink on your way out will wear on a member after a while. Throw in being ignored at the front counter as you check in, paper towels on the locker room floor, sweat stains on the equipment, classes that start late and then run over their set time, and being surrounded by an entire team of staff that just grunts and who hasn't said thank you ever in an entire lifetime and you would wonder why anyone would sign up at a fitness facility, let alone stay any length of time.

Most members don't casually leave us at the end of their year. They're driven away every day by horrible member service. In this industry, you can provide better customer service than your competitors and still be lousy because, as an industry, our standards are just too low. As noted throughout this chapter, we are willing to deliver poor service because we operate under the belief that every member can be replaced and that new sales will outperform retention indefinitely. Because that has changed due to the increase of competition, we are now forced to live up to the fact that maybe we don't really know how to deliver customer service at all.

The lost rules of etiquette

The fitness business is at an unusual crossroads. On one side, we have the implosion of the box club concept as mainstream fitness centers struggle to stay relevant in a hyper-change business environment and where for decades the equipment has been the star at the expense of the membership. On the other side, the evolution of the training-centric model that puts the client back into the center of the business plan is putting pressure on how we do business and who in the fitness business will survive in the coming years.

The rise of the mainstream chain-style club during the 1980s also directly corresponded to the demise of most of what has passed as member service for the last 20 years in the industry. Chain clubs, along with the independent operators who emulate that business model, exist for one reason and that is to sell as many new memberships as possible each month. Membership revenue in these clubs is often 85 percent or more of the business's total deposit each month, and if there isn't heavy volume, there is no business. The problem is that volume and member service are mutually exclusive.

The rise of a training-centric, results-driven business model will perhaps be the most important breakthrough in the last 50 years of fitness. It sounds so simplistic to say those words that it somewhat negates the power of what is happening in the industry, but we are witnessing the end of the membership-driven model while simultaneously watching the return of the client-centered business.

Simply stated, fitness business owners have to figure out how to get the most results for the most clients or fail because the cannibalistic nature of the bottom-feeders is that the cheap eat the cheap, leaving little room to exist on volume alone.

However, this transition, is causing a number of problems, including the not-so-insignificant issue of the industry no longer understanding even the rudimentary points of supplying basic customer service. The volume sales approach negates the member as relevant because it is all about sell, burn up, replace, and sell again. Over the last decades, this belief that the member is forever replaceable has made us forget how to value and serve the clients we so desperately seek.

When you are struggling to stay alive in a crowded market, customer service is the one tool you can wield that gives you an edge at a low cost. As the mainstream box players live in the past, dreaming about the glory days of volume and how to recreate it, more progressive operators can invest in customer service training at a low cost.

Member retention

Members who feel they support a business where they feel valued will stay longer and pay longer and members who get results because the clubs touch beyond the traditional 3 to 6 percent of training clients will also stay at that club longer, generating more revenue than the club that lives to turn and burn its membership.

The following sections are a few simple rules of customer service we have lost in the years of seeking volume. Customer service is not a hard thing to master, and done correctly, true service is nothing but doing a lot of small things right every day. This isn't by any means an all-inclusive list, but these few points can serve as a nice foundation to build on.

❏ Start with the phone.

This is perhaps the most annoying part of any fitness business for the client. Trying to get information from a typical club employee over the phone could make a Southern Baptist minister down a pint of Jack Daniel's. Nothing should be this hard nor should anyone paying a monthly fee to support a business be treated that badly. The following are a few simple rules of giving good phone service:

- *Answer live by the third ring.* Do not under any circumstances—ever in your entire life and not even if you are a trainer in a small studio—ever rely on voice mail. Someone is already paying you or might be trying to give you money, so find a way to pick up the phone and say hello. There is no reason in any service business—no matter how big you are—to not answer live. You take their money? Then, you take their call.

- *Answer like you care, not like you are bored out of your mind or like someone interrupted your texting session.* Use a strong welcome statement each and every time the phone rings. For example: "Hi, we are having a great day at the Workout Company." Energy sells and is contagious and the transfer of this energy should start with the phone.

- *Learn to screen calls.* Do not say "Who is this please? Let me see if he is in." This is just another way of saying "Let me see if he wants to talk to your insignificant, worthless soul." It is always safe and sounds professional if you train your staff to say: "Fred is with a member (or is currently on another call). May I please have your name and number and a short message as to what the call concerns?"

- *Master appointments online to ease the phone volume.* Next generation software is a step forward for the members to be able to book online for training appointments and classes, easing the flow through the front desk phones. However, many of your older members will still pick up the cell phone and pound the buttons but keep the online registration option at the top of their minds, including Facebook and your website.

❏ Timeliness is the basis of respect.

Respecting someone's time is the first step in showing clients you value them as people and as paying clients. Failure to respect their time is failure to respect their money and you only need to do this a few times before you lose the client forever. The following are a few simple ways to look at time and clients in the business:

- *On time for a training appointment is 15 minutes early.* Trainers who have an appointment at 3 p.m. and show up at 3 p.m. should be fired. Respecting the client means the trainer is there at least 15 minutes early and has eaten, gone to the bathroom, brushed his teeth, and is ready to set the client on fire with energy.

- *Training sessions and group classes of any kind should be a maximum of 50 minutes.* Despite what the old-style aerobic divas say, there is no valid reason to keep a group class going beyond 50 minutes. Those who insist on going that extra five minutes into the next class's time because they think it is extra value are in reality annoying that member who needs to get out on time but is embarrassed to leave before the class is over. Many people do group because it is compartmentalized and breaking the rule of 50 minutes leaves a kid standing in the rain in the front of the school for another 20 minutes. This also goes for training sessions. If you can't do it in 50, you simply aren't a good enough trainer to do it at all. There is simply no valid training reason or service reason for a session or class to run past 50 minutes.

- *If you still have group exercise programs (aerobics for those of you older than 40), your instructor has to be part of the service act.* Instructors should walk through the club prior to their classes and invite people to join and the instructor should stand at the door and thank every single participant for taking part in the class today. Yes, you should give the instructor a few extra dollars for this, but this is not an option for the instructor. It is mandatory for the instructor who wants to keep the class.

- *End all group personal training with the official Todd Durkin "group hug," a move the master of energy uses himself after every workout.* At the end of the group session, he calls everyone in, they give the group shout, and then Todd thanks them as a group: "Thank you all for being my clients and for supporting my business." Every group is thanked every time. If you take their money, say thank you.

❑ Your personal image is still important.

The trend today is to dress down, but in small business, you can create a stronger business environment by adding some style to your team. The following are a few points worth considering:

- *Wear real clothes, not baggy workout gear that always looks like you are an old crazy New Jersey lady walking the streets in South Beach.* There are so many uniform options now available that there is no longer any reason to rely on tacky T-shirts or golf shirts. Honor your clients by dressing a little better than you think. If you are a trainer, develop your own personal uniform that makes you look professional. Club operators are notorious these days for the jeans and shirt outlook, which is fine if you are trying to get naked with strangers on Saturday night but not so good if you are trying to build a business. Just remember that one badly dressed kid at the front counter is the image of your business when a potential member visits. Control your image by controlling the look of your staff.

- *Every member is thanked every time he leaves the club.* This isn't a hard one to master. Simply teach the staff to say "Thank you for stopping by today. We really appreciate your business." If the staff has an issue with this or is shy and can't say it, fire that person and get someone who is not afraid of saying thank you to a member who supports your business with his money and time.

- *There has never, ever been a club that is too clean.* Most of you spend so much time in your business that you become club blind. This means that you no longer see dirt, clutter, or decline in your physical plant. It is sort of like the middle-aged guy who drives a Porsche, wears his ball cap backward, thinks oversized basketball shorts are cool, and still wears the matching jersey. This is the guy who looks in the mirror and still sees himself as 21 and cool rather than 40 and pathetic. You see what you want to see and owners who are in a business more than they are at home stop seeing the business for what it really is. Dirty clubs cost you more female members than any other issue. Get outside eyes to look at your club. Get retired people to clean it constantly during the day to create the perception that it is really clean because your members watched someone clean it. Hire mystery shoppers or honest friends to visit the club and give you an opinion. The club is never as clean as you hope or as you think, so get some help here. One hint is that if you haven't used a piece of equipment or other clutter sitting in the corners in the last 60 days, then throw it out. Members equate clutter with being dirty.

- *Sometimes, problem members are what are helping kill your member service.* In some clubs, cliques form that destroys your image and work against your staff. This group of lifters or those group exercise people feel the need to control the club and will set other members straight if they don't follow the rules of the clique. The problem is that the rules of the clique often have little to do with the club rules. Mastering customer service for an owner comes from the understanding that you sometimes need to fire your members. Some just don't play well with others, and by letting them just carry on being a pain in the ass, you hurt the overall image of your club. If that member bothers you, he is probably irritating many of your members too and it might be time to walk him to the curb.

- *Start your service training with the thought that every member is not replaceable.* If you put this on the whiteboard at the start of your service training, you will realize that much of what we do in the business is not done to retain clients but merely to service the new ones before we run them out. The big question is: "If the member is truly not replaceable and you have to keep every member you have or fail, what would you do different in customer service?"

❑ Consider the total member.

A strong example of the lack of member support and member service in most clubs is the lack of a nutrition program. Everyone in the fitness business understands that working out is only a small part of the formula when it comes to lifetime fitness, and if you don't intervene in what and how the client eats, there won't be the results we need to drive retention.

Without an understanding of nutrition and its relationship to training, most members could work out for years and never get any great results. Without results, they lose interest and quit. They don't quit today but at the end of the membership. It's like we only give them part of the formula for success—and the smallest part at that. "Yep, I've worked out in this gym for two years now and not a damn thing on my body has changed except for a thinner billfold. Let me at that renewal."

How could an owner operate a gym without a nutrition program? The members are looking for a total support system and we're saying that all we offer is the workout part, which many training experts feel is only about 15 percent of the formula of what it takes to get into better shape. But a nutrition program is not writing out a program on the back of a workout card on a clipboard. Members expect more and will leave us without a solution. Without results, there is no renewal.

Many nutrition programs now have a strong online component that members can access themselves at home or work. Giving members free access to this web source will help keep a certain percentage inspired and educated and will help those seeking real change in their bodies. The emphasis here is that the club should provide free online support for all members and not just to a few for a fee. Remember that the goal is to keep members in the system longer and those who get results stay longer.

Mistake #5: The owner fails to reinvest in the business on a yearly basis.

It's common to visit someone's super club that everyone in the industry raved about several years ago and find it already starting to run down and only surviving off its old glory. Clubs are high-maintenance items that need attention daily, not yearly. Equipment changes, paint fades, good design ideas become stale, and even the most creative physical plants become outdated in a very short period of time. What once inspired is now tired and dated to the consumer.

Clubs go through three levels of maturation. Each level is driven by renewals. If an owner misses one level, it's hard to move to the next. The rule of thumb is that it takes the same amount of money every four years to keep the club competitive that it did to start the club, minus equipment and operational losses during the first year.

For example, if a club that was 10,000 square feet cost $60 per foot to build out when it was opened, or $600,000, that same amount of money would have to be spent over every four-year period to keep that club competitive in the marketplace. Where does this money come from? It should come from renewals. There is an adage that applies here that is worth remembering:

> Revenue from current members and new sales will keep
> the business running and pay the bills, but your next club and
> Ferrari will only come from renewals and retention.

Stage one level of maturation

The first stage of maturation comes at the 13th month the business is open or when the first round of renewals should kick in. If the club averages 100 new sales a month during the first year, then during the 13th month, it should do its 100 sales and realize additional income from its first wave of renewals.

For example, if the club renews 40 percent and has a loss rate of 12 percent from member moves and another 12 percent from nonpays (24 percent total), which are acceptable loss rates to be expected from 12-month contracts collected by a strong third-party collector, then the club should renew about 30 members. Look again at these examples from earlier in the chapter:

> 100 members – 24 percent losses = 76 members left
> at the end of year one

> 76 members left at the end of the first year (adjusted for losses)
> x .40 percent (realistic national average on retention) = 30

To further explain, the club could have had 100 members up for renewal during the 13th month but lost 24 percent, or 24 members, during the year. That leaves 76 possibilities for renewal. If the club renews 40 percent, it would end up with 30 members. This surge of renewals added to the new sales (100 new each month on average) should have increased the club's monthly revenue from membership income at no additional expense to the club.

Note here that 40 percent is a weak number and that you should be targeting 60 percent or higher as your retention number. By applying some of the strategies in this chapter, you should be able to move away from the industry low norm and into higher numbers. Look here at the difference 60 percent makes going into the second year:

100 members − 24 percent losses = 76 members left
at the end of year one

76 members left at the end of the first year (adjusted for losses)
x .60 percent (realistic national average on retention) = 46

This club would have a 15-member advantage going into the second year over its competitor through just one month of business or 180 members over a year. Compound this year after year and you can see why some clubs stay in business for decades and others fade away after three or four years.

Stage two level of maturation

The same thing should happen again at the 25th month as the second wave of renewals kicks in and members from the first year start their second round of renewals. This second wave of renewals should again affect the club's income without expense.

It is interesting to note that once members make the decision to stay after the end of the first year the continued losses from this population of members declines sharply from that point forward. For example, in the previous example, the club ended up with 30 members going into the second year, but if you track that group into the future, the losses will normally drop to only about 3 percent per year. In other words, you have to almost kill these guys to get them to leave after they make their first buying decision. This is why, in many cases, good clubs that have been in business for five years or longer will have 50 percent or more of their members in their second year or longer, making this business very hard to hurt in the marketplace.

Stage three level of maturation

The third stage of maturation is when the club would be fully mature with its membership. It is also the stage where the club continues to prosper or it starts to decline. This stage occurs at about 48 months and is the point where the fixed equipment and physical plant start to decay. The owner should have been reinvesting in the club all along, but if he doesn't reinvest at this crucial stage, the business starts to fade.

For example, a four-year-old club may have a lot of well-maintained cardio equipment that was in style when the club opened. Four years later, those upright bikes and all those stair-climbers still work and look great, but they're not what the members want anymore. The club would need to replace a sizable chunk of its equipment with whatever is hot in the industry at the time and with what will get the most members the best results in the shortest period of time.

Where would the money have come from to replace the old equipment and to update the physical plant? This money would have come from the stages of maturation driven by the renewals in the club. Without the renewals, there would be no surge in the income. Without the maturation effect in the club's revenues from the combination of new sales and renewals, there would never be enough money to continually reinvest in the club.

How renewals affect a maturing club

The following sections illustrate how renewals compound over the years to affect a maturing club. The sales numbers are not corrected for loss rates but serve mainly as examples as to how important renewals are to a club in today's market.

❏ Year 1

During the first year, the club signs up an average of 75 new members a month:

$$75 \times 12 \text{ months} = 900$$

At the end of Year 1, the club has 900 new members. During Year 1, the fixed equipment, such as the selectorized and cardio pieces, are new and fresh, although the club would already be adding functional equipment on a monthly basis, including kettlebells, bands, medicine balls, and other tools that wear out throughout heavy use.

❏ Year 2

During the second year, the club continues to average 75 new members a month for the year. The club also renews 40 percent of the members it signed up during the first year:

900 new members (75 x 12 = 900)
360 renewals from Year 1 (900 x .40 = 360)

At the end of the second year, the club would have 1,260 active members.

❏ Year 3

During the third year, the club signs up 75 new members a month or 900 for this particular year. The club also renews 40 percent of the members it signed up during Year 2. Members from Year 1 also continue to renew for another year. These members are in their third year and will renew at about a 60 percent renewal rate:

900 new members (75 x 12 = 900)
360 renewals from Year 2 (900 x .40 = 360)
216 renewals from Year 1 (360 x .60 = 216)

At the end of Year 3, the club would have 1,476 active members. At the end of Year 3, 39 percent of all the members in the club are renewals.

❏ Year 4

Year 4 is where the club starts to really benefit from the compounding effect of the renewals.

Note that as members stay longer in the system, they renew at a higher rate:

900 new members (75 x 12 = 900)

360 renewals from Year 3 (900 x .40 = 360)

216 renewals from Year 2 (360 x .60 = 216)

173 renewals from Year 1 (216 x .80 = 173)

At the end of Year 4, the club would have 1,649 active members. At the end of Year 4, 45 percent of all the members in the club are renewals.

❑ Year 5

Year 5 shows the transition where half the members in the club are renewals:

900 new members (75 x 12 = 900)

360 renewals from Year 4 (900 x .40 = 360)

216 renewals from Year 3 (360 x .60 = 216)

173 renewals from Year 2 (216 x .80 = 173)

138 renewals from Year 1 (173 x .80 = 138)

At the end of Year 5, the club would have 1,787 active members. At the end of Year 5, approximately 50 percent of all members in the club are renewals.

There is a simple rule that might help here, although this can vary greatly from club to club. Plan to reinvest about 8 percent of your gross revenues each year back into the club to keep it current and plan every fourth year to reinvest the equivalent of 15 to 20 percent of that year's revenue to redo the big issues the club will face. The downside of this business is that it is capital intensive, which is why the trend toward smaller clubs will have such an impact in the coming years.

Mistake #6: The club does not offer trial periods.

Retention will be higher if all potential members go through a trial period first. This was lightly discussed in an earlier point, but it is worth mentioning again separately. Giving trial periods does not obviously appear as something that would help your renewals 12 months into the future but a solid initial trial period where the member can actually try before he buys cuts your losses and increases your renewals. Even shorter trials, such as 14 days, lead to the only people you are signing up are people who truly want a membership and are fully aware of what they are buying. These members weren't drop-closed or beaten into submission in an office but rather had a chance to experience your club and meet the members and staff.

Pressure sales, meaning sales that are forced during the potential member's first visit, often lead to hidden losses later. While it looks good on paper that you wrote a large receivable total, in reality, it means little if you can't collect any money from those memberships.

Old-style salespeople can close and can talk—by the use of old pressure sales techniques—many potential members into signing up today. The clients who respond to this pressure are often the ones who later fail to make their first payment or are mad when they leave and simply cancel or start the membership but refuse to support the club or bring a guest. Pressure sales can generate a lot of good-looking numbers, but at the end of the year, it only really matters as to how much money you have in the bank.

If you use trials, the goal is not how many you sign up today but how many you sign up by the end of the trial period you are using. For example, if you are using a 30-day paid trial, the important number to track is how many you converted within 30 days of the member's start date. You overall goal should be a 60 to 65 percent conversion rate compared to the true national average for closing, which is about 38 percent.

The higher conversion rate can only be generated by good follow-up, good customer service, and good results for the client during the trial period. The key, though, is that if this number goes up, your overall retention rate will probably also go up because so many of your new clients are getting started properly rather than being left to fend for themselves in the club.

But the trial period has to be a real one. One workout or even one week isn't enough to base a buying decision on for most members who look at the membership as a long-term investment. Before a member will invest, which is how most see joining a club, and before they reinvest as renewals, they need to understand and feel comfortable about the product. Once they make the decision, instead of a drop-closing, ex–used car salesperson talking them into it, they are reluctant to walk away because the responsibility belongs to them instead of blaming someone else for forcing their decision.

Mistake #7: The owner fails to keep the club competitive.

This is different from reinvesting in the club in that a club can be clean, freshly painted and improved, and have new carpet and even some new equipment and still not even be close to being competitive.

Much of the failure to stay current comes from repeating an extension of the past, especially from owners who build multiple clubs over a number of years. For example, a club owner builds his first club in 1995—a solid little multipurpose gym as part of a national franchise—and has great success. Three years later, he builds again. Will he try something new or will he just repeat past success?

Five clubs and 15 years later, he builds his sixth unit, which is the ultimate investment, rolling all his hard-earned assets and cash into the new venture, and gets his ass destroyed. He can't figure out what's wrong and blames the economy, the location, or the new competitor who isn't playing fair and opened a club in "his" territory.

The failure is none of these factors but in reality is simply that he has gone one club too many without changing the concept. The new club is almost identical in concept to the first club, but it is shinier and had different equipment brands and a higher degree of finish because the owner has more money, but technically, it is the same club done again and again.

Concepts change, technology changes, and how we train and entertain the member has to change too. Staying competitive is more than just buying new treads and putting them into the exact spot the old treads were in the club. Staying competitive means you and your team just spent a year researching new training techniques and you now reinvent your entire concept from the floor up, replacing lines of static equipment with functional cable-driven styles, eliminating dead group rooms, and changing your entire pricing system to match.

To understand the theory of keeping clubs competitive, you need to understand how the nightclub business works. A club may be extremely popular, packed for six months straight with a line and mega-monster doormen guarding the entry. One month later, no one visits anymore because the patrons have all moved on to the next club of the moment.

The fitness business should try harder to emulate part of this theory. Most clubs stay static too long. The equipment never changes—either by additions or replacements or by simply moving it around once in a while. The walls may be repainted but always in the same colors. The owners invest in some artwork, but because they paid a lot to have it done the first time, it stays on the walls year after year. Even the staff wears the same uniforms for a year at a time. Everything in the business changes yet nothing really changes at all.

What does all this mean to the members? You have members not renewing simply because they are absolutely, positively, incredibly bored beyond the human capacity for tears. The members wanted to stay—they really did—but they need to be challenged, entertained, and fussed over much more frequently than most owners are willing to do. Reinvestment by the owner proves to the members that you are taking them seriously and that you are using the money they gave you wisely.

Cardio equipment may be the best example of what it takes to stay competitive in the fitness industry. When cardio first started to gain acceptance, all anyone had were old-style mechanical bikes. Then, came the upright electronic bikes and every person in the gym was fighting over whose turn it was. The bikes shocked a complacent industry because for the first time, owners had to part with the real bucks for cardio equipment.

Before a member will invest, which is how most see joining a club, and before they reinvest as renewals, they need to understand that you are reinvesting in your own business.

The bikes were the members' rage until the stair machines entered the stage. They were new and fresh and the members could cheat beyond belief. The first StairMaster brand machines stormed the industry not only because the machines provided a great way to do cardio, but for the lazier members, they were also great triceps machines.

Extend those arms, lock those elbows, and wiggle those ankles. The members not only looked good, but they could actually stay on for an hour at a time. This gave those members great status in the gym. And some were even reportedly seen sweating, but that was only in the southern states.

Still, the members needed more change and stair machines gave way to elliptical machines, which gave way to treads, which led to treads that do steep incline, which led to who knows what is coming next?

The members seek change. They are aware—through magazines and by visiting other gyms—of what's hot and what's coming next. Change makes it more fun and maybe that next machine will be the one that gets that particular member in shape. At least he thinks so.

Mistake #8: The club fails to target renewals.

Eighty percent of your business is derived from 20 percent of the customers and the Pareto principle holds true here as it does in so many other businesses. In any club, there is a small core of members who generate an overproportional share of the club's revenue.

This core of members brings in the most referrals, supports the profit centers in the gym, and usually spends the most money overall throughout the year. In relationship to renewals, this means we need to learn to target the renewals we really want and not necessarily broad-based programs that chase all members equally.

Yes, we need to concentrate on all the members' first 30 days because many of the members set their perceptions of what the club is about during that time and few clubs put enough of their resources into that time frame. But we also need to be aware of the period at the end of the memberships and then spend our time and energy on the members we really want to keep and who we depend on for the money they spend with us. For example, a member who participates in the club's nutrition program, trains regularly, makes a few pro shop purchases on a frequent basis, and participates in the club's social events is more important to the club's revenue stream than a member who rarely trains and is frequently late paying.

Some gyms develop special teams to chase renewals. This could be a small group of the best employees or just one key employee in the smaller clubs who dedicates special time to contacting and surveying targeted members up for renewal.

The focus of the renewal team is to learn how to identify and fix the problems the potential renewals present when they are contacted. Many members who do decide to leave could be saved if someone contacted them for a different reason than to just get the person to renew. These members may have small problems they have never had a chance to express to anyone in any authority on the staff—usually problems that could be solved simply.

When chasing lost renewals, try to talk to as many as possible about why they didn't renew. What went wrong? How could the staff have gotten involved earlier to save the person? Talking to lost customers can help you figure out where your business has failed in the past, where it is today, and where it should go tomorrow.

Mistake #9: The club does not contact members on a regular basis.

You have to keep the members part of your family and make them feel they belong. The web and all its derivatives, such as social networks, allow us to touch each member weekly without incurring any expense. These weekly touches keep the members connected to the club even though they might not work out that week.

The following are the basics as of today that you should do to keep the members in contact. Keep in mind that by the time this sentence was finished, it might be outdated, but at least look at the general concepts here and apply them to whatever media you have available at the time:

- *Your web site should be entirely video driven.* Videos are the new words and even your introduction to the club should be a short video clip by someone on the staff.

- *The first thing a member should see on your website is a sizzle clip, which is a 30-second to 90-second montage of action going on throughout the club.* This should change several times per month.

- *You should post a "Fitness Tip of the Week" every Monday in the form of video.* These clips are then moved to your YouTube channel, where they are archived for people who start their search for a fitness club there or for those who hear your name and simply want to see what you have posted.

- *You should post a short clip daily on your club's Facebook page.* This doesn't have to be professional, but it should be exciting and consistent

- *You should use an electronic format to send a newsletter from the club monthly or twice a month if you can.*

- *You should also have everyone's email to keep them informed of specials in the club or specials you arrange with merchants in the area.* For example, you could go to a sporting goods store and ask it to run a special on workout gear for your members who present their membership cards on Friday from 3 to 6 p.m. You email your members (think flash sale here) and get them into the store. Never under any circumstances let anyone else have access to your list. If it works, go back next month and offer to do the same thing for $500. Do one free email to validate the process and then charge the merchant for repeat mailings. This especially works well with restaurants in your immediate area.

One thing to avoid is any type of "You haven't been in and we miss you" cards. We don't want to remind members that they aren't there, but instead, we should try to give them motivation several times a week to get into the club. The goal here is to keep touching the member throughout the week or, in the case of the website postings, give him a reason to click on something while he is sitting at work. These touches keep the members as part of the family and keep them tied to the club longer.

Summary

Remember, if given a choice, people always prefer to do business with a friend, even if they sometimes can make a better deal elsewhere. If we lost a member, it's because we didn't make that person a friend. This sounds simplistic, but you see it all the time at the best restaurants. People like to be known and they like to feel they belong to something bigger than themselves.

Even that one really fat guy who has been in the club for years and who never gets any results at all likes to hang around if he feels welcome and accepted. If a member doesn't renew with us—and remember the financial implications of that situation—we have to assume it's our fault and do whatever it takes to get him back.

Final points on retention

- *Renewals will be one of the most important issues you have to deal with in the fitness industry in the coming years, meaning that part of your ongoing business plan includes sections on how to exceed the national average in your business.* Your target is 60 percent after adjusting for losses.
- *Track and be aware of the renewal average in your business.* This is one of the most important numbers you need to know because it reflects how your business plan and member service plan are working. You should track this monthly and then compare annually.
- *Remember that the members are a lot like you.* They get bored easily, need to be challenged, seek new and exciting things, and don't like to be taken for granted. For more information on being taken for granted, see your spouse.
- *Renewals will take the pressure off new sales in a fitness business.* Eventually, in most marketplaces, you will run out of new sales.
- *Put together a system that increases a member's chance for success during his first 30 days.* Keep the rules flexible and do whatever it takes to get the member started correctly and confidently. Remember that no one rule will work for every new member.
- *Member service starts at the front counter.* Hire older, more mature front counter people who have good communication skills. These folks set the tone for member service in the club and directly affect the club's renewals.
- *Clubs are extremely high maintenance.* To stay competitive and to keep renewals, the owners need to continually reinvest in their businesses. One rule of thumb is to budget $150 per thousand square feet per month for repair and maintenance, with a minimum of $1,500, and another $150 per thousand square feet for capital improvement, with the same minimum. If the money is not spent that particular month, it should be moved to an accrual savings account for the club because it will be needed eventually.

- *Everything changes, including what members want and expect from a gym.* Great equipment that is still working means nothing if it's outdated or out of style. The members seek change and know what's coming next in the industry. Everything that is current is online at the training sites or featured in the popular magazines. If you want to stay competitive and keep those renewals coming in each month, your gym has to change to reflect the current trends in the marketplace—and not just the latest and hottest piece sold to you at a tradeshow.

- *Move away from the emphasis on first-visit closing.* You still have to sell memberships in this business, but *when* you sell can change. Move toward a trial membership system that truly allows a potential member to try before he buys.

- *All renewals are not equal.* Track and document how members support the club. Target renewals that are the best members, meaning those who come regularly, come to the social events, bring guests, and spend money in the club's multiple profit centers.

January 17, 2014
One of the hardest things to grasp as a consultant …

One of the hardest things to grasp as a consultant is how many people I meet that are in their 30s or older who are so unhappy with their lives. Many people get trapped on someone else's path and you can't be happy living someone else's dream. We start out on our own journey but then get hit with "Why don't you do the right thing here?" or a family person throws "It doesn't matter what you want, this is what you should do." Anytime someone says do the right thing, it means do what that person wants to control your life and it is seldom about what is right for you. Happiness is an art, much like advanced fitness, where you have to study, think, and work to stay on the right path. This weekend, make a list of the top 20 things that make you truly happy. Then, list 20 things you are doing that don't make you happy but that you do to please someone else. Finally, list 10 things you are going to start doing that make you happy and are all about you, your life, and your career. Yes, I am giving you permission to be selfish, but if you aren't happy, it is pretty damn tough to make others in your life happy.

January 20, 2014
Personal pride is personal belief in yourself.

The most successful people take pride in everything they do or touch. If you own a business, you should have deep pride in what you own, how you run it, how the staff treats others, and how clean it is. If you work for someone, you should always bring a deep pride to the job, which is reflected in your refusal to do anything but the best work you are capable of each day. People who do less than they are capable of lack pride in themselves and value themselves poorly. Who at the end of the day can take pride in work that was far below your potential and how can you think so little of yourself that you don't even care how you are judged by that work? Pride is the driver behind personal growth. Pride is the driver behind personal achievement and pride is what separates the average from the great. If you are not accomplishing what you want in life, maybe you just don't care enough internally to take pride in who you are and what you do. Don't worry about what others think about you and care more about what you think of yourself.

10

Short-Term Debt Has Killed More Fitness Businesses Than a Salesperson With Bad Breath

A fitness business can only handle a certain amount of short-term debt at any time during the business's development. When short-term debt rises above a defined percentage of a club's monthly base operation expense, the club is in trouble, although the owner may not realize it until it becomes too late to fix.

In the old days, everyone thought the absolute kiss of death was a salesperson with really bad breath. There was just no other way you could hurt a fitness business worse than by having your lead salesperson slam down three slices of garlic pizza and then tour prospective members. The prospect's reaction was always the same: disbelief, shock, and then maximum distancing.

As the fitness industry has matured, the newer generation of owners with better business skills has identified and is dealing with a new killer. This killer is not just in the fitness industry. It is common to almost all small businesses in general. This hideous beast is too much short-term debt—a killer that slowly chokes a small business to death over time through the restriction of cash flow.

A simple definition of short-term debt is garbage debt. This is high-interest, short-term obligation that is easily obtainable by most owners and is often sought because of this ease and because by using it the gym owner can solve a pressing problem. For example, an owner begins to get a steady stream of complaints from his members about the age and functioning of the club's cardio equipment. The owner instantly reacts first of all because he hates the complaints, and secondly, the treadmill rep is visiting the club that day, so he grabs 10 new treads leased for three years. The problem is solved, but the owner just added yet another big payment to the club based on an aggressive three-year payback. This type of debt is seldom acquired all at one time. It sneaks up on owners over a year or two of normal business, accumulating into a heavy monthly toll on the cash flow.

Equipment leases are a good example of short-term debt because most leases in the industry are for a three-year period, although there has finally been a trend toward five-year financing. The three-year lease is a very aggressive payback at usually a very high interest rate, and although interest rates did fall during the economic turn, most were still much higher than a typical five-year bank loan or more conventional financing. Other examples of short-term debt are car leases, credit card debt, short-term bank notes, and other borrowed money that has a high interest rate attached with a three-year or less payback.

This hideous beast is too much short-term debt—a killer that slowly chokes a small business to death.

High interest and short-term debt hurt the business.

The two negatives that most affect an owner are the interest and the payback period. In almost any state of the economy, interest can be defined as high if it is 10 percent or more. It's not unusual for an owner to have two to three leases at 12 to 18 percent and higher, plus a credit card or two at 18 to 21 percent. Short-term debt is defined as any debt with a payback period of three years or less. Car leases that are run through the business are a perfect example of a three-year, high-interest obligation.

The reason so many owners get buried by so much short-term debt is that the loans and leases are so easy to get and so logical to the owners. Almost any vendor at any trade show can get an owner a quick three-year lease on a pile of equipment. A few papers and a quick pulse check and there you go— new equipment for the gym delivered in 30 days.

From an owner's viewpoint, these leases make so much sense. Pay them off in just three years and own the equipment free and clear. Suffer a little now and make money on the back end after the equipment payments are over.

The problem with this thinking is that it breaks a basic tenet of owning a small business. Stated clearly: There will always be debt if you are running a competitive fitness business. If you want to continue to grow the business, eventually take money out of the business for yourself, and stay competitive in the marketplace, you will always have some amount of debt. The key is not the debt itself but how the debt is managed so it fits your operational plan yet still allows the business to become stable and remain competitive in tougher markets.

Another lesson to learn here is that the majority of owners of any type of fitness business are reactive, which means they only make changes in their businesses when they are forced to by outside entities. For example, the reactive owner is the one who hangs on to his equipment a year or two too long, puts off painting until next year, adapts slowly to new ideas and tech (such as the advent of functional training), and might run a clean, decent club, but that business is always just a little outdated and a few years behind on what is happening in the market. Due to the fact that their businesses are almost always a few years outdated and usually somewhat run down, reactive owners attract competitors into their markets because a competitor always knows that the reactive owner will be slow to update his facility and slow to react to serious competition.

The more rare breed of owner is the one who is proactive. The proactive owner anticipates the market and is always making changes that are ahead of the market curve. Keeping the club several years ahead of the average market keeps competitors away from this market because a current, up-to-the-minute gym is much harder to compete with compared to an older, dated physical plant with older technology.

There is a family-owned licensed gym in Florida that is virtually debt free and is the perfect example of an owner who is totally reactive in his business planning. The owner has an 8,000-square-foot gym with about 1,200 members. The gym's base operating expense is about $40,000 per month and it deposits around $43,000 to $45,000 in a typical month and up to $50,000 during a few of the happening business months of the year. The club is a little more than five years old and is a very clean and organized business. It also has 30 pieces of cardio equipment that are completely paid off. However, the club doesn't have any functional equipment that is accessible to the members except through a trainer. For example, the club does have ropes, kettlebells, and suspension trainers, but it doesn't let the members use them because the owner hasn't been to a workshop in years and he feels he can exploit these tools by forcing the members to go to a trainer to gain access to them. He also feels that the members might not use the tools correctly and may hurt themselves. This same owner has four bench presses on the floor and dumbbells that go up to 100, but he feels the members can handle these without any problems.

This club will start encountering some severe financial problems during the next few years, especially with the addition of new and brighter training-centric competitors, unless the owner rethinks his debt-free plan and decides to reinvent his business.

In this club, the colors are outdated and the physical plant needs quite a bit of upgrading. The cardio works, but it's not cardio anyone wants to use anymore. The members want what's next and what's hot, not eight upright bikes that are at least five years out of style. The club is also a 1995 version of a shrunken fitness center with several lines of fixed-plane equipment that are no longer competitive in the market. Everything is clean and well maintained but also old and not desirable by potential members. Today's members want space, functional tools, and access to all the new training trends they see on TV and in magazines. This club can't survive in a competitive market unless it repositions itself as a training club rather than fighting the bigger chain clubs that have moved into the market by offering a lower monthly price for essentially the same service.

The club owner needs to reinvest, but he is living off the net each month. He and his wife have saved about $50,000 over the last three years, but they could reinvest the entire amount and still not bring the club back to a competitive position. Besides, a typical club should have at least one month's BOE (base operating expense) in reserve and preferably two months' worth if the club is mature, meaning it is at least three years old.

*The only solution is to get in debt: They need to acquire
controlled, managed debt.*

A rule to follow for planning is that every four years, you have to spend what
you spent to build out the club when you opened. For example, if you spent
$40 a foot to build out an 8,000-square-foot club, or a total of $320,000,
you would have to spend another $320,000 during every four-year period to
keep the club competitive. The original $40-per-foot build-out didn't include
equipment, but the reinvestment money that needs to be spent every four
years includes equipment purchases and upgrades.

The fitness business is a lot like the nightclub business. A nightclub may
be wildly successful for two years and then fade away as some other place
becomes that month's hot spot. When this happens, the owners rip out the
old look, give it a new theme, and go again. One year, it's a heavy metal dance
club, and the next year, it's a sports bar. The owners simply changed the decor
to match the changing needs and wants of the market.

Most fitness owners don't understand this concept. Once the gym is
built, it becomes part of the family and there isn't much you can do to get
them to make major changes on a regular basis. That's why you see so many
pathetically old physical plants and equipment in the industry. It's theirs, it's
paid for, and they're going to keep it like that forever. This is also the reason
so many chain box clubs have fought against the advent of functional training.
If you have $500,000 of equipment that is only a few years old sitting on your
floor, then you are not likely to embrace the fact that most of this equipment
has been invalidated by a kettlebell and a 50-foot rope.

Besides, just last week, a prospective member told the owner that his
club is the best club he's ever been in. It may have been the only club he has
ever seen or he may have been working out in even a worse dump, but the
comment is enough to keep the owner going for another year or two without
having to fix up the club. This owner refuses to meet the changing demands
and wants of the consumer, and eventually, the business will suffer because
of this attitude. In other words, this owner will never change until an outside
force, such as a new training club down the street, forces him to change. Lose
200 to 300 members, and suddenly, new paint and a weekend training course
sound a lot more attractive.

The vehicle for this change is controlled debt. Controlled debt means there
is a balance between short-term and long-term debt and between short-term
debt and the monthly base operating expense. The pivotal point in a gym's
development is the five-year mark. All the original short-term debt the club
owner acquired to get his dream started should be paid off and the club's
first bank loan or investor note should be dramatically reduced by this point.
Keep in mind that most investor paybacks and bank loans that don't include
real estate should be 7 to 10 years in length. This is the optimal length that
ensures decent principle payback, coupled with a reasonable monthly payment
that allows the gym to get healthy.

A club can only handle 10 percent of the BOE in short-term debt during the first three years.

As for short-term debt, the club can handle up to 10 percent of monthly base operating expense during the first three years of operation. For example, if a club has a BOE of $50,000, it can handle up to 10 percent, or $5,000, in monthly principal and interest payments. Remember, short-term debt is defined as equipment leases, credit cards, short-term bank loans, car leases, and any other debt that has to be paid off in three years or less.

Anything more than a 10 percent mark starts to choke the club due to the high interest and aggressive payback, especially from the credit cards, personal bank notes, and accelerated payments. Because too much money goes toward interest and accelerated debt reduction, the business is unable to get healthy because the owner has no money to spend on profit center development, keeping the club competitive with equipment and staff education and developing a two-month operating reserve.

After the third year of business, the 10 percent short-term debt ratio should start to decrease. For example, during the first year, the owner buys five treadmills and puts 10 percent down on the lease. At the end of three years, the owner now wants to add four elliptical machines. But this time, the owner puts 30 percent down and has a much smaller monthly payment than the old treadmill payment. Therefore, the owner has reduced the short-term debt ratio.

By the fifth year, the short-term debt ratio should drop to a maximum of 5 percent of the BOE. For example, by this time, the owner should have a stronger equity position in the equipment or should have refinanced all the short-term debt into a long-term obligation, which again is 7 to 10 years.

The club also probably has a long-term note as part of the debt structure for the first five years. In the family-owned club in Florida, it had a five-year note for $250,000 as start-up and build-out capital. The owners also had about $150,000 cash to put into the project.

A five-year note for $250,000 would have a monthly payment of about $5,000, which would be another 10 percent of the BOE. Depending on the short-term debt, this club might have a total debt percentage of 15 to 20 percent of the BOE for the first three years of operation.

The goal is to lower the overall debt percentage to 10 percent of the BOE, meaning 3 to 5 percent short term and the rest long term, which is the percentage the club will probably carry forever as it remodels, upgrades, and trades equipment over the coming years.

One primary tool to reduce the total debt ratio is to refinance all club debt with long-term debt every three to five years using the 7- to10-year position as the target period and the longer 10-year period makes business sense if the interest rate is 8 percent or less.

For example, if a club has a five-year $100,000 note at 10 percent, the payment is about $2,100 per month. If the long-term debt ratio drops to 5 percent of the BOE during the fifth year, the club could simply borrow another $100,000 and maintain the same payment, which is built in as part of the club's BOE. If the club needed money earlier, it could refinance sometime during years three to five, allowing the club to take out and reinvest whatever money it has previously paid down on the note.

Summary

Short-term debt probably kills more small businesses than almost anything else. Start-up gyms are notoriously undercapitalized, so most owners fill the gap by taking on too many high-interest, short-term obligations. The most a club should have in short-term debt during the first three years of operation is 10 percent of the BOE, which is the club's base monthly operating expense, and it should reduce this percentage to 5 percent by year five.

Your goal is to lower the overall debt percentage to 10 percent of the BOE, meaning 3 to 5 percent short term and the rest long term, which is the percentage the club will probably carry forever as it remodels, upgrades, and trades equipment over the coming years.

Year five is pivotal for a club business. The club's total debt structure should be refinanced or restructured during year five so the combination of short-term and long-term debt is no more than 10 percent of the BOE. Preferably, this ratio should be in the 5 to 8 percent range of the BOE, but again, it should cap at no more than 10 percent of the club's base monthly operating expense.

Every gym owner will always have debt if he wants to keep growing and stay competitive. Controlling and understanding this debt and how it affects the business is what sets successful clubs apart from nonproducing businesses.

Consider these points for your business

- When you open a new business, analyze how you are going to capitalize the business. If you depend on too many short-term leases and loans to get started, you will eventually encounter some tough spots in years three to five of your new business.
- Put together an aggressive plan in years three to five to refinance and restructure your business to bring down the total debt ratio. Don't forget traditional bank financing and Small Business Administration loans as sources of revenue.
- Build a set amount of money into your BOE that's used for retirement funds. Don't put all the cash back into the business forever. Everything eventually ends, and when it's time to walk away from your business, you should have money you've put away outside of what the business is worth.
- Set up a capital purchase accrual account for the business and budget about $150 per 1,000 square feet per month for future capital purchases. For example, if you have a 10,000-square-foot gym, you should be saving $1,500 per month for future equipment purchases, which will eventually drive down the debt ratio as you start to pay cash for your equipment

additions. Get into the habit of moving this money into the account each month, even if you don't have any immediate equipment needs. The money will then be there when you need it.

- Don't become a fanatic about reducing your debt. Some owners are so aggressive about paying off loans that they hurt the business. If you have a little extra money each month, pay a payment and a half toward your notes. Much more than this starts to work against you because it's usually at the expense of building a reserve fund, taking money out of the business for the owners, or building up an accrual account for future purchases. Also note that the extra money you pay on notes may be considered as phantom income or profits you have to pay taxes on at the end of the year.

January 7, 2014
Sooner or later, one of the big four will kick your ass.

Life is tough—and especially the fitness business—and no one can hold it together for too long without blinking. The big four are death, divorce, distress, or drugs. You can't live for long without one of those things affecting your life, someone you care about, or your career. It is how you handle these issues that defines your life and who you are as a man or woman. The people with strong core values, such as personal strength, integrity, and the willingness to fight back, always come through the other side. You can't hide from any of these and it is inevitable that one will find you at some point. Remember that these issues may set you back or damage you for a while, but none of them can change who you are and what you believe or take away your belief in yourself and what you want from life.

January 10, 2014
The most important question you can ask the person sitting in front of you ...

The most important question you can ask someone sitting in front of you seeking change is "Why are you doing this and who are you really doing this for?" Unless the person can clearly express the answer to this, he will most likely fail. Most of his friends and alleged support groups really don't care if that person drops 20 pounds. People have their own lives and won't put much effort in helping someone else lose weight or get healthy. If change is going to happen and you are the one who is going to guide this change, then you need to get the client to clearly express why this change is important, and most importantly, you have to get him to find his own private reason to stay with the goal. Self-image, personal confidence, lose weight or die young, be there for your children in the future, or simply achieve a level of health that allows you to be an active participant rather than a passive person watching life go by are all examples of internal generators that keep people coming back every week. Have your person write it down and make him carry it with him every day. Your job is to help him find his reasons to live at a higher level and to accept fitness as a forever lifestyle.

Section 3

MANAGING
WHAT
YOU OWN

11

Making Money in Any Type of Fitness Business Depends on Your Ability to Stay Focused

Stealing a famous quote, many owners in the fitness business lead lives of quiet frustration. This frustration stems from the owners' inability to know what to do each day to make money in their business. If you are slowly starving to death in a business you loved at one point, any idea—even if it is terrible—can seem like the one that can change your fortune. In the world of the lost and ineffective business owner, any bright and shiny idea looks good and these owners will often make bad business decisions because they depend almost entirely on having someone else tell them what they should be doing each day rather than learning the business and learning to make decent decisions themselves. If you don't have a tight focus on what you are trying to accomplish each day, you become like the four-year-old who spends the day chasing bright shiny things and who has the attention span of, well, a four-year-old.

In almost all small businesses, owners fall into two categories: the ones who simply focus on hanging on to what they already have and the ones who seek growth and are willing to accept a little risk in the process. The first category is called *maintenance people* and the second group is called *risk-takers*.

Maintenance owners focus on just one thing: keeping what they have already achieved even if what they have is not enough to be successful over time. Owners who plan their month by just matching the same numbers as the club did last year are examples of a maintenance management style. Owners who hang on to equipment for an extra year past its life span, put off painting their facility for another six months, rip off programming instead of buying proven systems, and hire the youngest and dumbest staff because they can be hired cheaply are all signs that this operator is more focused on just keeping things going rather than trying to grow the business.

Risk-takers are much more rare in small business and are willing to take a little risk if it will give them an advantage in the market or if that risk will allow them to grow their business to a higher financial level. These are the owners who market each month, invest early in proven programs, have a more mature and better trained staff capable of generating income, and are willing to sacrifice a little now in the business, such as painting the club as needed each year, in order to achieve higher retention numbers later. Risk-takers are willing to gamble a little if it will improve their business and are the ones who seek growth rather than taking the chance of becoming stagnant in the market.

The breakdown in the industry of these owners matches the numbers in the previous chapter. In any small business, only about 20 percent of the players make money, about 60 percent just do enough to stay in business, and the bottom 20 percent need to get out and get a job somewhere because they should have never, ever opened their own business. Risk-takers are included in the top 20 percent and maintenance people are the 60 percent and perhaps a small percentage of the bottom-dwellers.

Perhaps the biggest problem with developing a hardcore maintenance management style is that you end up relying on tools and techniques that are no longer effective. There are the guys still out there in the marketplace who keep doing what they did 10 years ago and now wonder why it no longer works. For example, in today's market, there is pretty good evidence that most of what worked in the 1990s doesn't really work today for the club or the member. Long, slow cardio has been proven ineffective for weight loss, crunches destroy your back, circuit training has about a six-week window and then fails for the client, and most standard club business practices, such as the pursuit of pure membership volume, is getting harder to do because so many owners are now flocking toward low price and there are now too many fighting for a shrinking segment of the same market share.

Staying focused on what is important in your business is the foundation of what it takes to be financially successful over time and is often what separates the maintenance people from the risk-takers who make money. The key to developing a focused management style is learning how to keep your business focused daily on creating revenue as well as learning how to project your business into the future over time. Focused management helps you avoid the new, bad idea and makes the need to chase the bright shiny distraction less appealing.

Part of a risk-taker management style is learning to be proactive in your business instead of operating as a reactive to your competition and to what they are doing in the market. To become proactive, you need to understand the importance of planning. Every owner should have the following planning tools in motion at all times:

• A plan for the coming month
• A plan for the next 24 hours for your staff
• A plan for the next 90 days for growth

Other planning tools you will need in your business include the following:
- A 12-month marketing plan
- A staff training plan
- A member service plan

Most owners are totally reactionary by nature. If the guy down the street runs an ad, you run an ad. If the guy down the street lowers his price, you lower your price. If sales slow down for a day or two, you panic and run crazy price specials, hoping you can pack the club overnight.

The guy down the street is not any better of an operator than you probably are, but he is trying to move forward and even a weak plan is better than no plan or no action. He is also running ads under the same conditions that you are in your business—without a long-term plan and probably in reaction to current market conditions or to what he views his competitors are doing.

There are many problems with being a reactionary manager, but perhaps the main one is that you let business happen to you—you don't make it happen or create the business you want. This means you're not creating or growing your business or your revenue by a plan, but instead, you're letting your business be dictated by the surrounding short-term market conditions. Another name for this is *situational management*, which means you react to whatever situation or catastrophe that is in front of you at the time rather than working off a set, well-thought-out plan that keeps you focused on what is important in your business over time.

For example, let's say a club owner wants to generate 60 new memberships a month. Most club owners do set a sales number they would like to achieve that month and most do some random marketing and then hope for the best. Their salespeople may be given a few quotas and the owner may increase marketing that month, but there is still no actual plan in place to generate sales. Setting a number is just a small part of focusing your business. Remember that it is not just setting the number that is important but the "How I will make money and make that number happen?" and the "What is my written plan to make money?" that are really the most important parts of the equation.

There are several problems with this scenario that work against the owner's success. First of all, the sales goal is too short term. Are the 60 sales part of a year-long sales goal based on last year's numbers or is that number just what you happen to need this month to cover the operating expense? Most of the time, a goal such as the 60 sales is totally reactionary, meaning it's based on what you have to have this month to survive and not based on any long-term growth formula for the business. Basing numbers one month at a time keeps your perspective too short term. In other words, you lose the focus over time to project your business ahead and then you fail to create steps that will keep you growing over time by projecting your business into the future. This ability to visualize your business at some stage of success in the future is replaced by "What are we going to do this month to survive?" which blocks you from investing in a plan that ensure the sustainability over time of what you own and have created.

In the previous example, you also need to know how many potential members (leads through the door) the club would need to generate to end up with 60 sales. If the club has a 40 percent closing rate for sales, then it has to have 150 potential members come through the door to end up with 60 sales. The 40 percent closing rate is an almost insurmountable problem for your business because 60 out of every 100 potential clients are walking away. Very few small businesses have the financial resources to continue to market when your sales team can only convert 40 percent of your traffic into new business. The minimum goal for conversions, which will be stated throughout this book, is 60 percent. Anything less than a 60 percent closing rate over time means that the business has a higher likelihood of failure and is harder to sustain in the market.

You also need to know in this example exactly how much marketing to run. However, before you can determine a marketing budget, you first need to know your average response rate for the last several months as well as your cost per lead for potential members.

If the club has had a 1 percent response rate from its marketing, which is good in the real world these days, then it would have to run at least 15,000 pieces in the club's immediate five-mile ring. It is important to look at response rate as a gross average rather than a direct derivative of the marketing itself. For example, if you send out 15,000 pieces, you may only get a small number of people walking in carrying the cards. The important thing to track is that you sent this number of cards and you had 150 potential clients in the clubs from all sources that month. It is getting harder and harder for a club to directly attribute a lead to a specific piece of marketing and you are safer just looking at gross averages, especially because few owners just do one marketing piece at a time.

Keep in mind that 80 percent of a club's membership comes from a three- to five-mile ring or 12-minute drive from the club. Specialty clubs, such as sports performance centers, women-only clubs, and most personal training businesses draw from a larger ring because of their uniqueness and may have drive times (total market availability) of up to 30 minutes.

If the club in this example is using a direct mail tool, such as a flyer insert, and is paying 30 cents for each piece, it would have to spend $4,500 for its marketing that month. This works out to $30 per lead if you divide the 15,000 needed pieces by the 1 percent response rate, reflected by the total leads from all sources through the door for the month, and then divide that number (150) into the $4,500:

$$15,000 \times .01 = 150$$

$$\$4,500/150 = \$30$$

For these numbers to make sense, they need to be part of an annual plan and budgeting process for the club. When annual plans are used, another big problem of reactionary management is covered, which is a lack of consistency in your attempt to create new business for your club. Consistency in marketing in any small business has to be defined as chasing new business and building your brand every single week and every single year you are in business. As the old saying goes, you need to constantly feed the pig because the pig is always hungry for more new business.

In the previous example, the club will probably not be successful in attracting its 150 potential members because it has done nothing to create consistency in its marketing. Most marketing takes at least four months to get any type of traction and then it has to be maintained every month to keep growing over time. If you need 60 sales this month but you don't start your marketing until this month, then your marketing doesn't have time to work, so you probably won't get the desired results.

The goal of all marketing is to develop a recognition factor in the market. Most club businesses of any type need to have a consistent presence in the marketplace. Consistent marketing develops that "top of mind" recognition factor that is so important to any small business. In our case, the need for fitness happens 365 days a year. We simply never know when a client living within our businesses' competitive ring is going to need fitness. Joe Average gets up one day, his pants don't button in the front due to too much beer, pizza, and lousy living, and he at that moment wants to join a club now, today, before he goes home after work. Top of mind means that when this trigger occurs, your club pops into his messy head because he has seen your ads and other marketing every week, every month, every year since he moved near your club. You don't know when the moment is going to happen, but when it does, you want to be in the guy's head at the top of any fitness list he might know.

If the club in the example was using a consistent 12-month marketing plan, it would have real numbers and percentages to work with each month rather than becoming trapped by short-term decisions that might force mistakes. If this owner were making long-term decisions, he could then increase the number of pieces and then anticipate some type of expected result because that month's marketing would be related to all the marketing the club has done over the past 12 months.

In this case, knowing his response rate and cost per lead would allow him to project a higher expected lead base that depends on the increase of his marketing budget. If it costs me $30 per lead to get 150 leads and I am spending $4,500 now, increasing my marketing to $6,000 should correlate to a proportional lead increase. This owner should also work daily on his closing percentage (conversion of leads into new members) because his current rate of 40 percent is not acceptable or sustainable over time. As stated earlier, most clubs of any type have to master at least a 60 percent overall closing rate to be successful or to even stay in business.

Another problem with no long-term planning is that reactionary management simply wastes a tremendous amount of money. Using the previous example again, if a club starts and stops its marketing, it would receive no cost savings from its printers, its newspapers, or its mailing costs if it doesn't run enough pieces to qualify for bulk mail rates and, most importantly, the business has no chance of establishing a recognition factor in the market because it has an erratic brand image.

You can't budget and negotiate long-term discounted rates if your marketing plan is only by the month. For example, with typical newspaper inserts, an owner can save as much as 40 percent of the cost if he commits to a 12-month sales contract. However, most owners won't commit to any type of long-term plan because they don't know what kind of marketing they will be running next month, let alone six months or a year from now. Why? Because they never built a plan that would project their business beyond the end of this month.

Keep in mind that a reactionary management style is not limited just to marketing. Most reactionary managers are reactionary in all aspects of their business. A proactive manager would be watching the trends in the industry and making changes in his club before the market forces him to react.

An example here is the advent of functional training in the first decade of this century. Members were seeing kettlebells on TV; athletes were doing articles in the major fitness magazines on their new approach to building speed, agility, and quickness; and such gurus as Todd Durkin, Mike Boyle, Brett Jones, and Alwyn and Rachel Cosgrove were writing books on how they were getting results based on the new rules of lifting for strength and fitness.

Everything about what we thought we knew about fitness changed except that the owners of most box fitness centers clung to circuit training and other dated ways to get members in shape. Risk-taking owners would have spotted the trend, gone to educational events, and installed everything they needed to be the source in the market. Reactionary owners simply sit and wait to see what will happen, waiting to change until someone or something forces it to happen.

Reactionary managers kept trying to fix the same old problems and kept circuit training as their core offering no matter how much money they were losing or how many members they were losing to the competition. For many owners, it is easier to ride the club down to complete failure than it is to admit what they are doing isn't working and then try something new. However, in clubs run by proactive/risk-taking management, failing programs would be replaced with next generation equipment built on a new training-centric culture in the club.

A reactionary/maintenance manager also encounters problems when it comes to staffing issues. Most major staffing issues start as little problems that could be handled early. For example, a club has a uniform policy backed up in writing in its employee manual. However, the club manager has a maintenance mind-set and just doesn't want to approach an employee who has been with him for a while because it is easier to ignore a problem than it is to correct it. The employee shows up out of uniform and the manager grumbles a little but basically ignores the problem. The employee has now been taught that small deviations from club policies are acceptable.

Most reactionary/maintenance managers ignore things until they get so mad that they go from being quietly reactive to totally proactive, meaning somebody is going to pay and it's today. In the case of the employee and the uniform, by not being proactive and addressing the issue before it becomes a problem, the manager has left no out for himself, except to overreact later when the employee's minor transgressions accumulate into something bigger.

The employee who was taught early that minor rule breaking is acceptable becomes the same employee that drifts in 15 minutes late for his shift. This is also the same employee who will always have problems with the uniform policy because there is no consistent, proactive stance from management. When the big day arrives that the manager is so upset that a confrontation takes place, the damage is already done. It would be very hard to retrain this employee to be any good, and in many cases, it would be easier to replace the manager than it would be to replace all the employees.

The same holds true for member transgressions. The small, constantly grating things members do, such as the guy who drops the dumbbells and then screams, are usually ignored by a maintenance manager whose viewpoint is short term and who is afraid of losing even one member. However, these irritating members cost the gym money in the long run because they damage equipment, scare off the softer members who are intimidated by their rude and dangerous behavior, and may eventually injure other members by having those dumbbells land on someone's feet. In other words, saving a single member payment now might cost the club thousands of dollars over the next year in losses that are based on one nasty member who should have been tossed out.

If such members were corrected the first time or simply removed from the club, all these problems would go away. Proactive managers live with more peace of mind. Reactionary managers are constantly in agony because they only make decisions in a crisis mode.

For an owner to move into a proactive style, he should have a number of plans in place that help project the business into the future. Plans are really guides and goals that keep the business moving forward instead of sideways, away from the ultimate goal of profitability. Being a proactive risk-taker also means that sometimes you have to deviate from your plans. If a club fails down the street and you have a chance to pick up some used equipment at a good deal or can take over its membership, being proactive means you should move on it.

Being proactive in this case means there is an accrual fund for capital improvements and a set financial plan to understand the risks of taking in a large number of members at a price that doesn't jeopardize the business. Being a reactive/maintenance owner means quickly reacting and grabbing the members from the failing club and buying all the used equipment without understanding the ramifications for the rest of your current business.

Business Planning for Fitness Business Owners

In the fitness industry, it's easier to think of business plans as a number of distinct types that have different applications depending on what you are trying to get done in the business.

The following are the plans most owners would use in their businesses and when you would use them, followed by how to implement each in your business:

- *A plan for the coming month:* This plan establishes goals and a plan of action for the coming month. In many ways, this plan may be the most important of all the plans because it keeps you focused on making money during the next month.

- *A plan for the next 24 hours for your staff:* Staff members don't do well with "big" goals that lay out targets for the next quarter or year. Effective owners break down the numbers they are trying to hit for the month into bite-sized chunks that staff can handle mentally. Take care of the next 24 hours and the month's goal will take care of itself.

- *A plan for the next 90 days for growth:* Writing a fresh 90-day plan each month helps you anticipate the bigger issues you might be dealing with, such as planning special promotions or events, making major renovations in the club, or planning an extended marketing campaign.

- *The one-, three-, and five-year business plans:* The one-year business plan might be the most underrated tool in small business. Many owners write a business plan once, which in reality is usually written by their accountant, and then throw it in the desk drawer once the bank has given you your first money. Good owners will update their one-year plan monthly forever and good owners have been known to adjust their plans 30 times or more a year as competition changes, as they add new programming or if their numbers change dramatically. Keeping your business focused into the future, as opposed to being trapped in the present by short vision, is perhaps one of the most important things you can do. The longer plans are really two different ways to look at your business. The three-year plan keeps you focused on operations and the five-year plan is always a version that keeps you thinking about building value into your business so at some point you can get out. Good owners always know how they are going to get out before they get in and a long-term plan that keeps you focused on building up the working value of what you own is part of that process.

- *The 12-month marketing plan (included in the one-, three-, and five-year plans):* Marketing is the area of almost any small business that highlights the maintenance/reactionary management style. Few small business owners plan their marketing in advance and instead rely on panic marketing that is done when the owner becomes desperate for traffic or new sales. Marketing should not be the last thing in the budget but rather the first thing and good owners would fire staff, sell their car, or do almost anything they can do to keep from not marketing. If you are hungry, you buy food first with whatever money you have. If your business is starving, reflected by the need for new sales or business, you have to feed it and the small business version of fresh meat is leads generated by your marketing. Planning out marketing, even if it is low-budget, person-to-person handouts at the mall, will keep your expenses down and keep you focused on the need to keep working every month forever to keep the pig fed.

- *The staff training plan (included in the one-, three-, and five-year plans):* Blocking out set times, such as Friday afternoon from noon until 4 p.m. (yes, we really do work like a real businessperson in this industry), and then projecting your staff training into the future overcome many of the weaknesses a typical small business suffers from daily. For example, lost

Making Money in Any Type of Fitness Business Depends on Your Ability to Stay Focused

clients many times stem from bad customer service and inexperienced or out of touch owners blame their staff for these lost clients when in reality the staff person standing at the front counter answering the phone and servicing members has only been trained about an hour a month and has only had a few days of training combined during her entire tenure with the club. You cannot train staff once and then expect them to get it. Staff training is every week for as long as you own the business. Your staff will slowly develop into effective workers through the constant repetition of what is important to you and your business. This takes time and planning and setting aside a weekly block of time ensures you stay on task with your team.

- *The member service plan (included in the one-, three-, and five- year plans):* Member service is not accidental or random. It is not hiring a bunch of smiley people and putting them at the front desk. Good service is a written plan of attack that covers everything from cleanliness to how to handle complaints. Service has to be planned for, taught to staff, and structured as part of the business plan to be effective.

Your plan for the coming month

The most important week in the month for most fitness business owners should be the last week of the month, which is when you set your financial targets for your business for the coming month. The unbreakable rule here is that you never start a month without a clear plan to make money. This plan has to not only reflect the actual dollar amount you are projecting for the business, but it must also include a detailed assignment of every dollar projected to an individual on your team.

For example, if you project a total deposit of $70,000 for the coming month, that number then has to be broken down by department and then by individual. Remember the fundamental rule of creating staff performance: There is never production unless there is individual accountability. Everyone on your staff has to be involved in the moneymaking process as an individual with a defined responsibility as to how he contributes to your business and to the overall revenue.

However, just knowing the number is not enough to be successful. You must also establish the "what" and the "how" if you want to hit that number. The what and the how refer to what are we going to do and how are we going to do it to turn this number from a projection on paper into a real dollar deposited in the bank. The number is not relevant unless there is a plan that states how you are going to do it and what has to be done by the team to make this number become real. It is a good habit to start writing a three- to five-page mini business plan for the coming month, with a separate page on all the key anticipated revenue sources in the club. Too many owners talk about numbers, but few can explain just how those numbers are going to be reached.

Most small business owners start the month with a hope that something good will happen. They hope the business will pick up. They hope summer will save them. They hope that last month's weak numbers were just a weird one-time happening that won't be repeated this month. Hope is not a business plan.

A business plan is a business plan. Hope is how you run your business when you don't have any plan whatsoever in place to create revenue. Good owners project every dollar they want to make in the coming month and then assign that dollar to someone on the team who is now responsible to make it happen.

Learning to project your monthly revenue

The first projection number you need to master in your business is the target deposit. The target deposit (TD) is the total of all revenue that runs through the business for a given month. For most fitness-related businesses, this includes the recurring net receivable base, the income from new sales, and the income from the business's profit centers. Let's define these terms further before we apply them to our calculations:

- *Target deposit (TD):* This is the money from all sources that is generated by your business that month and then deposited that month. This is the actual cash deposits (cash, credit cards, checks) made that month and not the value of a membership that will be collected in the future. If you have extra sources of income beyond that related to memberships and normal business operations, such as rental revenue from a subletter, you may choose to add this revenue or not. Just be consistent each month by doing it the same way each time. Broken down even deeper, the TD includes the net check you receive each month from the total of your member/client payments, any day-to-day cash generated from such things as drink sales, shakes, or training paid for by credit card, and new sales cash, such as down payments on memberships or a daily workout fee.

- *Net receivable base:* Most fitness business owners let their members pay for their membership each month using a contractual obligation. Some use contracts for 12 months or others just go month to month. (Pricing systems are discussed later in this book.) Most aspects of training, such as personal training or group personal training, are also now being done using monthly payments over time (mostly 12 months) rather than the dated style of just sessions or packages, which fail to establish any stability for the business. Successful clubs also usually farm out most routine tasks that get in the way of daily production. Therefore, most use a strong third-party financial service company to collect the monthly member payments directly from the members/clients. The amount returned to the club each month is the net collected, and if the club is using 12-month memberships, this number reflects an amount of the club's outstanding receivable base.

- *Income from new sales:* Most club owners collect a one-time membership fee when a new member joins the club. The club will also collect daily fees, short-term paid-in-full memberships, and other various fees that are classified as new income from sales. This number usually represents about 10 to 12 percent of the total deposit for the month. Few fitness businesses still expect members to pay in full for the year. If the business does collect for a year in advance, which is not recommended, the amount is usually in the $99 to 199 per year range.

- *Profit center income (nondues revenue):* Any money a member pays that is not related to working out or for a membership is usually derived from a club's profit center. These might include but are not limited to supplements, munchies bars, training revenue, cooler drinks, tanning, day spa, specialty classes, or any other offering the club has that allows a member to make a purchase that day in the club not related to working out. In recent years, another source of income has developed for fitness businesses through online sales. For example, some training clubs now offer workouts online for members to use when they travel or for virtual members who want help from that club but who also might live too far away to visit regularly. It is important to note here that progressive club owners separate their training revenue from their membership income. This has especially become important because most training facilities and mainstream clubs have now replaced their short-term training tools, such as packages and sessions, with extended programming, including group personal training, small group training, and unlimited one-on-one pampering memberships that include everything the client would need to be successful. The goal of this business shift is to establish a recurring income stream from training that surpasses the club's established membership revenue, which in effect gives the club a huge competitive advantage in the market because it is generating more revenue from members already in the system than it does from just its membership. As a side note, if your club's total training revenue is less than 20 percent of your net receivable base, you are just in the membership sales business and are leaving an enormous amount of monthly income on the table. Your goal again in a progressive club is to get your monthly training revenue to an equal or greater number than your membership revenue.

The projection concept

Owners not experienced in projecting revenue all make the same mistake: They look at what they did the same month last year and then either try to match that number or slightly beat it. This is not an effective way to project revenue for several reasons. First of all, using prior history can be restrictive in making a projection for this year.

For example, let's say that last year, the club did $67,000 in total revenue deposited for the month in question. Most owners will look back at that month when they are approaching the same month this year and decide that if they just beat or at least match that number, then they are doing good work. However, this is a very poor goal for the owner because it does nothing to reflect the current state of the business.

In the same month this year, there might be an extra Monday, which is always good for any type of fitness business, and also this year, you have a new manager, you started marketing again, you added functional equipment, you did extensive customer service training, and you had a competitor fail. Your business this year looks nothing like the one you were running last year. In fact, you might leave thousands of dollars left untapped if you do nothing more than put together a plan to just match last year's performance.

And don't forget that the cost of running a business has also most likely increased in the last year—at least by point or two. The number that will be mentioned often in this book, as well as in all the other books I've written about the business of fitness, is that you must continue to grow your business by at least 3 to 5 percent per month every year.

Every component in the business can continue to grow each year except for new sales, which will always top out in your market due to the length of time a potential member will drive to be part of your business. Each market has natural limiters based on population, competition, and affluence, which all affect your ability to continually drive up new sales each year. However, you can continue to drive up total revenue by learning to chase a higher return per member rather than just chasing more volume.

The following sections define some key terms that will be used in learning to project your income efficiently.

History

History is a comparison of the coming month with the same month last year. History is the most used method of projecting future revenue but is the least effective because so many things change in a business from year to year. If you based your projection for this year on just history, you most likely would be looking at a lower number than you should achieve. Keep in mind that a variety of factors, such as an extra Monday in the month, new staff changes, the loss or addition of competitors, more marketing, or a change in the economy could all affect how the business is performing this year and last year's reference point has little value this year.

History is almost always a limiter for your business because just matching or slightly beating last year's numbers is almost always less than you should be doing. An example of a simple history comparison would be to look at whatever month you are targeting this year and compare it to last year's number. For example, last June, the club had a total deposit of $67,000, which becomes the historical reference for this June.

On the other hand, if your market has declined, a historical reference at least gives you a minimum target, although this target is probably no longer valid because there is always more than one factor that changes in a business. In the case of a declining market, you may need to build a new projection from scratch using current trend lines, which are discussed next.

Trend lines

A trend line is more effective for projecting a target deposit because we are using history as a mere reference point, but we now add the percentage of change using comparable time periods. In essence, you are replacing a single reference point (history) with a much more dynamic view of how the business is performing over a certain time period. For example, if you looked at a still photo of someone doing a golf swing, he might look like he is performing the swing well, but if you replace the swing with a short video clip, you then might see that the guy has a terrible swing and that the single still photo was a poor representation of the actual ability of the athlete. In this case, history is the single picture and the trend line represents a dynamic look of how your business is performing overall.

Let's look at an example of projecting the target deposit for a fitness business. The target deposit is the total amount of money the business will deposit from all sources for the month. Most fitness facilities only have three sources of income for the business:

- *New sales money*, defined as any new money that arrives as part of the sale of any type of membership or to simply workout in the facility, including membership fees, short-term membership money, daily drop-in fees, or paid-in-full memberships of any type
- *Multiple profit center money*, defined as any new money that is derived from someone who is already a member, such as revenue from supplement sales, training packages, or perhaps spa services
- *Receivable base income (recurring income)*, defined as the net collected from all your members who make payments each month to belong to the facility. It is recurring because most clubs use some form of membership that allows the club owner to project income into the future, such as a 12-month membership. If you just let the members pay month to month, you have cash flow, but that is not as secure as having members on contracts/membership agreements, although cash flow can still be projected into the future.

The goal of any type of fitness business should be to build up an as large as possible recurring income stream. The most effective way to do this is to develop one stream of income based on memberships to your facility and a second that represents your training revenue. The current trend is to do away with short-term sessions and packages for training and replacing them with longer-term commitments that help the owner develop this second stream of revenue that can be projected into the future.

The target deposit for the club is the combination of the income/revenue from these three groups. The formula looks like this:

$$\text{Target deposit} - \text{EFT average} = \text{daily needed cash through the register}$$

The EFT average, or the net proceeds from all member payments collected from the club's third-party financial service company or your own system, can be projected using a three-month average. Remember that EFT stands for electronic funds transfer, or the ability for the club to automatically deduct membership payments from a member's credit card or checking account.

To project your net EFT from membership, simply take the net checks from the last three months and do a simple average.

Example: During the last three months, the net collected from the third-party financial service company checks was:

- May: $40,000
- April: $39,000
- March: $38,000

$117,000 (three-month total)/3 = $39,000 average

This simply means that the club can count on approximately $39,000 per month on average from the net proceeds of its current member payments. This is money that is part of the target deposit, but because it is somewhat automatic, the club's manager or owner only has to concentrate on generating income through new sales revenue and through the club's profit centers, such as training.

The following is an example of a typical club's projection for total target deposit using history as a reference and a trend line as the key indicator:

Month	Last Year's Total Deposit	This Year's Total Deposit
May	$60,000	$64,500 (9% increase)
April	$58,000	$64,380 (11% increase)
March	$55,000	$60,500 (10% increase)

This club is showing a 10 percent average increase over the same three-month time period last year. Using the trend line method, the club should be able to maintain the 10 percent increase for the coming month of June this year. Obviously, if we based this projection on just history, the club could beat the $67,000 target by a few thousand dollars but still underperform in comparison to its trend.

During June last year, the club deposited $67,000.

Projected total for June this year = $73,700
(illustrating the current growth trend of 10 percent
for the last three months)

$67,000 (June last year) + 10 percent (trend line) = $73,700
as a total deposit for the club

As you can see from this projection, this club is trending at a 10 percent growth rate for the last three months. Most owners in this situation know and understand that the business is having a few good months or a current good run, but very few owners take the time to establish a performance trend and then apply this number to projecting the business into the future.

This formula can also be used to project any other aspect of the business, such as sales or training revenue. The key concept here is that what you did in the past is not nearly as relevant as how the business is performing in the present. By basing your future revenue on what happened a year ago, you will most likely limit the potential of your business.

24 hours at a time

Now that you have this projection number, what do you do with it and how do you get your team engaged in helping you generate this revenue each month? Effective owners understand that most of the people they hire in their businesses are usually good people willing to work hard, but few have a great deal of business maturity, meaning that your team will usually not respond to goals that involve yearlong work. For example, in the real business world, many companies work off of year projections and quarterly goals, but keep in mind that many of these companies are usually stocked with a more sophisticated workforce.

The teams we usually hire, except for our management team, just do not have the business experience necessary to stay focused on numbers projected so far into the distance. Therefore, the most effective way to motivate a hard-working but inexperienced business team is to break all the numbers we need to hit into bite-sized 24-hour chunks.

The daily focus meeting

In the previous example, the club needed $73,700 to hit its target deposit. Knowing that number is important, but just knowing the number without a plan to generate that revenue is worthless.

We also know that the club is expected to receive $39,000 net from its third-party financial service company.

$73,700   (the club's total target deposit)
– $39,000   (the expected net from the club's receivable base)

$34,700

This club must do $34,700 through the register that month to meet its goal.

$34,700/31 days in the month = $1,119 per day

In this example, the club owner and manager have to get the team focused on generating $1,119 per day for the month. This number has to serve as a focus tool to keep the management team and, therefore, the staff always concentrating on doing what is important in the business on a daily basis.

It is worth noting here that many owners confuse busy with being effective. Your day can be filled with trips to the accountant, bank deposits, staff issues, toilets that are clogged, disgruntled members, and other busy work that gets you into the club early and out at dinnertime. You had a really busy day, but you forgot an important point: You didn't make any money today. You were undoubtedly busy, but you were not effective. Busy is busy, but effective is something entirely different.

One of the most important things you can learn early in your business is that if it gets in the way of production, get somebody else to do it. The saying that is used often in a productive gym is that 95 percent of what we do every day in a fitness business is to sell somebody something. We are a production-based business, meaning our job is to create fresh revenue every day. If something gets in the way of that production, get an assistant, farm it out, or simply don't do it.

For example, many owners want to collect their own memberships, thinking they will save a few bucks. Why would you create a bureaucracy and try to collect locally for a single club when you can hire a third-party financial service company with thousands of clients and that has been in the business of servicing memberships for fitness businesses for over 30 years? The same question applies for such club processes as payroll, accounting, and marketing. Why do it yourself when you can pay professionals to do it better and more effectively, allowing you to focus on the most important thing in the business, which is selling somebody something every day?

The $1,119 number we created in this example represents your business plan for the week. Your goal is to put together a plan representing the "How are we going to hit this number?" and the "What can we do to make this happen?" Remember, it is not just knowing the number that is important. It is the "how" and "what" that will make it a reality.

You should really write a business plan for the week even if it is only one sheet. Use this mini business plan to answer the big questions, such as "Where will those leads really come from?" or "How many guests will we convert to a higher priced training option and how will we get this done?"

This mini-plan allows you to stay focused on one day at a time and then extend it slightly to a full week. Once you get focused on the daily number, stated clearly in your plan, you will slowly learn to do the big things first in the business and delegate or eliminate the other things that get in the way of production. Remember, not every activity in the business is equal, but when you don't set priorities by focusing on the things that make you money, you can easily fall into the trap where going to the bank to make a deposit looks just as important as a 10-minute staff training or closing a sale. Knowing the difference and creating a plan to focus will be what separates you from the businesses that don't really make any money.

Running your business from Monday through Sunday

This might sound obvious, but if you aren't doing this yet, it is a good habit to get into early. Setting goals starting on Monday and then running the goal through the close of business on Sunday allows you to take advantage of Mondays, which are usually strong, as well as allowing you to adjust the numbers to reality as the week progresses.

As shown in the earlier example, we seldom make money at an $1,119-a-day clip. In reality, you will probably have a heavy early week and then things will slow down on Friday, followed by a strong early Saturday and then a flat Sunday. Effective planning and projection recognizes this fact:

$1,119 daily number needed x 7 days in the week =
$7,833 goal for the week

On Monday, the club does $4,200 through the register.

$7,833 − $4,200 = $3,633/6 days remaining in the week =
$605.50 (the adjusted daily goal)

Each day, you keep adjusting the needed daily cash down. The somewhat funny way to look at this is that on Monday in this example, you need $7,833 for the week, and by counting down each day, the Sunday staff person, who is usually the team rookie and not always that productive, might only need $12 to finish the week and help the team make its goal.

A plan for the next 24 hours

So far, we have figured out how to project the number and we have discussed the importance of knowing how and what you need to do to make those numbers a reality, but we still haven't made the transition from establishing the numbers to what it takes to get the staff involved. Getting the numbers to your staff and getting them involved takes daily effort on your part. Don't forget that we are trying to get a typically young and not always business experienced staff to buy into the club's mission for the month, which is to generate revenue resulting in a profit.

Translating the numbers for the staff involves two separate tools:
• Visual management
• The daily meeting

The skill of visual management

Visual management has been around for a number of years, but it is one of those skills that seem to have been lost somewhere when owners and managers fell in love with their computers.

The temptation in this business is to turn everything into a high-tech solution, including workouts and daily management. However, there are a few things that should not be relegated to the world of sitting at a desk behind your computer screen.

The daily operational things we do that benefit from technology are usually the processes in the business, such as the collection of member payments and most reporting and member scheduling. Technology has made these once a nightmare jobs highly efficient and doable by the most naive tech operator in the world, freeing up owners and managers to escape the trap of sitting in an office and believing you are making money.

On the other hand, there are some processes in the business that become more ineffective when more technology is supplied. One example is paying bills. Computerizing bill paying by a bookkeeper and even eliminating checks altogether by using online banking can streamline your operation and shorten a once time-consuming and boring activity, but by doing this, we have also lost one of the most efficient teaching tools for staff, which is the bill paying committee.

Establishing a bill paying committee is an easy thing to do. During the last week of the month, give each key member of your management staff (or those who you think someday might become a manager) a simple folder with a single sheet of paper stapled inside. Divide the paper into three columns: one for projecting all the bills for the coming month, one to list the actual bills when they arrive, and a third for plus/minus that determines if the actual bill came in over or under your projected amount.

The bill paying committee meets every Tuesday morning at 8 a.m. to review all the actual bills that have arrived since the last meeting and to then make adjustments on their sheets, reflecting if the bill was as budgeted or if it came in over or under the projection. The goal of the committee is to come up with ways to save money for the company by figuring out how to reduce the operating expense. Each bill should be discussed and compared to the projected number from the start of the month and then the team should come up with ways to cut that bill or eliminate it if possible. Offer a $50 to $100 bonus for every idea that saves money that is big and be open to any idea that might work.

The team does not pay bills in this case. It is recommended that you only pay bills twice a month—usually on the 5th and 20th or on the 10th and 25th. Paying bills every day ruins the budgeting process, as do CODs, which should be turned into net 30 terms as soon as you establish that you pay your bills on time.

The purpose of the team is for the members of your team to understand what it costs to run the business and how they as a group can affect the numbers. This is a low-tech solution, but it is still a great way to get the team focused on the business. Managers simply do better jobs when they have a greater knowledge of what it takes to run the business and how they affect those numbers through their daily jobs.

The real concept to explore here is developing the skill of visual management and using this skill to keep your staff focused on the numbers they need to achieve today, this week, and for the month. This is also a low-tech but effective way to manage the business and your staff.

Visual management centers on focusing on the key indicators of the business and then tracking those indicators daily on a wall in the manager's office or in the employee room. These numbers are tracked by either the manager or by the department heads depending on the size of the club. You should still do this, though, even if you are a one-person club. As noted earlier, no matter how big or small your business, you will always have the pull toward equating being really busy with being effective. The numbers on the wall are there to keep your head in your business and on hitting the key numbers daily that will add up to a successful month.

Key indicators are numbers that are important to our industry but may not have much relevance in other small businesses. For example, food costs in the restaurant business is one of the most important numbers to track but has no value to anyone in the fitness business. On the other hand, average EFT per client sale is an important number for a fitness business owner to track, but it is a worthless number for any other small business.

Key indicators can be defined as numbers that immediately tell you how you are doing in the business, where the weaknesses might be, and where you should focus your energy. For example, if you are tracking leads, which represents the amount of potential business you have coming through the door, and that lead number is good based on your need but your conversion rate from potential client to real client is weak, then you don't have a lead problem, but you do have a sales training issue that has to be addressed now, today, because your business can't overcome too many lost leads.

The following sections detail 10 key indicators you should be tracking now. There are many more numbers you might eventually end up tracking and it is not uncommon for an experienced owner to track up to 90 different numbers visually flowing down the wall in the office throughout the month. Start here, though, with the basic 10 and add more as you gain experience and confidence:

#1: Leads/tours

This is the number of qualified potential buyers you have through the door each day. This number does not count phone calls. Only count butts in seats with your sales team. The following chart shows what the leads might look like flowing down the wall in your office.

Leads/Tours Target for the month = 150 Target per day = 5 (30-day month)			
Day	*Today*	*Cumulative Total*	*+/- Target (Cumulative)*
Day 1 (Sunday)	3	3	-2
Day 2 (Monday)	2	5	-5
Day 3 (Tuesday)	0	5	-10
Day 4 (Wednesday)	7	12	-8
Day 5 (Thursday)	6	18	-7
Day 6 (Friday)	5	23	-7
Day 7 (Saturday)	4	27	-8
Day 8 (Sunday)	9	36	-4
Day 9 (Monday)	9	45	0

#2: Conversion rate/closing percentage for the team

How many potential clients became real members? Only count long-term memberships here. Inexperienced staff usually takes the easy way out by selling the shortest-term membership on the list. Your goal is to convert at least 60 to 65 percent of all potential members into long-term memberships (defined as at least six months or longer).

#3: Conversion rate/closing percentage for each individual on the sales team

New salespeople should be closing about 40 percent during their first three months of work. After that point, everyone needs to be at the 60 to 65 percent mark, and if an individual is not hitting that number, he needs to get some spot training to bring his numbers back to the target. Tracking individual rates also keeps a little peer pressure on because all these numbers are posted on a wall for everyone to see.

#4: Annual sales

This number is referenced as part of the conversion rate mentioned earlier. Your goal again is to convert at least 60 percent of all qualified leads into new members during a 30-day period. Most people reading this book will probably be using some type of trial membership, such as a paid trial (for example, 30 days for $39) or a risk-free trial (21 days free). If you are using a trial membership as your primary marketing tool, do not worry about trying to sort the person by the month he signed up in. For example, if a trial member signs up for his trial at the end of March but becomes a real member in April, do not try to go back and count him in March. Simply count his membership in the month he signed up and figure his membership against all potential members that are registered that month. It all averages out, and by doing it this way, it keeps the paperwork much simpler.

#5: Average EFT per sale

This might be one of the most important numbers to know about your business. For example, in a club with a single membership of $39, if you averaged the payments from the last 50 memberships sold (disregard the membership fee or any money taken the first day), you would find that practically every club you would review would have an average monthly payment that is less than the single monthly payment, which in this example is $39. The average number will usually be less because most clubs offer discounts for so many types of memberships. For example, a club might have discount for couples, discounts for students, discounts for seniors, and discounts for corporate memberships. Look closely and you will find that most clubs that list their membership price at $39 in reality average about $27 to $32 per true monthly average. (Divide couples by two if they are on the same membership agreement.) Your goal in this system is to get your average EFT/monthly payment higher than the price for a single member. The only way to do this is to add a layered pricing system to your business plan. This will be discussed in depth later in the book, but for now, look at this example. This club sells memberships for a $49 membership fee and has a simple access membership to the club (floor and cardio access only/no classes) of $39. This club also has additional 12-month memberships for training layered on top of the regular simple access membership.

Sales for a typical day:
- $39 x 12 (simple access membership to the club)
- $39 x 12
- $39 x 12
- $39 x 12
- $79 x 12 (group personal training done with one trainer and in groups, sharing the cost of the trainer with up to 12 clients; offered 8 to 12 times per week on a schedule; normally a structured workout done for the entire month)
- $39 x 12
- $129 x 12 (semiprivate training done in groups of up to four; more instructional than the regular group personal training; offered 20 to 30 times per week depending on membership. The workouts change daily. It should be noted that the client for semiprivate small group training is a different person altogether from the large group personal training: normally older, more into the coaching rather than the music and energy, and usually more affluent.)

In this example, the club sold seven memberships for the day and has a monthly EFT/payment average of $57.58 ($403 total of the monthly payments divided by seven memberships sold). The important thing to note here, of course, is that the club's membership for a single person with simple access to the club is $39, but the club sold seven memberships on a single day and obtained an average of more than $57.

It is also important to note that this system allows you to show a low entry point in a competitive market—in this case, the $39—yet generate a higher return per membership sold by using a layered pricing system.

#6: The daily number/total deposit

This is the number that was calculated in the earlier example illustrating how to project revenue for your business. In that example, the total target deposit for the club was $73,700 and the daily number—after adjusting for the net receivable check from your third-party financial service company—was determined to be $1,119. The following chart shows what tracking that number would look like flowing down the wall in your office.

The Daily Number Target for the month = $73,700 Target per day = $1,119 per day			
Day	*Today*	*Cumulative Total*	*+/- Target (Cumulative)*
Day 1 (Monday)	$3,800	$3,800	+$2681
Day 2 (Tuesday)	$2,460	$6,260	+$4022

#7: The usage rate

The usage rate represents the amount of money spent per member in the club each day per member visit on the club's profit centers. For example, let's say the club has 500 visits on a Monday and the members spent $1,500 on nondues items, such as training, supplements, and spa services or at the sports bar. In this example, the club's usage rate for all profit centers is $1,500/500 = $3. In other words, members spent $3 per member visit that Monday on stuff in the club that wasn't related to paying to work out. The goal is to establish a baseline for each profit center and then work to increase those numbers each month. The higher the usage rate in the club, the higher return per member you are generating, which lowers the club's vulnerability in competitive marketplaces.

You should track all the profit centers as a combined number, but you also have to track each one separately. If you just combine them, you will often find that one strong one will mask the ones that aren't performing and that need work.

#8: The number of visits the club gets monthly, weekly, and daily

These numbers have a number of uses in the business. As noted earlier, daily visits are the key to determine the effectiveness of your club's profit centers and their penetration rate into your membership. These numbers can also be used to determine the effectiveness of new programs, times of the year to raise or decrease staff, and how badly a new competitor might be dinging you. The number of daily visits is a solid example of a number your accountant might never mention but is a key indicator of performance in our business.

#9: The number/percentage of conversions

Most of you will at some point be using a layered pricing system. As referenced earlier, most clubs in today's market seek to show a lower entry point in order to attract a wider range of clients but then build a series of layers on top of that low price designed to meet the needs and wants of the widest range of clients possible. Pricing will be covered in depth later, but it is necessary to illustrate a sample structure here so you can grasp the idea of conversions. The following is a sample structure for a typical mainstream club. This concept was originally developed for training clubs, and then after several years of validation in that environment, it was tested and then broadly applied to the mainstream market:

- *$19/$39 x 12 months for simple access to the club:* In this example, this would only include access to the training floor and cardio. The club owner would choose either $19 or $39 as his low price depending on the market.

- *$69 x 12 months for unlimited entrance into group personal training:* This category attracts a group of members that most mainstream clubs don't normally get as clients. Group personal training is normally restricted to 12 to 15 people maximum and is led by a personal trainer, not a group exercise person. There is also normally a fixed structure for a 30-day period involved as well as good music. Most owners using this format follow some form of this structure:

  - ✓ *The one-minute meet and greet:* Everyone in the group gets a chance to meet each other prior to the workout beginning. This is a tool used to build individual relationships in the group, which leads to increased retention over time.

  - ✓ *A 12-minute dynamic warm-up:* This is done as a group.

  - ✓ *A 20-minute strength segment:* This is traditionally taught in a two-minute on/one-minute rest format that allows the coach to mix levels by either reduced time or decreased load or both.

  - ✓ *The three- to five-minute big finish:* This is the metabolic crusher at the end, sending the group home sweaty. This is normally done in a group, but it can also be done in stations too.

  - ✓ *The group hug:* Everyone is brought together at the end and thanked for being a member and for the good work he accomplished today. No one ever leaves without being thanked for being a client.

  The club would offer 8 to 12 group personal training sessions a week depending on the number of members, time of year, and experience with the program. The target market for this group was originally the 24 to 44 age group, but this is proving to be somewhat on the young side and many clubs have seen the average age of this group climb as the members get more experience and more confidence in their ability to do it.

- *$99 to $149 x 12 months for entrance into unlimited semiprivate small group training:* This is smaller groups limited to a maximum of four, but experienced club owners will sometimes extend this upper limit to six. These are offered on a set schedule each day, although many clubs just start groups on the hour once they get to a certain number of members, who then just drift in at the start of each hour throughout the day. The main difference between the small group offering the large group experience is that large group is a structured group usually taught the same for the entire month based on progressions and music. The semiprivate group is based on the workout of the day idea and usually written on a large chalkboard in the club's training area and the coach will stop and teach new moves and concepts without worrying about stopping music or disrupting the energy of the large group experience.

- *$299 to $499 x 12 months for five sessions a month for one-on-one training:* This is more toward the traditional model of training, but the main difference is that a long-term agreement replaces the normal sessions and packages, which are limiters in your ability to attract more clients. In this example, the client can use these five sessions anytime during the month, but the sessions do not roll over into the next month. If the client wants to come more often, he can double the price paid per month or buy five sessions for $299 to $499 (depending on the market) with no discounts for a higher number purchased all at one time. In this program, the coach would design a program specifically for the client. Most clubs using layered pricing will find that they will do less than 15 percent of their training revenue through one-on-one clients. You don't necessarily get fewer clients, but instead, you dilute the number your currently attract in your business by adding categories you might not have attracted prior.

- *$799 to $1,999 x 12 months for unlimited one-on-one training:* This is usually referred to as a pampering membership because the client can have unlimited access to training as well as added value perks built in, such as supplements, spa services, massage, munchies bars for the month, and protein powder. Most clubs offering this restrict the actual one-on-one training to two to three times per week for the overzealous who want to come almost every day by guiding the client into using the other offerings a few times per week, such as getting him into the group personal training. It is important to note that in a layered pricing structure, the member gets everything noted included as part of his membership as well as the membership to the club itself. It does not make sense to charge a client for a membership to the club when he is paying you a $100 a month to be a training client.

Based on this membership model, the owner/manager would need to track daily the total number of clients who opt to either take one of the higher-priced offerings or who starts as a regular member and then later exchanges that membership for a higher-priced one. Conversions in this case means that the client converted from a lower-priced membership into a higher-paying one.

Your goal for conversions would be to convert 40 percent of all new members for that month into buying a membership that is priced higher than the simple access, low-priced membership. Compare this to the 3 to 6 percent penetration rate that a typical mainstream club achieves for the amount of members involved in training when only using the old-style one-on-one model. Layered pricing will simply attract a wider range of clients to your training program—either due to the more affordable pricing and the ability to share the cost of the trainer or due to the different offerings that appeal to totally different clients than the club is currently attracting to its training program.

#10: Retention numbers

There are a number of ways to look at this depending on your type of club. Mainstream clubs should be tracking the total number of members retained adjusted for losses. For example:

100 new members – 24 percent due to losses = 76
members left at the end of the year (assuming all 100
members are on a 12-month contract)

76 x .65 (targeted retention rate) = 49.4

In other words, this club signed up 100 new members on a 12-month contract/membership agreement in a typical month and by the end of the year retained 76 after normal club losses. The losses are defined as the following:

- About 1 percent per month—or 12 percent compounded annually—will leave a typical club by simply moving throughout the year over 25 miles from the club, which in most states results in a legal cancellation for the member.
- There are also loss rates associated with each type of membership. For example, twelve-month memberships usually have loss rates (the person doesn't pay for financial or personal reasons) of a little less than a point per month or about 10 percent per year. In the previous example, we used 12 percent as the annual loss rate, reflecting in a total loss rate of 24 percent for the year for the sample club.

The 76 members at the end of the year won't all stay, of course, but the club should target 65 percent as its retention goal. In this example, this club started with 100 members and going into the next year has 49 left, which is an example of good retention with minimum losses for the club.

The national average for retention is hard to factually determine. For example, many clubs report numbers that are unusually high and are often in the 80 percent range, but this is a virtually impossible number to achieve due to clients moving away, dying, not paying, or simply disputing their memberships.

These clubs get to the higher number because they seldom adjust their numbers for any type of loss at all. If you start with the 49 number and then count renewals from that point forward, then it would be easy to show a much higher retention number, which is better for the ego but not so good for your business. Keeping all this in mind, it is relatively safe to state that true retention as a national average is less than 40 percent, which is the number you should be using as the minimally acceptable number for your business.

Showing unrealistic retention numbers is also where so many new owners destroy their projections in their business plans for their first clubs. It isn't uncommon for a new owner to show 100 new members and then show 80 or more sticking around for the second year, which is wildly unrealistic when compared to the 49 highlighted. It is a fact of life in the fitness business that people move, get divorced, lose jobs, or simply stiff you on the payment and that volatility has to be built into the plan. When you build your plan, use 40 percent as the conservative number, but target 65 percent as your operational number once you are open.

Training clubs should try to target 80 percent retention over a 12-month period. Most training clubs claim this number, but in reality, few attain it over time for many of the same reasons, such as moves or divorces, but they should overall keep more because they have a limited clientele that is fundamentally more stable in most markets.

These are the basic numbers to start with for visual management. There are 10 on the list, but if you break down the categories, you might end up with a large number of sub lists from each one. For example, if your business has four profit centers, you might end up tracking at least four different numbers under that category as well as the overall usage rate for all profit centers.

Some of the other indicators you might begin to track over time include the following:

- Attendance per program
- Retention per program
- Potential member sources
- Revenue per short-term membership
- Average EFT growth per month
- Percentage of coverage of monthly expenses by the net receivable check and the day each month the club goes into profit mode, meaning the date where the club has completely covered its operating expense for the month, with the intent of moving that date backward toward the first each month

The key is to start small, master what you are doing, and then add more as you progress.

React to red

The first indicator on the previous list referred to leads/tours in the club. As noted in the example, the club does not get on track with those numbers until the 9th of the month. When you track those numbers on your wall, get into the habit of writing any negative number in red chalk. In this case, the club was projecting five needed leads per day but ran negative until the 9th, when the team managed to get the plus/minus total back to zero.

Do not wait to see if these numbers correct without help by the end of the month. If you see red, react now and react strongly. In this example, the owner should get the management team, which might include the manager, the lead salesperson, the lead trainer, and the lead counter person, together for a 30-minute jam session and put some ideas together to get the numbers on track.

Many people use the term running a business and it means just that: You take a proactive response to things that aren't going right for you. In this case, you aren't getting enough leads in your club, highlighted daily by the red chalk flowing down the wall in front of your desk, and you need to do everything you can to correct those numbers now rather than waiting until later in the month to see if they correct without your help.

Keep your staff positive and don't just chew their collective asses for the entire meeting. Instead, ask for each one's best idea to fix this problem, give them a firm timeline, and do something even if it might not work.

Action is fixable, but inaction is the death of all small businesses. For example, you might have the training department open up for guests for the entire month. If you are any type of client, you can bring a guest for the entire month free. Post it on Facebook, send a tweet, create a script for the trainers to use with each client, and get it done today. It may not work, but at least you are in motion and trying something.

The daily meeting as a focus tool

Perhaps the hardest task a manager or owner faces is keeping his staff focused on the daily tasks that lead to increased revenue for the club. It is very easy in this business to spend the day running flat-out busy and then at the end of the day realize you didn't really make any money.

The strongest method of keeping everyone focused is to break down big numbers into smaller chunks that make more sense to the team. This might sound like: "Don't worry about those big numbers out there, team. Let's just worry about what we can do for the next 24 hours, and if we hit today's numbers and tomorrow's, then the big numbers we need to hit will be there for us at the end of the month. One day at a time is our goal."

The tool to use to accomplish this is the daily meeting. This is where you get your management team or full-timers if you are a smaller club together for 30 minutes and then focus on what they need to accomplish as individuals and as teams between now and tomorrow's meeting. Realistically, this really is about what will happen tonight in this business, but there will be an overflow into the next morning and this keeps your momentum going in the right direction.

The following are the keys to the daily meeting:

- Have the meeting exactly the same time every day in the same place and for no more than 30 minutes at a time. The most efficient place to hold this meeting is in front of your visual management board. This also forces you update the board every morning and getting the numbers current should be the first thing you or your managers do every day. The smaller club operators often think that managing the board and tracking their numbers isn't as important, but in many ways, keeping current and focused may even be more important for you because at any given time, you might be selling a client, working someone out, answering the phone, or cleaning the toilets. Make sure these meetings are held standing up and do not allow this time to become group chew-ass time. Keep the meetings focused and positive, with the primary goal being figuring out how you are going to generate new money now.

- The meeting is mandatory attendance for all managers or for all full-time staff depending on the size of your facility. This will take some discipline to get these started and to keep them going, but once you feel the effectiveness, they will become easy to maintain. Those owners who are time challenged (habitually late for everything in their life) have to step up here. The staff picks up their cues from you, and if you are not on time and don't take the meetings seriously, neither will they. Staff members mirror their owners at a level way beyond most owners' comfort level. If you are attempting to lead a young team, it is less about what you say and more about what you do that they mirror. For example, you can talk all you want about uniforms, but if you show up dressed in old jeans and a badly fitting shirt, your action said more than your words could ever convey.

- The primary goal for a focus meeting is to set your numbers for the rest of the day, tonight, and through tomorrow morning and then assign those numbers to an individual or team. Remember that knowing the number is an important thing, but just knowing is not enough by itself. Setting a number and then writing a short plan on how to reach that number and what you need to do make it happen are the most efficient ways to create new income for your business. Put another way, it is not just the number, but it is also the "How are we going to do it?" and "What are we going to do to make it happen?" that are the way to work.

- Break the entire meeting into five-minute segments to establish a set meeting routine. Many owners fear meetings because they often struggles with content, leading to a meeting that feels random and unstructured. Segments keep you focused, keep the meeting from straying to crazy member stories, and establish a consistently that will allow others to run it if you might not be available or have multiple units. Once you master the format, all you have to do from that point is just fill the slots. The following is a proven sample meeting format you can use to get started:

  ✓ *Where are we right now in the business (one segment)?* The visual management tool is the most efficient way to remind the team about the goals we are trying to hit this month and where we are in that chase as of today. Spend five minutes reviewing all the goals and the status of each on the board and how the team is progressing in meeting those goals.

  ✓ *Set a goal for each team or individual (two segments).* Everyone in the meeting should leave with a specific, verifiable goal, a plan of attack as to the how and what, and detailed instructions. Never accept a staff person saying "Well, I can do about four sales tonight." Teach them to frame their answers in positives, such as "Put me down for $2,000 in training revenue tonight. I have five assessments and we will convert a minimum of three into programs." This is the part that will take some practice. Be sure everyone knows that the first month you try this that the team can be really off in some of its estimations. Allow for a one-month practice, but after that first month, hold everyone accountable. You have numbers to make, meaning revenue to create, and "It is my responsibility" should be the staff motto.

  ✓ *Review something that can be done more efficiently (one segment).* There is always something in the business that gets neglected, such as closing procedures, paperwork, or customer service. Use one segment to review something that needs to be fixed, but review it as a positive. As a side note here, make sure that when you review things or try to teach the staff something new, you always tell them clearly what to do, but you also need to spend a lot of time on how to do it and why it is important to the team and the company. Many owners have a lot of combat business experience, so throwing out a quick fix for an issue that it took that owner 20 years to learn leaves the staff dazed and confused. Never tell them what to do without reviewing how to do it and why it is important and always assign a timeline if that applies. You also need to always assume that they do not have your experience or frame of reference, so patiently give background as to why you want something done to help educate the team person and to bring him to a higher level of understanding.

✓ *Teach them something new (one segment).* This 30-minute focus meeting is the perfect format to keep people current. For example, assume you are adding a new boot camp format to your summer schedule. Use this segment to have the lead trainer review what the camp is, who it is for, how you are going to promote it to the members, and how much it will cost. Most staff people want to do a good job for their owners, but that is hard to do if they aren't aware of what is happening in the business. Members always start their inquiries at the front desk and an ill-informed staff can't help you sell. This segment done daily allows all the key people to know exactly what is going on and the part they play in it.

✓ *Review the goals one more time at the end of the meeting to check for understanding and commitment (one segment).* Start every meeting with the goals and end each meeting with the goals. Make the last segment a review of what needs to be done, who is going to do it, and what everyone needs to make sure it happens.

✓ *Gather everyone at 5 p.m. to set the tone.* Exactly at 5 p.m., gather everyone back into your office for the one-minute meeting. "Okay, team, we are going to have a lot of guests (members/clients) in the house tonight. Time to show these people a good time and don't forget about our goals." Just one minute is all it takes, but this short burst of energy is always a reminder to take care of the guests and to stay focused on what counts in the business each day.

✓ *Ask the big question at the end of the day.* There is only one big question that counts at the end of the day: You just put in eight hours today, so what did you do to make this company money? This is a lot more efficient question than merely asking how the day went. It is also important to understand that when you begin asking this question every day, they will soon understand that they are being held accountable for their time and their jobs. This is a difficult question for many new owners to grasp and many feel uncomfortable about asking it, but it really is the most important question you can ask a staff that just took your money for the job and was there for a full day. Don't be afraid to hold people accountable and don't be afraid to ask people what they did today to be productive.

The daily meeting, along with the visual management tool, is nothing more than a simple focus tool that not only keeps the staff on track but you too. The fitness business is heavily customer service driven and it is easy to spend your entire day going from one problem to another. Throw in the routines of the business, such as deposits, accounting, payroll, marketing, and staffing problems, and you will find it easy to put in a 12-hour day and still get nothing done that affects the bottom line.

Force yourself early to use tools that emphasize the production aspect of the business. Things that get in the way of production should eventually be given to others or delegated to service companies so you can spend your time managing results rather than doing the work. Your job is to produce fresh revenue every day in your business and this takes a tight discipline and hard focus to make it happen.

A plan for the next 90 days

The nature of the business often forces owners to shrink their world down to living within just a one-month period. We have this month's bills, we have to meet payroll for the month, we have to track sales a month at a time, and if we are lucky, we survive another month and get to keep going in business.

Being trapped in the monthly perspective often results in a reactive management style where we live within the month and fail to project the business ahead in time. For example, we need leads for the month, so we meet with the local paper, run an ad that is heavy on instant incentives, such as extreme price discounts, and then hope that it works and the club is filled full of potential buyers the day the ad appears.

The pitfall in this is that we limit the growth of the business because we fail to make long-term plans that would increase the revenue and value of the business over time. In the earlier marketing example, the club owner also probably pays full retail for the ad because it was not part of an extended marketing plan. This owner also had to offer deep discounts, which eventually fail to work because discounting burns the market so quickly, to drive traffic into the gym because random reactionary marketing does nothing to build a consistent brand over time.

One way to break out of this trap is to project your business ahead 90 days at a time each month. Doing this is easy, and as you sit down at the end of the month to plan for the coming month, just add two more months to your projection. The following are the key things you should include in your 90-day projection:

- *All marketing for the next 90 days, including traditional sources, such as newspaper inserts, and a detailed plan for electronic marketing, such as posting your fitness tip video of the week on your site.* In this model, you should have an idea 90 days in advance of what your video tips will be so you can keep them sequential and tie them to your other marketing if needed. Planning your marketing this far in advance—and for a year in advance as you get more experience—allows you to make better deals with your ad sources because you are committing for a longer period of time and can then sign contracts if needed.
- *Staffing and scheduling needs for the next 90 days.* For example, you might be coming into summer, where you might be able to cut hours and classes, therefore saving money.
- *Equipment needs and how you care going to pay for them should also be included in your 90-day projection.* Knowing that you might need $5,000 in kettlebells in three months allows you to start putting a little cash away each month into the savings so you don't take the hit all at once. Equipment maintenance should also be included in any 90-day projection.
- *Large repair and maintenance projects should also be included in any type of longer-term projection.* Very little repair and maintenance in this industry is pre-emptive, meaning that replacing tile, flooring, failing air conditioners, or other fundamental operating needs is usually something we do when it breaks and is beyond repair. Again, money is wasted here because instead of anticipating these needs and then seeking multiple bids

or alternative solutions, we end up spending too much money now because we are desperate and the members are pissed because the water heater broke down yet again this week.

- *Special events and promotions should be on a schedule for at least 90 days and, if possible, at least six months out.* Many owners have good ideas about promotions that will either increase revenue or drive in new traffic, but these ideas fail because the time it takes to execute a good promotion is usually much longer than clubs allow. For example, if the club is launching a new programming idea, most owners wait and start blasting it to the members a week or two prior to the launch, which practically guarantees it will fail. On the other hand, starting several months out allows for a consistent message to be created and delivered to the members through electronic sources, in-house promotional tools, and direct delivery through the front desk. It is easy to develop this habit by simply planning the event 90 days into the future and then working backward.

The real concept behind projecting your business ahead for 90 days is that you move from being reactionary to proactive by anticipating the bigger issues in your club and then building a plan further in advance. There will always be surprises in your business, but you can minimize these by anticipating your needs and budgetary concerns further in advance.

Other Planning Tools You Will Need in Your Business

Here are a number of planning tools you will need in your business at some point. Most owners are notorious for never committing anything to paper until forced to by a bank, the IRS, or an investor and the only planning they ever do is to submit a business plan, drawn up by their accountant, to the bank whenever they need a new loan.

The big idea behind planning, as has been noted a number of times in this chapter, is to move an owner away from a reactive management style into a proactive position. Another way to explain being proactive is that you drive the business and market, forcing it to react to you rather than you constantly reacting to whatever is front of you at the time.

The story about the little Dutch boy from your childhood is a great example here, and no, you most likely won't find this done as a video game. In this story, a little boy discovers a hole in the dike and he is terrified that it will grow and harm his town, so he puts his finger in the hole and stands there all night until the town's people find him and he becomes a hero. Sadly, this is how too many owners run their businesses.

Reactive management in this case is the kid, who represents the owner, walking by and is shocked to find a hole in his dike. He immediately reacts and puts his finger in it. In our owner's version, he walks into his business and spends his day plugging holes until he runs out of fingers, toes, noses, and anything else he can poke into the hole to temporarily fix the problem.

See a problem and fix it and then he equates this method of management as having a successful day, when in reality, this owner wasted an entire day fixing problems he should have anticipated.

This same owner demonstrating a proactive management style would have been looking at the dike routinely for years, anticipated the wear and tear, budgeted for a new dike, and then had it repaired long before he needed to shove a finger in a leaking hole. Proactive management allows you to spend your days working on your business rather than being the little Dutch boy who spends the night shivering in the dark because he wasn't smart enough to plan his business any further than the end of this month.

All these plans are just tools to help you become the proactive manager that projects his business into the future rather than suffering the limitations that come with being a reactive owner/operator.

The prospectus plan

The prospectus plan is used to raise money for a new business. Most business rookies make their first major mistake here by confusing a brief but thorough prospectus with a lengthy development business plan for the new business.

Investors and bankers are busy people normally. They don't usually have time to peruse 150 pages of wishful thinking, which is what most business plans resemble, to see if there is a business opportunity buried somewhere inside. Perhaps the best quote from any banker concerning new businesses is: "I have never seen a business plan or pro forma I didn't like," which means most of the endless plans always look good on paper, but the reality of the plan often crumbles when it meets the reality of the real world. The typical plan most inexperienced owners submit is normally too long, too detailed in the wrong areas, such as including class schedules, and not grounded in the realities of the investment world. Few investors or bankers really want to see a sample class structure or the description of your Friday night sweaty yoga class.

Serious investors normally want a brief plan—usually no more than 12 to 15 pages—that gives them an overview of the project, who is behind it, where the money is coming from, and how they, as the money people, will benefit if they invest. Most importantly, they want to know what is in it for me if I give you the money you need to do this project? Even bankers have the need to understand that your business can perform and that it can repay the loan, along with the interest the loan generates.

Contrasting the two is simple. The prospectus is a short look at the business concept you are proposing. The typical business plan submitted by someone who most likely has never gone through the process before is usually an operational plan that details how the business will run with too much fluff and not enough of the basics of business, such as who will run it, how much experience does that person need, and can the business repay its loans to the investors or the bank.

A prospectus plan should include the following sections:

- *A one- to two-page overview describing what the project will entail.* "What it is you are going to do?" "Where will you locate this business?" "Who will this business serve and is there a need for this business in this market?" "Who will run it, why are you opening in that particular area, and how long it will take to get the thing going once you receive the money?" are all basic questions that are typically addressed in this type of plan.

- *The second section should be a one- to two-page projection describing the cost of the entire project.* How much is the build-out for that location, how much equipment do you need, at what cost are you going to get this equipment, how much reserve money is allotted to sustain you during the first months of operations, how much for fixtures, desks and programs, etc.? This section would also include anything unusual for this project in the way of expense, such as the cost of land, permitting if it is out of the norm, or nontypical build-out expenses, such as the demolition of a portion of the building to add a new addition.

- *The third section is usually only one page and describes where you are getting the money for the project.* Are the banks putting up the money? How much equity, meaning his own capital, does the potential owner have invested? How much money is expected to come from investors? And where is the project financially at this moment in time?

- *The fourth section is the most important because this is where you build a financial projection that shows the ability to repay the banks and investors.* How does money arrive each day, each month, and over several years in the business? Is there enough left over for investors to reap a reward? How does the business grow over a two-year period and how much will it need in reserve before it shows a profit? What does it really take to run this business? And what's left over after expenses? All this should be addressed in a formal two-year financial projection. This section should also include a breakdown of a typical month's expenses, a typical month's income stream, and a sample price structure.

- *The next section shows what's in it for the investors.* If our friends, family, or other investors put money into this project, what kind of return on investment or equity is the owner offering? This section should detail what the owner is trying to raise and from what sources as well as what is being offered in return—be it a fixed return, equity, or both. Basically, the investors want to know: If I put money into this project, what do I get back besides the satisfaction of helping a young businessperson get started?

- *The next section should give a brief resume of who is going to put the project together and who is going to run this business on a day-to-day basis.* Investors want to know if there are any special qualifications, skills, or experiences the owner and key people possess that might guarantee this project has a chance. Experience in business counts for a lot when you borrow money for the first time. Experience in this business is even more important. Potential owners without real fitness experience who take time out of their lives to work in a club and attend workshops and training seminars and who are willing to sacrifice a portion of their lives to learn about the business they are opening are more likely to get money than someone who is merely interested in fitness. For example, just because someone likes to cook for his friends on Saturday night does not mean he will be successful in the restaurant business nor does losing 50 pounds make someone qualified to run a fitness business. But this same person who takes a year out of his life and works at various jobs in local restaurants or in a fitness facility has increased his chance of not only getting money but also in being successful in the business.

- *The final section is a summary of the entire plan.* Tell the reader again briefly what the project is about, where the new business will be, how the money is going to be raised, when the project will open, and who will run it. Keep it brief and simple here. If the investors want more information, they will ask. This section should be at a maximum of no more than two pages and it would probably be better in just one page.

In summary, keep this type of plan brief enough where the reader can handle a first look through it in just a few minutes. Investors are busy people who won't sit and read a 150-page bound document. However, these people might sit and review a 12- to 15-page prospectus that simply and briefly states what you are doing and what you want and financially why it might work.

The development business plan

This is the masterwork plan that creates the business on paper before it exists in real life. Most people trying to start a fitness business for the first time spend way too much time writing and rewriting this plan, but despite the hassle of doing this, it is something worth doing. The best way to think of a development plan is that it helps to make sure you have at least a working understanding of what the project will take before it is created. In other words, it forces the potential owner to look at all aspects of the business and then think through how that segment will operate once you are open.

Existing owners who are opening their next unit should also write one of these operational-based plans because many times, a project that looks good in your head won't look so good when you take the time to write out a development plan. For example, a common mistake owners make when they open a second unit is that they don't put any operational systems in place. They've run their existing club by their personalities, with minimum paperwork, and with a hands-on style rather than with actual systems that can be easily duplicated or sustained by others if the owner is not on-site. A written development/operational plan helps determine whether a system exists and if that system can be duplicated in another location.

The development plan should have the following parts (length is irrelevant in a development plan—write what it takes for you to understand your project).

#1: The overview

The overview should tightly define the scope of the project, the proposed size of the new facility, the location, why putting a club in the area is a good idea, who the target market will be, and an approximate target date for the completion of the project.

#2: What the facility will look like

The second section is a physical description of the proposed fitness facility. How big it will be, who it is for and why you made that choice, what niche it will fill in the community that is neglected by current competition, and how it will be different than your competitors should also be addressed in this section.

#3: Demographics

The third section should be a complete demographic breakdown of the proposed target market. Pay special attention to the 12-minute drive time rule, which states that approximately 80 to 85 percent—and even up to 90 percent in some markets—of all our members will come from a 12-minute drive time from the club, established during prime drive hours, for mainstream fitness centers. Specialty facilities, such as training businesses, sports performance centers, or women-only clubs, usually draw from a little farther away from their locations due to the specialization of the product. Good demographic studies should clearly illustrate how many people there are in a three-mile and a five-mile ring from the proposed site. These lists are usually broken down by areas of town and can be further defined by affluence, which is a key indicator in determining if someone will join or support any type of fitness facility.

#4: Target market

The fourth section is especially important because it is where you define your true target market. Most fitness projects are too broad in scope and many business plans state that the new club is for everyone in the community. Keep in mind that 80 percent of your potential members will probably come from a specific target market segment, which is usually defined as two-generational, and by affluence. Another simple way to state this is that "likes attract likes," which means people like to hang out with other people who are similar to themselves and that it is hard for an owner to build a club that provides the equipment, energy, programming, color, and right staff that pleases everyone in that town.

For example, you might choose a high-energy, music-driven atmosphere for your gym—similar to many of the original franchise-style facilities. The target market in this example would be people within three miles of the gym who are 24 to 40 years old. Once this facility is established, the club would then attract other people in that age group, and eventually, about 80 percent of the members, which is the target market, would all be from one defined demographic.

The common mistake made in this section by new owners who want to someday develop multiple facilities is to try to be everything to everybody in the community. You have to be able to clearly define who this club is for, what the demographics are for that group, where they live, and how you would market to them. Knowing this going in gives you a huge advantage once you begin the daily operation of your business.

#5: Defining capital sources

This section should detail the needed capital for the project. Be sure to include a detailed equipment list not only for the workout equipment but also for support of the profit centers, such as computer needs and license fees. Before you write your plan, be sure to get an idea of what the build-out costs are in your area. Also be sure to include a reserve of at least two to three months' operating expenses.

The reserve capital is not a luxury but rather a fundamental part of opening a new business. Most new businesses need time to get healthy and to be able to stand on their own financially. In the fitness business, the new business should be able to cover its own monthly expenses somewhere around 9 to 10 months of being open, assuming that for most markets, you get it open between the end of August and no later than the end of February. Until the breakeven point, you will normally burn up about two to three months of reserve capital to cover expenses until your business can stand on its own.

This is also the section where you would detail the start-up costs for the business. This sounds obvious, but many start-up people fail to get down deep enough into what it really costs to start the business of their dreams. This failure is often because the potential owner hasn't done his research and really doesn't know what it takes to get a facility open and this same owner will often fail to dig deep because he knows what he has in money isn't enough and if he continues to research he will realize he shouldn't do it, therefore ending the dream before it began.

Few owners open any small business with the proper capitalization. Most have enough to get open but not enough to cover operational losses until the business can stand alone. The reserve capital that is discussed in virtually every business book ever written on opening your first business is usually used about two months prior to opening to cover the overage in build-out and other start-up costs. There is a basic rule that is talked about often by experienced owners who have done their own projects in the past called the 20/20 rule. This rule states that your new project will take 20 percent longer to open than you were promised and that you will be at least 20 percent over whatever cost you anticipated.

These owners justify opening anyway by creating pro formas that are too good or just borrow what they can and then hope the bank or a parent will bail them out if they run out of cash. It is surprising here how few potential owners seek out the information that is so readily available to them that would help create this plan. For example, it is not unusual for a new owner to get into the business without ever working in a fitness business or without ever talking to a successful owner to determine how he got started, what it costs to really open a club, and what kind of mistakes and pitfalls the new owner should expect.

Do your homework, attend seminars and workshops, talk to a number of successful owners, and then use all this information to build a realistic plan based on the facility you can really afford to own rather than the one you talked yourself into emotionally.

#6: Financial plan

This section should be the financial section and should include the same type of financial information that is included in the prospectus plan, such as two-year financial projections, a sample month's operating expense, and a sample month's revenue projection. However, when you build an operational plan, you should go beyond the fundamental information in a prospectus plan. Use this section to add estimated payroll breakouts, including what your management team will consist of and how they will get paid, sample monthly class schedules for your first few months of operations with pay rates for the instructors, and a detailed plan for your training department.

The key here is to create a separate sheet for every area of the club so you start to understand how everything in the business ties together. Most owners usually just go with their strengths and virtually neglect the other parts of the business. For example, a trainer will build a detailed plan for his training department and equipment list and then just throw together a few basic numbers for the group exercise component.

#7: Raising money

If you have to use investors or the bank for the project, this section should detail how you will raise the money and what you will give up in the form of ownership or return to get it. Remember that investors are seeking either a return on their investment, equity, or a combination of both. Banks want to know you are building a business that can handle the debt service. Investors want to know what they get for what they give and how that investment compares to other options they might be considering for their money.

There is a short lesson to learn here. Long-term debt is better than short-term debt. Long-term debt is defined as anything five years or longer. For example, if you borrow $100,000 from an investor, you would be better to pay this back over a period of 7 to 10 years rather than trying to get him his money back in a shorter period of time. Yes, you would pay more interest, but you and the business are safer because the cost of servicing the debt is lower, giving you a chance to build up a decent business that isn't starved to death early due to so much short-term debt.

Short-term debt is defined as debt that is three years or less and is usually coupled with higher interest rates and an aggressive payback. This rule also applies to mortgages. If you are given a choice, take the mortgage that gets your payments out to 25 to 30 years and then check to make sure there is no prepayment penalty for making extra payments. Start with the lowest expense you can establish and then you can always pay extra if the money is there after you pay your bills.

#8: Marketing

Research and include a 12-month proposed marketing plan for the business. Be sure to cost this plan out so it may be included as part of your projections.

Start with a marketing budget for the first year of about 10 percent per month of your base monthly operating expense (BOE). For example, if it will cost you $60,000 a month to run your club, budget about $6,000 per month for marketing. The minimum any club or training facility should spend each month is $3,500. If you are hungry, you buy food. If your business is starving for new leads, you have to feed it each month. Marketing is a 52-week-a-year proposition and is not the first thing you cut in tough times but rather the last.

Marketing is usually broken down into two distinct parts: retro marketing for a target market that is usually 40 years old or older and electronic marketing for those who sleep with their phones, use their iPads before getting out of bed, and live and breathe everything gadget. These are two distinct groups within your market area and you have to chase both equally. The cost of retro marketing, such as full color flyers stuck in a newspaper, is the most expense side of the formula, while a lot of the marketing you can do electronically is either free or fairly cheap.

Even websites—still a staple for most small businesses—are coming down in cost in huge steps as more and more are becoming template driven and as the tools you need to make one efficient are becoming more readily available to the average guy who isn't a programmer. For example, posting videos once took a resident webmaster to do and now any five-year-old kid with a cell phone can shoot and post a decent video in minutes.

#9: Staffing

The staffing section should be broken down into two parts. First, you need to project your staffing needs for a typical month's worth of coverage. Break this coverage down to daily staffing costs, including salary and hourly costs. Include payroll tax projections as well as proposed commissions and bonuses. Second, develop a staff training guide you can use for the first six months you're open and for each job in the gym. What you want people to know, how and when you will train them, and how much training you will provide before an employee is allowed on the floor are all considerations that need to be addressed before you hire your first staff person.

#10: Member service

The member service plan should also be included in your development plan. You should cover how to handle member complaints, surveys and information-gathering materials, items or services that could be added to the club the first year to increase member service, such as amenities in the locker rooms, and daily staff training procedures that increase your member service response. Customer service is not random. It takes a plan and it has to be taught. Basic procedures, such as how to greet the guests each day, learning and using their names, and thanking every client every time he leaves are not something the average front counter employee is going to bring to the job. If you want it to happen, you have to teach it—and you can't teach it effectively if it isn't in your staff manuals.

You should also open with employee manuals detailing everything from vacation days to the things you can get fired for in the job. Your local attorney can help you with this and a basic one can be purchased and then adapted to your business. It may be small when you first get it started, but over time, these manuals usually grow to fit the uniqueness of your business. You must have one when you open and there is no exception to this rule. If you have one employee, you should have an employee manual.

#11: Profit centers

Multiple profit centers, or nondues revenue, are a vital part of any club's business plan. Include an entire section to the profit centers you will feature, especially how these profit centers will be promoted on a daily, weekly, and monthly basis. Include the start-up cost of each profit center. Be sure to include staff costs if they are separate from your staff projections.

#12: Staff needs

Resumes from the owners and all key staff should also be included in the plan. What type of expertise do you really have to make money in the fitness business? What types of training, such as accounting classes or certifications, should you seek before you open? Any weaknesses should appear when you gather your resumes from the key players. Be honest at this stage. For example, if no one on the staff has ever done a payroll, then someone needs to meet with the accountant, master the software needed, and then learn enough to become the point person for the team. In small business, what you don't know might just kill you, so be realistic with the players involved on the actual skills each one brings to the table.

#13: Moving on from your business

The final section should be a fairly detailed plan as to how you will get out of this business. Getting into any business is fairly easy, but getting out is the tough part and you should never get in without a plan to get out at some point.

A summary sheet should be thrown in at the end. Because this is a development plan for your own use, the summary should be used to focus the entire project down to just a couple pages. If you can't focus the entire project to two pages, you may not yet have a project clearly enough focused to work. Plus, if you have to show this plan to anyone, most people will start with the summary and only read selected sections anyway. Make this finish strong and concise. In other words, if you can't simply explain the project, you most likely can't build it either.

Operating Plans Help You Keep Your Business Focused Ahead and Competitive

One-year, three-year, and five-year operating plans keep an owner who is already in business proactive. These plans also help keep you competitive in the market by helping you anticipate equipment and physical plant maintenance you will need to do to retain the members you have already obtained in the market.

When people first write business plans, they almost always start from today forward, working on paper toward a specific goal or idea somewhere in the future. However, the best way to write plans is start with the expected result in mind and then work your way backward. Start with the goal in mind, as it would look done correctly, then work backward, breaking it down into the doable working steps that it takes to get there. Each of these plans has a slightly different feel to it.

The one-year plan is considered a true operating plan. With this plan, you are addressing things that have to happen in a very short period of time in the business world. For example, what equipment do you need to add or replace in the next 12 months or what major maintenance issues do you need to deal with now before you lose members?

The three-year plan is a little more conceptual in nature. What programming may need to be replaced, what key staff will you most likely need to replace or develop more fully if they stay with you, or how can you refinance your business now that you've been around for a while to help reduce your debt structure and to free up some cash? These are all questions that should be addressed in a working three-year plan, which is written primarily to keep you constantly projecting your business ahead instead of merely reacting to market developments as they happen.

The five-year plan is primarily centered on long-range financial goals for you and the business. Where will the business be financially in five years? What additional debt do you need to keep the facility competitive? Where will you be financially in your own life in five years? Should you move the business into your own building or continue to rent? This type of question is primarily geared toward helping you make decisions that add value to your business over time rather than looking at just short-term ramifications that may work today but don't create long-term value that will help you get out at some point. For example, your landlord may entice you to stay another five years with a decent rent deal, which is easy to take because you are already in and have to do nothing but sign the papers. However, if you have a long-term plan that includes a projected exit strategy, you might instead want to buy your own building with the plan of someday selling the business but retaining the property and becoming a landlord.

The suggested components of a one-year operational plan

- The physical plant
- Equipment needs and changes
- The projected financial growth of the business for the coming year
- Individual plans, such as member service and a 12-month marketing plan
- Reductions or additions in your multiple profit centers
- Sales goals and renewal projections
- A staff development and training plan

You can use these questions to trigger your writing. The best time to write these plans is in November for the following year. Lock yourself away for several days and create a working plan. Do not worry about perfect, but concentrate more on just getting a working draft into your computer. There is a temptation to overthink these things, but you are always better to just write through the first draft and then go back and add or edit as needed. Remember the old adage: A good plan now is worth more than a perfect plan never:

- How much gross income can I project over the next year on an annual and monthly basis? How much money per month will the club receive? From what sources will this money come?
- How many sales does the club have to do on a monthly basis? What will the cost per sale be?
- What projected renewals should the club be doing on a month-to-month basis? How will that compare against last year's? What percentage increase is your goal?
- What's your target for total receivables growth? How much will you need to increase each month to reach that goal?
- What is your monthly marketing budget? What is your expected response rate from your marketing? What is your cost per lead and your club's monthly overall closing rate?
- What new profit centers will you add in the next 12 months? Where will the money come from for these additions? What profit centers need replacing?
- Where is your 12-month marketing plan?
- Where is your 12-month member service plan?
- What events do you have planned for the coming 12 months?
- How much should the club have in its regular savings account at the end of the next year? How much will be in the accrual account?
- What type of further development does your lead staff need? Who on your staff can step up as a future leader and what type of development do those people need?
- Who will be the manager for your next gym and what are you doing to get that person ready?
- What will you do over the next 12 months to improve yourself and your business skills?
- What is your educational budget for staff development for the next 12 months?
- What equipment will be outdated in the next 12 months? What needs to be replaced?
- What physical plant changes do you need to make in the next year? Where will this money come from? How will it improve your business?

The three-year operational plan

The same basics apply to the three-year plan, except they are extended further into the future. The difference, though, is that this plan should look more heavily at the overall financial structure of the business. For example, how can you reduce the overall debt structure of the business with the goal of freeing up more cash? Remember that you will always have some type of debt. But as the business matures, your goal is to reduce short-term debt, which is any debt that is three years or less, with cheaper, long-term debt, which is usually five to seven years. Having debt is not the problem and many old-time operators only had one goal—and that was to be debt free. These guys also have the nastiest clubs in town because they would never reinvest in the physical plant or equipment. Debt is part of owning a fitness business, but the goal is to have smart, manageable long-term debt rather than being choked with too much short-term junk debt that has high interest rates and an aggressive payback.

The five-year operational plan

The five-year plan should be the big picture plan designed to secure more equity in your business. Can you buy your building or build somewhere else in town? How many other units can you manage or how many do you want to own? How can you protect your business as your main source of income in markets that having rising competition? What major structural work does the club need to stay competitive and how will you finance this change? Be sure to include a plan that puts you on the road to retirement, which includes funding some type of personal IRA account. Remember again, getting into a fitness business is an easy thing. Getting out is where the money is made and where the better owners separate themselves from the ones trapped forever in a fading business.

Summary

Most small businesses are operated by owners who practice a reactive management style. This means decisions are usually made in a defensive mode, which is generally too late to do the business any good. Put another way, it is far too late to take self-defense lessons once a guy whacks you on the side of the head.

For example, you know you are getting a lot of complaints about a lack of cardio pieces. You put off the decision to add more treadmills, though, and just take the heat. Eventually, you cave in and add a few extra pieces after the complaints escalate and you start hearing that members are leaving you for a newer club down the street with more cardio. A proactive manager would have analyzed the initial complaints and acted before the situation turned into a defensive standoff between management and members, saving lost revenue and avoiding an image that the owner just doesn't care about how crowded it is or how little equipment the members have to use.

Proactive management can't happen without planning. Do you have plan to make money today, for the week, for the month, and for the next 90 days? Good owners will also sit down once a year and write a one-year, a three-year, and a five-year operational plan that projects the current business into the future. Future owners will create their new business on paper before it is created in the real world through the use of a prospectus, which is used to raise money, and a development plan, which is used to visualize the business on paper.

Applying this material to your business

If you haven't opened your first club yet:

- *Keep your business narrowly focused.* Most new owners want to open the perfect dream club with a little something for everyone their first time out. Keep your first project smaller, leaner, and less risky than that overbuild monster in your dreams.

- *Write the prospectus first before you write the development plan.* It helps you keep the project focused and narrowly defined.

- *Learn the numbers.* Start with projections, your average EFT per sale, monthly expenses, and the rent factor. These numbers drive the business and are the place to start for beginners.

- *Learn what you're really giving up to investors or the bank to open the club.* You have to give up something to get someone else's money, but learn what's acceptable and what isn't.

If you are currently operating a facility:

- *Start training yourself to think proactively now.* Weigh every decision, even the small ones, against what happens if you fail to act now, therefore putting off the problem or decision until you're forced to react.

- *Start your day by getting your numbers current for the business.* Set a plan with your team to make money during the next 24 hours. Keep your business projected out over 90 days, forcing yourself to see a bigger picture than being trapped in the month. Take a weekend away and write your one-, three- and five-year plans. If you have senior staff, get them involved in the writing process. Update the plans on a yearly basis and block out a weekend in November to create your plans for the following year.

- *Use the plans to force yourself to look at the big picture.* Most owners get so caught up in the day-to-day basis that they fail to relate the decisions they make today to the future of the business. Plans help you relate day-to-day decisions to a long-range look at your business.

- *Build your own future into the plans.* Nothing lasts forever, including businesses. Someday, you might want to get out of your business. Build a personal escape plan into the financial plan of your business.

November 29, 2013
The holiday rules of social behavior for fitness professionals

The fitness person's rules of social behavior for the holidays:

- Do not take the breadbasket, throw it on the floor, stomp on it, and launch into your Paleo diet lecture.
- Wearing flat shoes, a workout bra, and tiny little shorts is not acceptable church wear no matter how ripped you are.
- Forcing your family to do group burpees after a big meal is not socially acceptable.
- Kettlebells, while beautiful tools, are not appropriate holiday gifts for all your overweight relatives.
- Offering to take your mother out for a tattoo date is most likely not going to be well received.
- Replacing all the wine and beer at the family gig with bottled water will most likely end in your death.
- It doesn't matter how you sell it, 99% dark chocolate still tastes like crap.
- Ironing your best workout shirt does not make it acceptable for the big family picture.
- Yes, your uncle is fat and sleeping in the chair, but that doesn't give you the right to steal his keys and make him walk home.
- Shut up, sip on that glass of wine, and pretend that all those desserts everyone brought are well done and gracious. Lecturing family about fitness is like preaching to squirrels in the park: They appear to listen as long as the nuts are free.

January 24, 2014
The weekend mindbender

Here is this weekend's mind bender. Sit quietly and figure out all the money you spent on stuff last year (TVs, headphones, new cars, clothes, etc.). Then, make a list of your dream trips or experiences (surf Mavericks or the Australian coast, take a train across Europe, open a gym) and figure out what they would cost. The goal is to understand that you have the money to live your dreams, but you can get so caught up buying stuff that you deny yourself the experiences of life. Every year, you should plan at least one big, extraordinary, remember-for-ever experience. Stop putting off those things that can define your life, thinking there will always be time to do them later. You are alive now and should live now within your moment. It would also help to have a glass of wine and do this with someone you love or at least someone you want to love, having a really cool experience. Be peaceful this weekend and value yourself for a few hours.

12

It's a Business, Not a Baby

What the consumer demands from a fitness facility changes from year to year. Often, these demands are ahead of what the owners understand about their businesses or are willing to do in their clubs. The consumer reads a new book, sees something new and exciting about fitness on TV, or most likely reads something online and then wonders why his club hasn't embraced any of this information yet.

Perhaps the strongest example of this consumer demand came with the premiere of *The Biggest Loser*, which came at about the same time many mind-changing books were appearing in the marketplace, such as *Born to Run* by Chris McDougall, *The Female Body Breakthrough* by Rachel Cosgrove, *The New Rules of Lifting* by Lou Schuler and Alwyn Cosgrove, and *The 4-Hour Body* by Timothy Ferriss.

The Biggest Loser introduced millions of otherwise sedentary people to kettlebells, 50-foot ropes, and upright, functional-style training. For this group of viewers, what the people on the show were doing became their definition of fitness and many of these viewers came to the clubs thinking that this is what fitness really is about and not 1990s circuit-style training many clubs still try to pass off as current and effective fitness training.

These books also brought a unique pressure to the club owners and their training staffs. The consumer, armed with a book under his arm and 10 hours on the author's website, expects fitness to be something more personal and guided rather than merely renting the club's equipment for a low price. Through culture exposure and self-education, the consumer simply wants more than the clubs were currently offering.

Is this every consumer? No, of course not. There is still a consumer who wants to pay a cheap fee to walk on a treadmill a few times a week and call that fitness, especially during the era of the volume $10 membership clubs, but there is also the emergence of a new generation consumer that is smarter, better read, and, in many ways, more fitness experienced than many fitness business owners. For example, take any serious triathlete and you can bet he probably knows more about general athletic conditioning than most mainstream box fitness owners. We simply let the client get ahead of the business model.

But many owners still hang on to past trends, such as filling the clubs with a floor of bodybuilding and circuit-style equipment and then trying to force that vision of fitness on a resistant marketplace. Everything changes in time, but most owners are too emotionally tied to their clubs and programs to adapt to the current market conditions. What worked in the past won't necessarily work in the future nor will it keep you competitive in a volatile consumer market.

For example, have you ever been introduced to a friend's new baby, took one look at the kid, and thought to yourself: That just might be the ugliest baby I've ever seen. The kid is ugly and scrawny and has really strange alien ears, but the parents are telling you how beautiful the kid is. You can't believe you're looking at the same kid. One side sees nothing but yuck—the other sees nothing but precious.

The fitness business is much the same way. Physical plants wear out, such programs as group exercise (aerobics for you old-timers) run their course, and such hot trends as racquetball—now played by a handful of bald-headed old guys still wearing headbands—have faded to the history stage of our business. In this industry and virtually any other small business, you have to always remember that nothing lasts forever.

In the fitness industry, it's easy to get emotionally attached to a program or even to the gym itself. For many owners, it takes several years of planning and dreaming to get that first fitness business open. When it's finally done, a new owner may end up working about 100 hours a week for the first year or so in the business. It's easy to start losing sight of your gym as a business and to start thinking of it as an extension of yourself and your home. When you spend more time in one spot than you do at home, you lose your perspective. The term for this is *club blind*, which means you see something so often that you stop seeing it at all. The walls that need painting, the torn carpet, the cluttered front counter, and the dust bunnies running rampant through the club become your new norm and something you just stop seeing.

The same is true for programming. Your first fitness experience—the one that helped you get hooked for life—may have been, say, group exercise. You start your first classes and get hooked, and over the years, it becomes part of your life. It's what got you started and helped you get into your first real fitness shape and it's something that, now as an owner, you want to share with others.

The problem is that physical plants fade and need to be replaced. Programs hit a high in the market and then decline as consumers move on to the next hot trend. Our emotional ties prevent us from realistically evaluating our business and being able to make the right business decisions. Just because we love it, we think everyone will love it, but at some point, what you believe in no longer exists.

For example, look at this scenario from an actual operator. You visit the club and notice that the physical plant is really starting to show its age. The gym is about five years old, the paint is worn, the equipment is chipped and aged, and the design is no longer up to current standards in the market being set by newer, more aggressive competitors.

For example, the group exercise program was a central feature in the gym, with a beautiful glass room right in the middle of everything. The problem was that the usage in the program had declined over the years as the female members moved toward more strength training and the newer cardio equipment.

If you mention to the owners that their gym is looking sort of shabby, everyone becomes upset. "It's not worn out. We get great comments on this gym all the time." "Everyone who comes in the door loves this gym. They say we're the prettiest gym in the area." These are the typical defensive comments made by the staff and owners. It is as if you were looking at the baby in the earlier example and told the truth: "Hey, I hate to tell you this, but your kid is really ugly and, dude, what is with those ears?"

Most owners hear what they want to hear and have become emotionally attached to a building and its paint. At some point, they get a reality check—usually initiated by declining sales, a truthful member, or that epiphany moment where you see the business for what it really has become—and at that point, they finally agree to a remodel. Remodeling isn't cheap, and in fact, it is the capital-intensive nature of this business that makes it so difficult. In this example, these owners might spend $20 to $30 per foot to remodel—or more—and still have to replace cardio that is wearing out and perhaps a lot of their fixed equipment too.

One important trend worth noting going into the 2010 decade was that many owners were starting to realize that you no longer have to have such expansive physical plants to make money. For example, as functional training increased, club owners and operators were realizing that those big seas of equipment were no longer needed to make money. The harsh reality for many owners came when they realized that trainer specialists in 6,000-square-foot clubs were generating the same revenue that the 30,000-square-foot boxes were doing but with 10 to 20 percent more net profit. For example, training clubs generating $1.3 million a year with a pre-tax net of over 20 percent became a common thing and these clubs could be started and completely built at a high level for only about $400,000, which is what a 30,000-square-foot box operator might pay for just equipment.

In this example, if owners moved and shrank the group exercise room into a back area, added a functional training area, upgraded the cardio, replaced some of the outdated equipment, and gave the place a fresh look with different colors and paint, they would most likely find that sales will increase, but more importantly, renewals will increase immediately and probably stabilize for the next two years. Members like to see reinvestment and most know when what you have is no longer current or serviceable.

Everything in the fitness industry seems to change on a fairly consistent basis. In fact, it changes roughly about every 10 to 12 years. These changes can be divided into two categories, with each category having its own distinctive characteristics. Another way to look at these changes is that what is old is often new again and most of what we do in this industry is we have done before during a prior incarnation of the product or service.

Microtrends

Changes in this group are better known as cycles, which simply means that some program, activity, or piece of equipment gets hot, fades, almost dies out completely, and then comes back with a new repackaging. Perhaps the most relevant example of a microtrend is group exercise. Group exercise/aerobics had a strong following in the 1970s and was a primarily women-only activity relegated to church basements and grade school gyms.

During the 1980s, group exercise was without question the hottest activity in the country. Your fitness facility was defined by your instructors, the depth of your program, and which guru you followed. Aerobics was on TV, national contests ruled the major conventions, and you weren't anyone unless you were wearing leg warmers and spotless white shoes.

Eventually, the sport faded, and by the early 1990s, it was virtually gone in most mainstream fitness centers—only to get another rebirth in the late 1990s through the advent of the infomercial and kickboxing. It developed slowly, hit full force, faded quickly, and then disappeared for a few years. It was still out there, but as an activity in fitness, it was struggling for an identity and it took an entirely new angle, such as the kickboxing component, to make it relevant again. Group exercise—except for cycling, which is being adapted by the training population as a way to increase general athletic conditioning—is currently trending downward despite a brief resurgence of dance-based programming from South America.

Another prime example of a microtrend that seems to regain strength every decade or so is the low-priced business model based on a high-volume membership approach and a membership price point of $9 or so. The reintroduction of this model by the Planet Fitness gym chain—just one of a dozen chains trying the same approach—in the early part of this century started almost a panic in the industry as established clubs, which were charging $49 or so for a membership but in reality offered nothing more than renting equipment and were doing exactly the same as the low-service models, cried foul and unfair competition.

However, the low-priced model is nothing new to the industry and many companies still in business, such as Lucille Roberts in the Northeast, have offered a price below $10 since the late 1960s. The cycle, though, is never complete until it starts the fade and the low-priced business model is already showing signs of becoming another trend that will come and go over its 10- to 12-year cycle, primarily due to the fact that it is not sustainable as a business model because competitors can easily match or beat your price offering.

The real defining characteristic of a microtrend is that it usually has a set cycle with a ramp up period, a hot period, a quick decline, and then a period of low usage, but the activity usually comes back at some point. For example, roller-skating represents an activity that started with wheels strapped to shoes in the 1800s and has evolved through a number of different configurations, including rollerblading. As of now, it is dormant as a popular activity in the fitness world, but roller-skating in some form might rise again and catch fire for another cycle.

Other microtrend examples that tend to come and go through the years are tanning, running (which as of this writing is going through a rebirth due to the interest in triathlons as a fitness goal for novices), and the advent of barefoot running and the minimalist shoe and racquet sports, which are currently in the decline stage in the fitness business.

Macrotrends

Macrotrends are unusual in that they affect how business is done in the industry. The strongest current example of a macrotrend is the reintroduction of functional training as a training philosophy, which is really a retreat to where the fitness industry started. Physical cultural training originated in Europe in the 1800s and was created by people seeking total body development through the application of fitness and a healthy lifestyle. Look through the old books—first magazines and then classic pictures and illustrations from the 1700s and 1800s—and you will find early fitness enthusiasts climbing ladders and ropes, lifting kettlebells, and doing other "strongman" activities or calisthenics. This is a simplistic example, of course, but fitness in the early days was defined as full-body exercise with the purpose of developing your body and your overall health and well-being.

The fitness industry today is rapidly returning to its fitness roots, with strong long-term implications for the industry. Most innovation in today's modern society does not usually flow from the top down but rather from the bottom up, which can be seen in everything from the adaption of electronic goods, sports shoes, or design.

For example, the minimalist running shoe craze started with a book called Born to Run by Chris McDougall, a frustrated runner seeking a solution to his stream of injuries that seemed impossible to solve through normal medical channels or coaching solutions. He and his bands of converts started the trend to run barefoot or in flat-bottom sandals long before the shoe companies reacted and brought minimalist shoes to the market. In this case, the shoe wasn't a product of marketing but a result of a trend that started at the grassroots level and spread upward.

The same bottom-up approach is happening in the fitness industry, with the trainers leading the charge and followed closely by the consumer who is ready for a change away from traditional mainstream box fitness to the more organic approach of functional training. Training information has never been so plentiful and easily available through websites, literally hundreds of training workshops offered nationwide annually, and the advent of the "guru" concept in the industry, where such paradigm shifters as Stuart McGill, Bill Parisi, Mark Verstegen, Mike Boyle, Todd Durkin, and Gray Cook can build their followers through websites, books, and blogs available instantly online.

How we have trained the client through the last part of the last century is being challenged by the trainers at the ground level, and as this "return to what works" philosophy gains traction and we move away from the heavy emphasis on machines and isolation-style training, the very nature of how we do business in the industry will change. Most modern mainstream fitness facilities, defined as a large box-style facility that caters to a very broad spectrum of members, are based on principles made fashionable in the late 1980s and early 1990s.

These two decades were the peak years for yet another microtrend: the bodybuilding training philosophy that came, hit hard, faded, and then became a relic from our past. However, most clubs' physical plants are still built on that style of muscle isolation training illustrated by the lines of circuit equipment, the heavy emphasis on a certain type of free weights designed for the bodybuilder and not the athlete seeking full-body training, and a dependence on classic one-on-one training.

However, the advent of functional is not a microtrend but is a correction from the short run bodybuilding had in the industry. Upright, full-body training has been around for thousands of years and even the pioneers of bodybuilding, such as Dave Draper and Bill Pearl, were guys who squatted heavy, pressed heavy, and built their amazing physiques through more of a strongman approach rather than what passes for training in most of the current crop of muscle magazines, with the emphasis on six-day splits based on limited body part training.

It is interesting to note that fixed-plane equipment also emerged during the same time period as the bodybuilders. As the bodybuilders sought ever more infinite ways to isolate and develop individual muscles, the equipment manufacturers joined the trend by building lines of equipment that highlighted individual body parts rather than total body conditioning. Perhaps the biggest example of this type of equipment was the advent of the plate-loaded equipment that was such a rage for several decades.

The trend back to what works is important because of the effect it is having on the current industry and for the coming years. The following are just a few of the many changes this shift in training philosophy is creating:

- *Smaller physical plants:* If you don't need a sea of equipment, such as multiple lines of fixed-circuit equipment or plate-loaded machines, and if you don't need as much cardio to achieve a fit client, then you will not need as much space to house it. Many club owners who embrace a more functional approach also use group personal training or team training as part of their membership structure. This type of gym would offer 8 to 12 group experiences a week on a set schedule. The clients would sign up for 12-month memberships at somewhere between $69 to $149 per month depending on the market and be allowed to attend as often as they would like, which is generally two to three times per week. Owners who adapt this as a component of their membership offerings usually downgrade or eliminate most of their traditional group exercise programs (aerobics) because the club's emphasis on group training replaces most of what was accomplished in the group program. It is important to note that many owners are also frustrated with incurring a large expense for a group exercise program but then have to include it as part of the basic membership. Embracing a group personal training membership allows that same owner to now generate revenue from many of the same people who were once in the club at a much lower return per person.

- *Higher returns per member:* Functional-style training also allows the club owner to generate a higher return per client. Theoretically, this means that the owner can get more money from fewer people and, therefore, lower the need for extensive volume in memberships. For example, it is common now for a 6,000-square-foot training facility with only about 300 members to generate the same amount of total gross revenue that a mainstream box club might do. However, the key is that the training club was probably built for about $400,000 and the mainstream box club built at 15,000 square feet might have cost a million and a half or more to build in rental space and larger clubs in the 30,000-square-feet category could easily surpass $4,000,000 to build. Risk to return will be a key factor in how clubs will be built in the future, and if a new owner can generate a higher return with a much lower risk, you will probably see fewer chain-style clubs being built.

- *Better-educated clients who will seek results, not rental equipment:* The consumer has more access to more information about training than at any time in the past. He is coming to the club these days armed with more current magazines, research online, and often even his own equipment that the club hasn't gotten around to purchasing yet. This new generation client will not tolerate equipment that is 30 years outdated, and if you haven't got what he wants, he is gone. This issue will be how fast the chain-style clubs can adapt. Eliminating expensive equipment and replacing it with ropes, kettlebells, and suspension gear goes against every principle the box club was created on. Instead of self-service equipment that eliminates staff, these clubs will have to figure out a way to educate and support these new members, forcing a shift away from almost nonexistent member service and support to a results-driven business plan that forces them to change their product from selling just a membership to selling change and results.

What can you learn from this trend back to a results-first concept in the fitness business? We can learn that much of what we do in the industry is the result of a reaction to a microtrend that has a defined life span. There will always be hot trends in the business and every club will at some time embrace one of these trends, but the issue of major importance today is that the industry is going through a macrotrend and a return to our roots and the basic elements of what it takes to be fit.

Another example of a microtrend are the humble free weights, which were popular in the 1990s and which everyone thinks have always been a vital part of the fitness business, but this equipment was pretty rare in most of the 1970s when the must-have equipment was Nautilus. In that era of fitness, pools were a major part of your business and sales plan, but almost no one would consider putting them into a new midsized club in today's market.

And racquetball may be the best example of something most of the industry was very committed to in the 1970s, although it was very costly to build and implement. But who in the mid-1990s would build a 16-court racquet facility? The trend built slowly, became hot, quickly faded, and was gone maybe forever due to the cost and space requirements of offering this programming.

Why don't owners in the fitness business change to meet the demands of the market? Most people think that fitness owners, the franchise operators, and the national chains drive change in the fitness industry, but in reality, most change in our businesses comes from external forces and often from the ground up. An example of owners being the last to know would be the advent of kettlebells. The consumer saw them on TV, sports professionals were embracing them for years at the pro level, and even the national sporting goods stores were carrying them, along with basic DVDs on how to use them, all before most mainstream fitness centers even owned one.

Kettlebells are also a perfect example of change from the bottom up. The independent trainers, meaning the ones working in the small studios or freelancing by renting space, are the early adapters in our industry. The contrast is that most of the young fitness professionals spend all their time trying to determine what is coming next, what works with their clients, and where you learn to do this.

On the other hand, most mainstream fitness owners spend a lot of their time trying to figure out how to hang on to what worked in the past and most of these owners are very reluctant to embrace change. This is why the trainers at the park doing boot camps are usually using techniques and equipment the mainstream owners won't see in their clubs for several years. For example, why would that owner want his trainers to embrace new technology when he has $500,000 of equipment on the floor? Is this owner going to tell his members he has changed his mind and that all that equipment really doesn't work anymore?

There are several other sources that have major influences on the fitness industry and our offerings. First is the very low boredom threshold of our members. Many of our members in today's market love to work out and do so regularly as part of an ongoing healthy lifestyle, compared to the average participant in the 1960s who tended to fade somewhat quicker. In fairness to the member of the 1960s, most of what we offered in the industry couldn't really get you in shape anyway, so looking back, most probably left because what we sold didn't really help anyone get the results they were chasing.

But these new members also come at a high price. They get bored very easily and like to be entertained with newer and ever-changing equipment.

Let's face it: The caveman who first picked up a rock and moved it from one side of the cave to the other was doing a type of functional training. If we wanted to get basic, rocks would still get you in shape, provided you picked up enough of them often enough and pressed them over your head.

However, the members who work out on a regular basis want their rocks changed frequently. An example is the stair-climber. There was a time in the late 1980s and early 1990s when you could not get enough stair-climbers into your gym. The members would wait in line for them, ignoring the electronic bikes that were the rage the previous years. But the members' love for the stair-climbers soon faded—to be replaced by a new love for the treadmill and then on to the elliptical trainers.

As owners, we had rows of perfectly good stair-climbers probably still not paid for that we bought in response to members' demands. But they didn't want stairs anymore. They now wanted—in fact demanded—treadmills. Lines formed, sign-up sheets were hung, members stood at the desk complaining about how lousy the club is, and the race was on to add treadmills to the club's cardio repertoire.

Simply put, the members were bored with the stairs and wanted to get on the next hot product. They had tried treadmills elsewhere or had seen pictures and articles in the national fitness magazines that touted the advantages of working out on treadmills and cited the damage that might be done by doing too many stairs.

Seth Godin, a prolific writer on business theory and a must-read for any owner, stated in his book *Tribes*:

> Welcome to the age of leverage. Bottom-up is a really bad way to think about it because there is no bottom. In an era of grassroots change, the top of the pyramid is too far away from where the action is to make much of a difference. It takes too long and it lacks impact. The top isn't the top anymore because the streets (the heretic willing to learn on his own and introduce change) are where the action is.

Change in the industry is no longer what is hot at a national trade show. Now what is hot is what your trainer just learned at a three-day workshop on functional training, working out with his heroes, or a member who spends all his free time watching kettlebell videos online and now knows more about a kettlebell swing than the club's owner does. In other words, change is what is happening in your club while you are busy trying to make a dated business plan still work.

One form of change that owners do inadvertently create is change by default. This method of change was one of the prime reasons that aerobics faded from its once prominent role in the fitness industry. Owners themselves stopped doing aerobics on a regular basis and the programs faded. As long as owners participated in aerobics classes, they were willing to keep working toward keeping the classes fresh.

But as the owners stopped supporting the classes, support for the programs soon faded. This lack of owner commitment signaled the end for many aerobics programs in the country because the owners, meaning the decision-makers, had already moved on to something else in the gym—primarily cardio equipment and cardio entertainment areas. This is true today, as many owners find that they own a heavy investment in traditional equipment yet they work with a trainer using bands, cables, kettles, and suspension tools. If you own it but no longer believe in it, you will eventually lose it.

Another example of change in the 1990s that caught many owners off guard was the difficulty in hiring, training, and keeping staff. Over a long period of time, from the mid-1980s to the present, staffing has risen to the number one problem owners list in running their businesses—just ahead of marketing. It's hard to find dedicated employees who will work for the wages the industry is used to paying. The fitness industry is also now competing for service employees against literally thousands of other industries who have the same employment needs and who are willing to pay more to attract a better class of worker.

Because owners didn't change to meet this shift in hiring and staffing, many have suffered in the business. The owners who prospered had to learn advanced hiring practices, be willing to pay higher wages, and provide stronger benefit packages and they had to learn to motivate and develop a new type of employee.

The nature of the employee had also changed. Look at any fitness business and compare the average age of the group exercise instructors and the average age of the trainers. In most clubs, the average age of the group instructors is often a generation or more older than the trainers. With the advent of functional training, many of the women entering the industry started to become trainers rather than pursuing the more traditional route of being a group exercise instructor. Owners can see this coming by just glancing through the window of the group room, but most refuse to deal with the issue that something that used to be a centerpiece in the club might no longer be viable in the near future.

How Can Owners Effectively Deal With Change in the Fitness Business?

First of all, realize that change is an inevitable part of the business. Everything changes in life and the gym business is no exception. Imagine this scene from a mountaintop in Tibet:

> The seeker of knowledge: Tell me, wise master, what is the secret of life?
>
> The wise man: The secret of life is change. Accept change, for everything in your life will change sooner or later.
>
> The seeker: Does that mean everything, wise one? My wife, my children, and my business will change?
>
> The wise man: Yes, everything changes. You will some day pass away, as will your family. Your business may go away. Everything

changes. Except, of course, if you're in the gym business, where most of you guys are five years or more outdated as to what's happening in the industry. There, nothing changes because everyone is so emotionally tied to programs, physical plants, and equipment. There is my wisdom, my son. If you don't want change to ever happen in your life, open a gym where you may spend your days frozen in the past and crying about how easy the business used to be.

To be a successful owner, you must be open to change. In fact, you must learn to seek change. To be competitive in the fitness business is to respond to the changing needs of the members. Members are bored and fitness aware in most markets and they want to be the first to experience the new and different. Keep in mind that working out is somewhat boring to most people and nothing represents this boredom more than endless time on a tread or going around like a hamster on a circuit. To keep it interesting takes a challenge, and if you as an owner don't provide it, another club owner will.

What Needs to Change to Keep Members Happy in the Future?

The best thing about change is that it can often be managed and planned in advance. For most owners, change is simply trying to look ahead and anticipate the needs of your members and your business. First of all, consider the physical plant. Physical plants wear out and usually do so at a much faster rate than is planned for by typical owners. The basic rule of thumb: To keep the club competitive, you usually have to spend the same amount of money over every four-year period that you spent to build the club in the first place.

For example, if you initially spent $50 per square foot to build your club and the club is 10,000 square feet, you'd have to spend the same $500,000 over every four-year period after you open to keep the club fresh and competitive. The initial build-out would not include equipment, but the reinvestment would. Treadmills are a prime example. The industry went from having practically no treadmills to treadmills being must-have items in just a few years. If you opened your club with none or just a few, you would have had to add some during your first four years of operation.

Even the training club owners who think they might be exempt from this reinvestment have to plan for the wear and tear of their equipment and physical plants. For example, a trend that developed quickly in the industry was the use of the large multipurpose racks systems that can accommodate 10 to 15 clients at one time, doing everything from chins to suspension training to almost any other functional exercise that can be done with a simple piece of bolt-on equipment. These racks are relatively inexpensive, with a working price of about $12,000, but once they hit the market, they became a must-have piece because a rack such as this solved so many of the problems a small operator will have finding space and equipment that can be squeezed into a smaller footprint.

Many owners also find that their existing physical plant no longer meets the business plan. You may have started out with limited cardio equipment and aerobics programs, but four years later, you find yourself with no aerobics and two to three times as much cardio. That type of change requires the ability to change the physical plant on a fairly regular basis as dictated by the microtrends in the industry.

Another type of collateral change that affects the physical plant is the member boredom factor or the "been there, done that" feeling of going to the same place several times a week for years. Fitness facilities are a lot like a good nightclub. They can be really the rage for a while and then everyone moves to the next hot spot down the street. People just get bored with the same look and feel every day.

It's sad, but some clubs never change. You can walk into a club one day and it looks exactly the same as it did several years ago. The same paint, same colors, same artwork, and even the same staff uniforms. Owners will change their cars, their homes, their spouses, their hair, and even their dogs before they realize they need to repaint the gym, give it a new look, move the equipment, or simply add a few pieces of new equipment. The side note here is that the members also like to see reinvestment, and if an owner is in business for a while and doesn't show that he is putting money back into the club via new equipment and programming, the members grow to resent this cheapness over time and will leave.

Three Factors to Consider When You Seek Change

The three most important factors to change and manage in a gym are color, light, and sound. These factors give the business depth and energy and are also the ones that get worn out most quickly by the members.

Colors become dated in as little as two years. That color combination that was hot when you created the gym often fades and becomes dated and boring in a short period of time. For example, it seemed that every club owner in America went through a phase where he had to paint the club emerald green and some shade of nasty pink. If you were really cool, you also added a few stripes in contrasting colors that circled the club, making you feel short and that the ceilings were dropping in on you. It came and it went for many owners, but there was always the owner who was too cheap to paint that left those colors on the wall well after they were fresh or new.

A good habit to get into is to paint a different wall every month and give the club an overall change in color scheme every two to three years. A wall that might have been white today and is some accent color tomorrow is noticed by the members and keeps the business fresh.

Light is the factor most often ignored by owners. They put the lights up and then that's the way they remain until the owner dies. By changing the placement and mixture of lights on a regular basis, you can control the energy and warmth in the club. For example, by adding bulb-type light fixtures over a juice bar that was previously only lit by the ceiling lights, you can add a center of warmth in the club that will draw the members to the area. For lighting to be effective in a gym, it has to be a mixture of your main lighting—usually some type of metal halogen fixture and incandescent light, which can give certain areas of the club warmth and atmosphere.

Equipment in the club is also a tough issue. The major problem is that most equipment becomes outdated before it wears out. You may have great cardio equipment, but it might be outdated by four years and the types that no one really wants to play on anymore. New equipment should be added and old equipment should be replaced on a very regular basis. If possible, a typical club should be adding a new piece of equipment as often as every other month. Most cardio has a working life span of about four to five years and the fixed equipment you have will only have a shelf life of about five years. Yes, the equipment will still function, but the members are bored beyond belief and need the excitement of new toys for Christmas. Still being in working order is a lot different from representing the best in field as of today.

A rule of thumb here is to budget a certain percentage of your monthly base operating expense each month for capital purchases. The recommended formula is $150 per every 1,000 square feet. For example, if your gym was 15,000 square feet, you would want to budget $2,250 per month for capital purchases. Even if you didn't spend the money that month, you would move it to a special savings account for future purchases.

A final point about change: Don't overlook the small changes. The small things add up over a period of time and mean a lot to members. A painted wall, changes in the staff uniform shirts every quarter, or the addition of a new rack of kettlebells gives the members something new and interesting to talk about when they come in for their workouts.

Summary

Everything changes. It's a simple fact of life. In the fitness business, it's vital that we learn to change to meet the changing demands and expectations of the members and to meet the changing nature of the business itself.

Most change can be planned for and managed. Such trends as the advent of treadmills and the shift toward women moving in large numbers to the functional training areas are easy to spot. These two trends could have been anticipated by simply responding to the requests of the members, attending a workout-based seminar, and watching the types of articles the national consumer fitness magazines are running.

A final note: Don't be afraid of change. Change for the most part is good in our business. And some of our old business practices, such as high-pressure sales in offices, need to be changed and done away with anyway.

One final point to keep in mind is that it's not what you want that will make you money—it's giving the members what they want. Without an openness to change, we usually make decisions based on internal factors and old habits that might result in pleasing ourselves but seldom result in increased revenue or more members.

Some rules for managing change

- *Plan and budget for change.* The money needed for change, such as ongoing improvements on the physical plant and capital purchases, should be budgeted for each month as part of your normal monthly operating expense.

- *Don't get emotionally involved with your business or especially the business concept you had in your head when you opened.* Just because you are a bodybuilder and love the old ways does not mean there are enough of you left to create a new business. It's a business, not a baby, and it will wear out, get ugly, and need to be completely demolished occasionally to make room for next generation changes.

- *Don't get emotionally involved with your programs.* Aerobics is a prime example of programming that ran its course but was hard for most owners to change because of the emotional attachment. Always remember that is it harder to be number one than to stay number one and owners who still have an attachment to old tools won't be able to match the current wants and needs of the market.

- *Survey your members often.* What do they want? What doesn't the club have enough of? What have they tried at other clubs that they might want to see added to yours? What hot new products have they tried? Remember that it's not what you want that will make you money—it's what the members want.

- *Be willing to say you were wrong.* For example, we were wrong on child care in the gyms. We always thought it would be a natural moneymaker with the types of members we had. It's not. It cost us a great deal of money to prove that we couldn't make money with it. The best solution was to cut the loss and concentrate on the things that do make money. The lesson to learn here is that anything that doesn't touch at least 10 percent or more of your members is probably losing you money. Using the child care example, most clubs have a penetration rate of only about 5 to 6 percent of their membership. This means that out of 1,000 members in a club, only about 50 to 60 would use child care over a 30-day period. Child care might seem crowded, but in reality, for most owners, it is the same small group of parents using the service over and over again during a month. If your penetration rate is as low as 5 to 6 percent, then at least 94 percent of your members have no interest in that program and didn't join the club because of that offering, although there are many old-timers in the business who would argue that the member may not use it but that it was what got him excited. The numbers don't lie and the only reality you can deal with in this example is the fact that about 94 percent of your members do not support something that might be costing you a great deal of money to offer.

- *If it's not making money, drop it.* Years ago, when the cost of starting a new club and the cost of operation were significantly lower, we could run such programs as child care. We felt we had to offer it because the competition did. No longer. It costs far too much to start and operate the typical club these days. Our rule now is: If it doesn't net at least 20 percent on a monthly basis and you can't fix it after a 90-day period, dump it and get on to the things that do make you money.

- *Get outside opinions.* Remember the ugly baby. Your club may be rundown and hurting, but you still see it in your mind as fresh as the day you opened. Get professional outside opinions on colors, light, and sound at least once a year.

- *Remember that it's easier to get to be number one than it is to stay number one.* Ask any National League Football team. Winning the Super Bowl one year doesn't guarantee the same will happen next year. Just because something worked in the past, such as pressure sales, going for cash memberships, circuit training, or extended group exercise offerings, doesn't mean it will work now. Technique and business strategies are also parts of the business that need to change and be reviewed on a regular basis. How you do things can become outdated as fast as that old piece of equipment in the corner.

November 21, 2013
Three things every trainer should think about

The following are three things I wish every trainer would think about:

- *If the client doesn't get results, you failed, not the client.* It isn't about you. It's about getting the client successful, and if he doesn't get it done, it means you didn't get it done and we can't blame him no matter how many potato chips he ate.
- *You have to live and teach in the client's world, not yours.* Just because extreme health and fitness is your life does not mean this approach works for the average client. His world is about modest goals met slowly, kids, and work and not committing to a six-day-a-week workout schedule and no alcohol—just roadkill and living to workout. We have to change him in his world, not drag him into ours.
- *Learn that there will always be that hardcore group that thinks you are a rock star and it will follow you to the grave, but that group will also do everything it can do to keep the group small and elite.* This group will drive out every decent member who "can't keep up." This is why so many CrossFits struggle and so many training gyms fail. You can't have the hardcore group dictating the atmosphere and constantly screaming for "harder and harder" when you are trying to make money in a real business.

November 14, 2013
Time is the enemy of fitness.

You never want to give any fitness client the "I don't have enough time" excuse. Try keeping most of your sessions, classes, or other offerings, such as cycle, to 50 minutes. This allows the client to park the car, walk in the door, do his thing, and get back to the car and head home in less than an hour. Most fitness professionals can devastate a client in six minutes doing nothing but body weight, but there is also a threshold where money spent equals value for the client and that magic number is 45 minutes, meaning the client has to be sweating for at least 45 minutes or he feels he isn't getting what he paid for no matter how badly he is getting burned at the time. You can offer special sessions that go longer occasionally, but it is important to keep the bulk of what you do less than hour—and this means not one hour exactly but 50 minutes. We have been researching this for over 10 years and the in-and-out experience in an hour is a powerful approach to retention and even makes the initial sale easier because you take away the time objection completely.

13

The Top 20 Percent Will Thrive and the Rest Will Struggle

The numbers you see presented about the financial success of the fitness business posted on the blog sites and in the magazines are usually misleading about what constitutes success in this industry.

When you read these articles by the industry pundits, the theme is usually ranting that so many gyms just aren't making money like they did back in the day. The more you read, the more you feel there seems to be a sense of entitlement attached to the chains and the old guard who own and operate the mainstream big boxes and independents. The harsh reality is that being in business and investing millions to get there does not give you any right, entitlement, or built-in guarantee of making money. You ante up your gym and all you get to do is get into the game and take your chances like the rest of the players.

Think about it: In what industry do all the businesses that comprise that industry make money? Is the fitness industry special in that we are entitled to be profitable because we are in the business of helping people? If there are 1,000 dry cleaners in Chicago, are they all entitled to make money and be top performers because this type of business also provides a service to a wide range of clients? As in any field, talent and hard work separate the weak from the strong and our industry is no exception.

Surviving in business for a long period of time, as have many of the old legendary gyms featured in the magazines, should theoretically give you an edge in the game, but as most of these owners have found out during the last decade, getting to be number one in your market is much easier than trying to stay number one for any length of time.

These owners, defined as ones who are already established in their markets for a number of years or who are part of a national chain or franchise, are usually the ones who cry foul and declare unfair business practices whenever any new player enters the market. This group of operators hated the small circuit gyms, hated the low-priced gyms, and is just now realizing that the real threat is from the small training gyms that drain their best and most lucrative clients.

All this is important because too many owners spend too much time copying what the other guy does in business, when in reality, few of those players really make any money. Knowing this gives you an edge in the game because you can stop worrying about what the competitor is doing, which is statistically most likely not working, and start worrying about what you are going to do in your business.

We always tend to focus on the other guy when we aren't sure we are doing the right things in our own business. The hardest advice to hear is that you have to find a method of doing business that suits you, your market, the type of business you want to own and operate, and the demographic in your market and then master the rules of that system better than anyone.

If you are chasing the higher return per member model advocated in this book, then master the components and build your entire culture in your gym around that concept, but understand that you will see competitors in your area doing the complete opposite—many of them big chains—and you will question the system and your own sanity. Keeping this in mind, you always have to remember that just because those other guys are doing it doesn't mean it is working for them. You can lose a lot of money for a lot of years in a big chain and still look good on paper. However, this doesn't mean that anything they do will work for you or should be copied.

In life and business, the best rise to the top of their fields and everyone else settles lower on the scale. The following list shows how almost any array of businesses grouped in an industry shake out financially over time. These are gross averages and every industry does have its stars that get the press and the losers that fail spectacularly, but the middle is where the sea of mediocrity exists and no one ever looks hard at that group. Again, this is important to understand for the next time you read about a CEO of a chain telling the reporter in an interview that every business he owns is killing it financially:

- *About 20 percent of any category of small businesses exceeds the average profit and this profit is what separates this group from the other 80 percent.* These are the superstars—the ones the franchises use as references and the ones the big independent chains use to get bank loans. In small business, defined as businesses that gross $10,000,000 or less a year, there is always a group of people that own a business in that class that simply work harder, have better locations, had more start-up capital, or are just plain the smartest people in the industry where they invested.

- *About 60 percent hit the average for that type of business.* The word average is defined here as people who make a little, lose a little, and generally run the world's greatest breakeven businesses. Fortunes aren't being made here, but money is also not being lost. This group will often live forever, but in capital-intensive businesses, such as the fitness business, the businesses in this class will eventually falter because at some point, it takes big capital to keep a big box gym current and functioning. You have to reinvest heavily in a box gym every five years or so and where is this capital coming from if the owner isn't making a sustainable profit? You can only borrow so much from the banks before the loans will overwhelm the business.

- *About 20 percent fall into the lowest performers for that particular industry.* One of the keys in the fitness industry is that you seldom fail during your first year in business, as do many retail businesses. Most fitness facilities that open can usually make it for about four years before going down. You cut staff, cut marketing, stiff the landlord, and basically run without paying anyone for a year or so, and when you go down, you take a lot of people with you. Many people in this class should have never opened their own businesses. While it is the American dream to do your own thing and own your own business, there are many owners who get into business who never have the money, patience, skill set, or talent to get it done.

This breakout is true of almost any small business concept you can identify. Look at pizza places, small retail stores, dry cleaners, restaurants, and most any other business concept and you can break them down into these groupings. The best make money, most people do just enough to stay in business, and the bottom 20 percent are wasting money when they should have jobs working for the city and leaning on a shovel.

This bottom group would go broke in a year or two in their own industries no matter how much money they started with and no matter where they opened. This group is in the bottom 20 percent because they deserve to be there, not because they are unlucky or surrounded by gifted competitors.

Fitness businesses fall into this same breakdown. For example, if half the clubs in a survey reported flat sales from last year or declining numbers, is this really unusual or is this report just a verification that the averages are holding? The top 20 percent will find a way to make money in good and bad times and the rest will fall into their respective categories as the economy and market dictates.

Opening a fitness business does not entitle you to make money. This is a fallacy that most new owners have to have beaten out of them quickly. "I have my life in this club and it's unfair that a new club is moving in and taking my business."

The same is also true of individuals. Only about 5 percent of the population in this country makes more than $205,000 a year. It is a very sharp point at the top of that demographic chart and gets sharper faster when you move up in salaries beyond this number. The best excel at what they do and everyone else works for someone else. You are seldom in that super wealthy group unless you had rich parents or due to luck and you survive at the very top because of many other skills in your life.

The best may get slapped around for a few moments now and then, especially those who rise to the top and then their company slides out underneath them, but most of the talented ones always rise again. The talented few that reach the top 5 percent are hard to kill no matter what they are doing or selling. Your goal, of course, is to prepare yourself to be one of the talented folks who figure out money and how to make it in almost any economy or business.

There has been a lot of discussion through the years on the economy and how it has affected clubs as it rises or collapses, but the theory expressed here holds true. For example, in the great recession of 2007, the owners who adapted to change (and broke away from the 1995 business model) and fought back hard by working their collective asses off not only survived but still made money. And this group made lots of money.

The good players still had great years, while the large group in the middle took the biggest hits. If you are barely making it, then even the slightest disruption will take enough cash flow away to finish you off. That middle 60 percent took a harsh beating and many failed, but the capitalistic system is unemotional and hard. You either adapt, change, grow, or die and the market will bear out your decisions. Failure is an option if you refuse to change how you operate because the financial universe will correct bad business decisions quickly and painfully.

If you sit on your ass and fail to react to everything and waste your life and business by complaining about the cheap competitor down the street, you probably didn't make much last year. You could have beaten him if you would have just shut up and gone to work. He didn't take your business. You gave it to him by not being aggressive in your own business.

The bottom 20 percent constantly disappear in the gym market and are replaced every year by another generation of people who feel they are a guaranteed success because they are great trainers or passionate people who lost some weight and now have to share their story with the world. Only the market will tell if they have the skill set to go along with that passion, along with the knowledge and work ethic to succeed.

Many of the people in this group are the ones who come into the industry thinking that running a successful gym is an easy passive investment. This is the group of novices that often buys franchises for a lot of money but won't take the time to go work in a working gym in sales or as a trainer before opening.

The attitude this group brings with it from the outside is often arrogance expressed by these thoughts: "If I am successful in another field, then how hard can this business really be? I mean, I made money in (fill in the blank), which was the hardest industry in the world, so running a gym has to be really easy. I mean, look at the people who run these things now."

The battleground is littered with thousands of out-of-business gyms opened by a group of very successful people who made a lot of money in real estate, hotels, software, retail, and financial services. The fitness business is a hard business in that it is capital and service intensive and the rules change as you change. There are some things that do stay constant across all industries, such as customer service, but there is always a set of ground rules in any new field that have to be mastered if you want to have a chance to survive.

This is an extremely difficult business to be in, especially now, but you can make money if you are willing to let go of what worked in the 1990s and embrace new ideas. The smaller clubs, which are more agile and more able to change, will lead this charge of new prosperity while the chains will slowly fail because they are not willing to admit that their business models are outdated by 30 years or more.

Build the big boxes and stock them full of 1995 circuit stuff and the market will judge you brutally, as it has most of those chains during the last several years. You simply don't want to be the last guy trying to sell a product that is outdated by 20 years. These players from the last century sell just enough memberships to give themselves hope, but the overall picture is grim and getting darker for the membership mills.

So, who does make money year after year in this industry and who makes money when the economy tanks? Most of the same people who made money in the good times just have to work harder to get it done. Good owners are good owners and will adjust as needed, buying the tools and education needed to keep moving and growing.

Who gets kicked during the lean years? The marginal owners who rode the good times but never really learned how to make money and just lived off the natural flow of their location and market. There are a lot of owners who have been lucky rather than good and the economy and full onslaught of new clubs saturating the market have edited this group down in size. Weak owners are weak owners, and while they complain that their numbers are down, if they really know their numbers, is anyone in those upper groupings really surprised?

One of the keys for breaking out of the rut of the average 60 percent is to master the key numbers and indicators in our business. Remember that numbers never lie.

Most owners, especially in the average grouping and always in the bottom 20 percent pile, make very emotional decisions and often make decisions that are wrong for their businesses. These owners use what is called a *situational management style*. Situational management means you base your decision on what is in front of you at the moment, and if that something is causing you a little pain at the time, the reaction and the decision are often emotional rather than what is best for the business.

Effective management is always number based. If you track the right numbers and understand what the numbers mean in relationship to your business, then you will make better decisions that will improve your business over time because the numbers never lie and will always point you to the decision you need to make to help the business grow.

For example, a typical owner who is not numbers driven is having a poor and extremely stressful sales month. He is sitting in his office when his local newspaper sales representative drops by to check in to see if he needs to run an ad. Our owner, who is frustrated that sales are slow, listens closely as the newspaper person paints a great picture of a new section coming out in the paper next week on brides and summer weddings.

The newspaper person tells him he just has to be in this section because it will be the best-read special issue of the summer, and if he isn't, he will miss out big time on a chance to get great exposure. Our hardworking owner—but dumb as a kettlebell—slaps together a special for a bride's boot camp, the paper designs the ad in about an hour with no thought to the club's brand or marketing look, and a few people drift in when the ad appears—but not nearly enough to justify the ad cost.

The owner had a frustrating day, makes a quick decision to solve that frustration, wastes some money in the process, and still hasn't helped the business. This is situational management at its worst because the decision was made through emotion and the day's frustration and not based on any real numbers that reflect the true financial situation of the club.

For example, most owners claim they track all leads or potential business through the door, but most owners lie in this case. Few owners really know the amount of qualified leads through the club over a typical 30-day period because they simply don't have a system in place that forces the staff to report correctly. Therefore, the owner always thinks he knows, but in reality, he seldom has a tight number. In the case of our kettlebell head, he made the decision based on frustration and not real numbers because first of all, he doesn't know how to gather real numbers, and secondly, he doesn't know what to do with them if he did have them.

In his case, if he would have looked at his numbers closely, he might have found something like this, which is often the case in a typical club. If he had control of his leads, he would have found out he really had 80 leads through the door and not the 60 the staff reported because there is really no incentive or punishment for not reporting true numbers every day.

He would have also found out that he only truly converts 35 percent of his total leads each month into new membership and not the 60 percent and higher his staff reports because what the owner doesn't know is that his sales team lowers the amount of leads it missed so the sales team looks better. The sales team might not really be trying to cheat, but they do find many reasons a person wasn't really qualified and dropped from the potential lead list and that eventually raises its closing percentage much higher than it should be.

If kettle head were really in the game, he would track his numbers every day for his team and for each salesperson and find out he doesn't have a marketing problem—he has a sales training issue because the numbers would have shown him that he is really closing less than 40 percent and no amount of marketing money can overcome a bad sales effort.

Training his staff would be far more effective than blowing senseless money on an ad. If he really wanted to do the ad, he should have his ad company do a real ad for the paper that reflects a thought-out special reflecting the club's brand, meaning the ad perpetuates the club's image in the market. A bride's boot camp might have been a good idea, but it has to fit the overall marketing plan for the business and the ad has to build a recognition factor in the marketplace.

The Most Important Number You Aren't Tracking

The most important number you aren't tracking right now is your average EFT payment. Typically, a gym might have a monthly rate of $39 for one person. If you break couples (two people at the same address) into separate agreements, you will find that if the club sold seven memberships on a Monday, the average EFT is always going to be lower than the single rate of $39. For example (ignore the one-time membership fees here):

- $39 x 12 months
- $34 x 12 (discount for second person at the same address)
- $29 x 12 (student discount)
- $39 x 12
- $29 x 12 (senior discount)
- $39 x 12
- $29 x 12 (corporate discount)

Total = $238

The average EFT payment—or average return per client—is
$34 ($238/7).

In our business, the average EFT has always been lower than the stated monthly single rate for one person—usually running at least 20 percent or lower than the actual stated monthly payment—which makes it hard to run a business over time because most owners base their success on the higher number. If you factor in all your discounts, you'll probably find that your number is actually lower than this example.

This lower number is what makes you so vulnerable in the marketplace to the lower-priced competitors because whether you want to or not, you are competing head-to-head on price. If the guy down the street is at $19 a month and your true average is only about $29 to $32 in this example, with a stated price of $39, you are in the same price game he is, except you are losing. Your true yield per sale price is too high to differentiate you from your competitor but not high enough to protect your business.

Your discounts reflect the only way most owners know to generate more volume in their clubs. You simply drop your price for every exception to the rule. Couples get discounts. Kids get discount. Seniors get discounts. Corporate people get discounts. Your business plan is to figure out a way to give everybody a discount.

What you should be working on is how can you raise your EFT average, not lower it. You can generate a higher monthly EFT average, especially if you switch your training away from session driven to monthly EFT.

Other clubs have also added weight management programs based on 12 weeks that is also EFT driven. But others have added programs, such as a sports performance school, that allow the club to drive more memberships by adding the children for just $15 per month per child and then upgrading the kids from that point into higher-priced sports performance training or one-on-one training.

Once your number goes higher than the one-person price, your vulnerability in the market drops because you are now making a much higher return per sale or, in other words, you are now making more money per club client. The following is what your sales for the day should look like:

- $39 x 12
- $89 x 12 (group team training)
- $150 x 3 (weight management)
- $54 x 12 (one parent with one $15 add-on for a sports performance program)
- $39 x 12
- $39 x 12
- $39 x 12

Total = $449

Average EFT for this club = $64 ($449/7)

Driving your average return per client served is one of the many things that separate the groupings listed earlier in this chapter. Your goal is to drive the average return per sale as high as you can go while still showing an entry-level membership that is competitive for the market.

Track this number every day and also get a monthly total. Your goal is to create programs in the club that allow you to seek a higher return per member and still get the highest number of new members possible each month.

This is just one of the numbers you should be tracking each month or each day. The secret here is to track the right numbers and then learn how to react to what you learn from these numbers. The numbers don't lie and they keep you from making kettlebell head emotional decisions based on situational management.

December 3, 2013
Want to lose clients today?

Try these surefire methods of frustrating and losing even your best people:

- *Talk on that cell phone and text during my entire session.* It's guaranteed to piss off even your most loyal clients.
- *Show up late for that session.* Nothing says professional like a coach who is always 10 minutes late. Thank you for being late and for pointing out that your time is more valuable than mine as a paying client.
- *Dress like a homeless person.* Your clients just love paying their professional trainer, who then totally shows disrespect by not even caring enough to put on some clean and decent clothes.
- *Go ahead—warm me up on that treadmill because you are too lazy or just too incompetent to take me through a dynamic warm-up that gets me up and moving.* Nothing says fun like spending 10 minutes of my session on a treadmill while I watch you catch up on your cell. Put the professional back in professional trainer this week people.
- *And put down that damn coffee cup too.* Carrying it around like you are worshipping the gods of Starbucks also makes them crazy.

January 23, 2014
We always enhance—we never discount.

The temptation for many professionals is to discount their service if the client buys more. For example, you see five sessions at $250 or 10 at $400. Do not do this. It lowers your credibility and return per client. Learn to enhance instead of dropping the price. Once you set your price, the price becomes the price. If someone wants to extend longer with you, add a few bonus sessions, a training journal, a T-shirt, or added supplements, but never come off the stated price. Treat people as you would like to be treated by rewarding choices that make you money. That client could have worked with anyone, but he chose you, so reward him for that gift. Always add more than you are expected to give. The old adage "Underpromise and overdeliver" still holds up today. "I signed up for training, but I never expected this bag or book." It doesn't have to be big, but it should be something the person simply didn't expect. Separate yourself from the herd by being the first kid in your neighborhood to show appreciation for every session you get. Reward the client, but never compromise your integrity by discounting your service.

Section 4

THE ART OF MARKETING

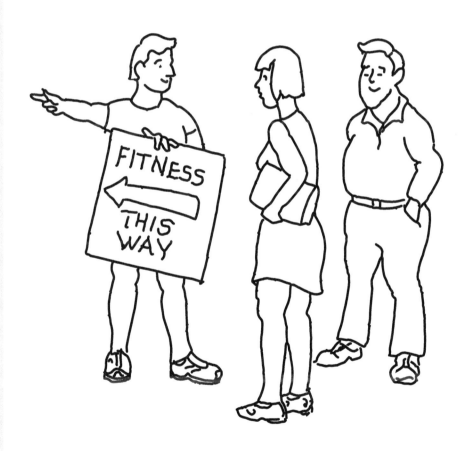

14

Even If You Give It Away for Free, You Still Have to Master the Art of Marketing

Even if you give something away for free, you still have to have a system to get new clients into your business and that system is called *marketing*. There can be no new sales and no new clients unless you develop a consistent way to entice potential business to inquire about what you do and why you do it. Good marketing has one purpose—and that purpose isn't to sell someone a membership but rather to create future interest in your business.

It is estimated that there are about 306,000,000 people in this country and only about 17 percent of this total population belongs to a fitness facility. Marketing to the 17 percent is a waste of your money. The people in this group "get it" and have already checked out every gym in their neighborhood and most likely have more than one gym membership. You can't do long-term effective marketing for this group simply because they have already bought the product you are trying to sell—just not necessarily your product and from you.

Price specials are usually not enough to pull a significant number of existing members out of other businesses. But this is one of the biggest myths in the fitness business—that a new gym can crush the older players by simply running a lower-priced ad. "Hey, I will drop my price to $10 and kill that guy's gym" has been said too many times for too many years. The reality is that a price war will pry a percentage out of existing gyms, especially if those gyms are charging more for the value they offer, but over time, the number of memberships drained in a competitive market over price—with the focus of chasing the members already in someone else's gym—is insignificant.

What this all means is that chasing the 17 percent will have no long-term success factor. Price is often of little concern for someone who is happy in his choice of business, especially when the price difference is only about $20 or so per month. People already using gyms are probably already in the gym of their choice and hoping that any price offer you can come up will tempt them to leave their safe and happy nests has never been proven to be sustainable business plan.

The future of marketing for you is going after the 83 percent who are not currently involved in a gym. Creating future business for your market is what you should be chasing and all our marketing over time should be centered on getting someone who has yet to make the leap to fitness interested in trying your product.

There are only two ways to attract new clients into your business. The first is based on putting your product on sale, thus lowering the perceived value of the product or service, and the second way is to entice people to try your product first before making a buying decision. The second method is called *exposure marketing* and means you are willing to let people try your business before they buy so they can gain the experience with you necessary to make that buying decision. Try the gym, meet the staff, and meet the members, and if we don't earn your business, we don't deserve to have you as a client.

In the "putting it on sale" method, you discount or reduce the price of your service or product to attract new clients. In other words, you put what you do on sale. Examples of this are discounted membership fees, two-for-one specials, buy one and get one free offers, and closeout specials where the price is dropped for a limited time. Many fitness professionals don't think they do this—and often feel they are above this type of behavior—but an offer such as "three personal training workouts for $99" is just another version of dropping your pants in order to attract new clients.

Price specials require one thing to work: The client has to have an already formed interest in joining your gym and is now spending all his free time scanning the papers and the Internet just waiting for a gym to put its memberships on sale. In other words, price advertising of any type of business assumes there is a prior interest for your product, but the potential buyers have been hesitant to buy just yet due to the price being too high.

This is a valid assumption if the client is buying something he is keenly aware of and understands the value and standard price of what is being offered. For example, if Calvin has been buying Bright White toothpaste for 10 years at $3 per tube and it goes on sale for $2, he is going to be all over that sale because Calvin is known as a cheap person and a bargain shopper. In this example, Calvin has previous experience with the product (prior knowledge) and a need for the product (have to brush those teeth every day), so this sale is relatively easy to make.

However, the fitness world is totally different. When a gym owner runs a price ad, he is assuming that every person in his market has enough experience with fitness and working out, understands the price of fitness in his market, and has the sophistication to decide if Club Cheapest is indeed worth the $10 price and is radically different from Gym Mainstream that offers memberships at $39.

In an era where obesity and being overweight account for almost 65 percent of the total population, it would be hard to makes any of these assumptions for the potential clients who receive the price-driven marketing. The people in this market don't respond because the price isn't right. They don't respond because they simply don't know anything about what we do or the product we sell. Hard to buy something if you really don't know if you need it and can do it or if it was really designed for you at all.

The exposure method of marketing is usually considered to be a classier way to attract clients, and more importantly, it is also the method that allows you to usually protect your integrity by getting full price for your product once the customer has some experience with what you do. The other way to think about exposure is: "Try it before you buy it." This style of marketing works especially well in our industry, where what we do for a living, meaning the delivery of a fitness service, is perceived as very complicated to the consumer as well as just plain scary to someone who is out of shape and thinks he will probably die during the first workout.

Modern fitness just has too many moving parts to be sold in one 20-minute session with a salesperson. If we are really moving beyond the age of circuit training and do-it-yourself-fitness, then explaining something as complicated as functional training, with all its full-body movements, just can't be done across a desk with a person who has no idea what those new "kettleballs" really do. If you want to understand how modern fitness works, then stop talking about it and get sweaty over several workouts and let the experience of fitness—done safely and with a master coach—sell itself.

Imagine walking into a nice nightclub and seeing someone interesting sitting on a bar stool across the room. You get a drink and start walking toward your new prospect, but just before you get close enough to talk, you trip and throw your drink all over the person. You panic at your stupid move and lean in, trying to help wipe the drink off the front of her shirt, and knock her off the stool. You then rush to help her up and bang her head on the bar while trying to get her off the floor. Finally, you get her back on the stool and there she sits: wet, bruised, and pissed. Is this a good time to ask her out for a date?

If this scenario doesn't seem like it would work, then how about this: Someone walks through the door of a gym. He is in his 40s, embarrassed about his weight, hasn't worked out in 10 years, and is a bundle of nervousness and fear. The salesperson takes him on a walk to the back of the gym, takes him back into the office, explains the prices, and then turns the guy over to a young, hard-bodied trainer who has never been out of shape in his life. The trainer takes the guy through a workout that is too hard and without any concern if the guy has any physical issues that are going to hinder success.

The session is long and difficult and the guy barely makes it through the 30 minutes. He is wet and embarrassed and now his doubt that he could ever get into shape is confirmed. Is this a good time for the salesperson to take him back into the office, which happens in virtually every mainstream club in business, and pound the guy to make a decision to buy a membership today—at his lowest point mentally and physically in years?

If a dealership lets you drive a new car for 24 hours, price will seldom be the deciding factor and "How did it feel, how did it drive, and how did your family like it?" are now the more important factors in the sale. Think about the puppy dog close from the 1950s where the pet shop owner says "Go ahead and take the puppy home for tonight, and if he doesn't work out, just bring him back tomorrow." What kind of heartless bastard ever brought back a used puppy? Other examples of this in the real world are extended 24-hour test drives of cars, free samples (including everything from cookie chunks to an introductory massage), and extended trial usage periods.

Perhaps the most well-known use of exposure marketing for those in the fitness industry is the paid trial membership, where the gym offers 30 days of fitness at a fixed price, such as 30 days for $30. This membership is not a reduction of service, such as three training sessions for $99, but rather a total introduction to everything you offer at a trial rate. If you treat them like a member and include everything in your gym for this price (training gyms might be 30 days for $89 or higher depending on the market), then the potential member has a chance to experience the product and service and can spend time with the other members prior to making a buying decision.

In the fitness business, we have a long history of usually taking the path of least resistance as owners and managers, and in this case, the easiest way to market a gym is to always just drop the price and then pound whoever shows up in response to the special of the week featured in your ads. There are a number of problems with this system.

Price Specials Assume Prior Interest

This means that reducing the price of your service assumes that somewhere out there is a client who is dying to use your service, but who hasn't yet responded because the price is a barrier. This sounds logical, but if it were true, why has the total percentage of people participating at a fitness facility only increased by 1 percent in the era of the low-priced gym? Currently, only 17 percent of the people in this country belong to a gym—up a whopping 1 percent since the last survey done about 10 years earlier.

You can make a case that the total population in the United States is up. Therefore, this number is higher in relation to the total it represented just a few years ago. While this is true, it still points to the fact that we don't do much of job as an industry when it comes to penetrating the percentage of people who are not yet interested in fitness and who haven't decided to join a gym. If sales and low price were the answer, we should have been overwhelmed by millions of new members who were patiently waiting for someone to offer a $9 membership. Someone did offer it in the industry and the people didn't come. So, maybe there just isn't enough prior interest out there waiting for the magic number.

Price-Related Sales Devalue Your Business

Putting something on sale means you couldn't sell it at full price, so you have to dump it at a lower price. You know that, they know that, everyone in the world who has ever shopped knows that basic rule of life, but why do we think the potential client doesn't know that reality? Once you start down the eternal "selling by discounting" road, it becomes almost impossible to change direction. The verification you need to prove that sales drop the perceived value of your business occurs when someone calls the gym and asks "What kind of sale do you have going this week?" Selling by price special and discounting lead to more selling by price special and discounting, and eventually, the process erodes the perception of value entirely.

Price-Based Advertising Eventually Fails

The longer you run price-driven ads, the less effective they become. Try running one year for $199 as an experiment. Let's say that this campaign brings in 100 new clients that month for your gym. Everyone is excited and the owner can't wait to repeat it again next month. The problem is that each successive time you run a price-driven ad, this leads to a further erosion of the market.

The term applied to this occurrence is the *law of diminishing returns*, which states that an act repeated over and over again will produce a lower result each consecutive time. For example, if you plant a field of corn and get 50 bushels this year, you will most likely only get 48 next year. The same goes if you walk up to a guy in the bar and hit him 10 consecutive times in the head. The first punch will usually be your best and the tenth will most likely be of lesser force.

Advertising price works the same way. Over time, everyone who wants a membership for $9 in the market has bought one, and each time you run the ad, you will get a lesser response. Of course, the difference between corn and members is that if you live in a marketplace that has a huge turnover in the 20- to 40-year-old range, such as Orlando, Florida, you constantly introduce an influx of new potential clients who are now seeing your ads for the first time. But most markets are more fixed in nature, with a much smaller annual turnover, and these markets will show the constantly declining response over time to just running price discounting in your advertising.

Price Ads Force the Conversation Between the Salesperson and the Potential Member to Always Be About Price

Price ads also are built on the one-visit sales process, where the person responds to an ad and then gets pounded in an office with the "buy or die" sales approach during a 20-minute visit. The ad was used as bait for the real game, which is the office sale and all the old techniques that made this sales system so despicable to so many consumers.

If you can't talk about fitness and your product from a common position of understanding established through experience and success, then all you will talk about is price and then it becomes "Let's make a deal time." We force the price wars on ourselves because we just don't give the potential member any other choice.

Exposure marketing has two strong mechanisms going for it that price-driven marketing doesn't. First of all, this type of marketing—when done correctly—creates an interest in a product that wasn't there in the consumer prior to his experience. For example, a four-page newsletter featuring articles about fitness, how to get started, success stories and testimonies, and educational information on fitness will get people interested in eventually trying the fitness for themselves. In other words, you have to create interest in the 83 percent of the people in this country who have never been in a gym or who have and failed before price is relevant.

The second factor about using a trial, such as the 30 days for $30, is that it kills risk. Remember that risk is the biggest barrier to inquiry for most potential clients. Many people would like to try a gym, but they are afraid of getting signed up for something that is too expensive and traps them too long without a chance to really see if they might like it first. If this sounds like dating, it is. You would have to be one crazy person to get married the first date and then commit to years of time together. But wait! Isn't that what we are asking when we try to force a member into a commitment during his first visit to the gym? What about a cup of coffee or dinner? How about taking me to a movie before you have your way with me and I have to commit to a multiyear deal? Even the chains that offer open-ended membership options have this issue because the perception of commitment is still there, meaning I still have to sign up now during my first visit.

We have created this ourselves in the industry by using such practices as firs-visit pressure, double-teaming the potential client in an office, and cold-calling. Throw in the potential client's experience and knowledge of gyms failing in the news and in his town and you can see why anyone might be reluctant to commit to fitness during a first visit.

The second risk barrier is that the client doesn't know if he will fit into the culture. It is like being a 21-year-old female and walking into a bar where there are 100 old guys listening to Frank Sinatra and sipping on whiskey. The bar looked good from the outside, but it is horror-movie scary once she is in the door. Sometimes, you just don't belong in a certain business or setting, but in the gym business, it may take multiple workouts to discover this for yourself. Experiencing the product and the culture has to be the centerpiece of all marketing if you want to kill the risk that prevents people from even trying your business.

Trial memberships solve these problems. The risk is known and low—in this case, no more than the price of the trial membership—and you have a full

30 days prior to making the buying decision, giving you plenty of time to see if the culture of this business is right for you.

Trial membership advertising should have the following components to be successful:

- *You must use a reasonable testimonial.* Don't use someone who has lost 100 pounds in your ads. Very few people can identify with that client and he is not a role model. He is an entry barrier. Use someone who is a more normal weight-loss example—perhaps one who has lost 10 to 20 pounds and is someone a potential client can identify with as a role model.

- *Use a positioning letter to generate interest in what you do.* For example, a letter imbedded in the ad that talks about the five biggest myths of fitness would work nicely. Have it signed by you and include a picture of you and your staff at the bottom. This also personalizes your business in the market against those competitors that might be faceless or national chains that have no true local connection.

- *Include full service in the trial.* Give the potential client a strong overview of everything you do and spoil the person during the trial period. Remember that if you treat the person like a member, he will become a member.

- *Keep the price for the trial membership at about half of your lowest entry point—no matter what kind of gym you own.* For example, if your base membership is $39 a month for one person, your trial should be at 30 days for $19. This also applies to training gyms.

The goal is to expose the gym and what you do to the maximum number of potential clients who don't have current gym experience. Remember the 17 percent of the population that was mentioned earlier who are gym members. It does you no good to advertise to them. They have found their gym, have probably already been in yours, and are more concerned about service, equipment, and location than they are about price because they are experienced gym people.

Using a trial membership doesn't mean you just open the doors and let everyone try it until they turn themselves in at the front counter with their checkbooks in their hands. You still have to sell with a trial membership and this "try before you buy" method of selling still has to have systems in place that allow these sales to happen. The trial membership system is based on a 30-day trial period. During this time, the trial member has to be entered into a system, trained as we would a real member, followed up on by the sales team and the assessment team in order to get the sale, and then someone on the team has to convert the trial member into a regular member.

With a trial membership, the potential member is looking for a period of time to get to know the staff, see what kind of service the club has to offer, meet the other members, and grow comfortable to the point that he is ready to commit to a simple access or training-based membership. This prospective member may reach this comfort level at any time during his trial period, and sometime during the trial period, he does expect the gym's salesperson to ask him if he'd like to join.

In other words, every trial member understands that we are just letting him try it in hopes that he will like it enough to buy it. If you're an old sales dog, this is just another version of the puppy dog close mentioned earlier, where the pet store owner lets the family take the little puppy home for a couple of days to see if everyone likes it. No one ever brings back a used puppy and there are a lot fewer potential members who walk away from your business if they have had a true trial experience that gave them a chance to try before they buy.

We're doing the same thing with this tool. Try us for free to see if you like us, and of course, trying the club free for 30 days does build up a little obligation toward us in the trial member's head.

Treat Them Like a Member and They Will Become a Member

Trial members should be treated like real members because they are real members, although they're just short-term members there to experience your fitness business.

Your trial members may have visited other clubs before they found you. If this is the case, they are probably battle weary against salespeople. One of the keys to making trial memberships successful is to change their orientation. When someone first comes in to inquire about the trial membership, sit him down, register the person as a new trial member, and then tour him as someone who is already a member rather than a guest. This changes the person's orientation because instead of showing the gym as if we're trying to sell him, we're showing him the club as if he is already a member.

For example, instead of showing him the cardio area and pitching him on the number of pieces or brands the club has, you tell him this is where he will be doing his cardio work, here's how to use the machines, and, by the way, this is Anna—she's one of the trainers and she'll be the one who shows you how to get the most out of your cardio workouts.

By touring as a member, the prospect loses much of the defensiveness potential members usually feel around salespeople and he is much more likely to come back and use the trial membership if he feels he already belongs and isn't going to get endlessly pitched every time he walks through the door.

Trial Membership Procedures

The steps can be adapted to any length of trial membership. For sake of example, we're using the 30-day paid trial throughout the steps. When someone presents the advertising piece or as he inquires about the trial memberships he heard about from a friend, take the following four steps.

Register the person immediately as a trial membership.

The registration is important for future tracking. Most clubs get the same information you would need to fill out a membership contract. Then, as you close later during the member's trial period, you'll already have the information you need to get the person converted. Don't forget to have the person sign a liability disclaimer because he will be working out in the club.

Give the person a temporary membership card.

The membership card should be a bright, somewhat obnoxious color that works in the gym's computer system. For example, if you were using a third-party financial service company system, you would take the person's picture with the system's camera and give him a membership card that activates the computer system when he comes in each time. Anything that can be done to make the person feel like he already belongs is important to the ultimate number of trial conversions you can accomplish.

The card and the picture appearing on the screen each time he uses the card already make him feel that the trial membership is a serious thing instead of a low-rent giveaway. The card system also allows him to get that comfort level to start growing by understanding one of the club's procedures that every member must use.

Tour the new person as a new member and not as a guest.

Again, this gives staff members a position of power when they tour the person as a new member instead of as a guest. By touring as a member, the person loses much of his defensiveness because he now doesn't expect to get pitched. For example: "As a new member, Joe, let me show you your locker room and how you get a key and a towel when you come in to work out." We still have to tour—but from a different frame of mind and from a position of power now that the person is already a trial member.

Give them the tour and then present the prices.

To give the member added value on his membership and to help the salespeople get the sale, you still have to use some form of leverage. The suggested course of action is to track the trial guest for a week or so and then ask him to close and become a full member.

You will find with the trial that there is a high level of perceived value and many trial members will ask if they can finish the trial first so they won't lose the time they did pay for when they purchased the full 30-day experience. For example, you are two weeks into a trial membership for a potential member and the assessor sees that he is in large group for team training tonight.

If the assessor is doing the proper follow-up, she would find the guest at the end of the team workout and ask him how he enjoyed the group and if he is enjoying his trial membership. If the response is positive, the assessor would then say "Good—let's get your paperwork done tonight while you are here and get your regular membership started." The trial person will most likely respond by stating that he loves the gym but that he still has several weeks left on his trial and he doesn't want to lose the time he already paid for with that purchase. The assessor should then offer to add 30 days to the end of any membership the guest chooses as a way to buy back that time at a higher value.

For example, if the guest wants to sign up for the team training 12-month membership at $129 per month, the assessor could add the 13th month free as a gift and as a way to buy back the remaining time left on the trial. Everyone wins in that the gym gets a new membership and the new member gets a bonus for signing up today for $129.

Still try to close on the first visit. With a trial membership system, you can still expect to write about 30 percent of your business during the prospective member's first visit to the gym. Most of these early sales will be direct referrals, spouses or friends, or someone who is already familiar with what you offer and doesn't want to waste time with a trial membership. The 30-day incentive still works here and every new member should walk away with 13 months for the price of 12. Added value is a powerful tool and you want every new member spreading the word.

Set a Fixed Appointment With the Assessor and Give the Person a Formal Appointment Card

It's not unusual for a gym to have 40 percent or more of its trial members not show for their first workout after being set up as a trial member. There are several reasons why this might happen, but two important ones to consider are closing too hard during the first visit, which cancels out what the trial membership was designed to do in the first place, and letting the member leave without a clear idea of what's supposed to happen next.

Slamming too hard on the first visit sends a mixed message to the guest. He came in because he was responding to an ad offer that made trying your club feel safe and different from the other clubs in the area. We have in essence lied to the person when we use a trial to bring him in and then do a negative drop-close during his first visit.

The second reason is that he leaves without a clear idea of what's supposed to come next and what will happen to him once he's in the gym. Many also find that the gym was more frightening than they anticipated. If they don't come back, it's because they may have seen something that scared them out of their comfort zone. Constantly exam your trial rate, and if it is higher than 20 percent of the people scheduled that don't show, then you have an issue. Perhaps the biggest reason people do not come back after their first visit is that they feel they simply can't do it. The fear of fitness and the fear of failing at fitness are terrifying to someone who hasn't been in a gym in a decade—if ever. Because all the team members in a gym are usually fitness people, we forget about this fear, which can be fear of the physical or even the fear of looking bad and not knowing what to wear to the gym these days. Spend more time than you think during the initial trial sign-up to prepare people for their first visit with the assessor by anticipating the things that might cause them to not come to their first meeting.

An important point here is to understand that trial memberships often bring in a type of member that other gyms don't get and that you might never have had in large numbers in your business. These are the folks who would never consider even inquiring at your competition but felt safe checking you out because of the trial memberships. These folks need different handling than your regular workout people who have belonged to other gyms or clubs and they need a lot more personal attention during their first few weeks before they can be converted to a regular membership.

The trial membership system requires that you modify how you sell in the club. You still have to sell, but it's when the sale takes place that becomes more important in this system.

Because of the extreme pressure their sales teams exert to close the first visit, most gyms risk their entire chance to get a new member on a single encounter between a salesperson and the prospect. If the salesperson is that good, wouldn't he be more effective if he had a possible 15 chances to close the potential client instead of just one?

Trial memberships simply decrease the emphasis on the first visit by giving the salesperson more than one chance to close the member. In other words, we are going to close the potential client when he is ready, not when we think he should be forced to be ready. Doing this means you need to modify your sales system to one that has much more follow-up than a traditional first-visit system, and bluntly, you need a lot more patience to wait and give the person a chance to get acclimated to your gym, style of training, staff, and other members. People want to join a gym or they would not be there in the first place, taking up your time, but not everyone is able to, wants to, or needs to sign up during the first visit.

First-visit-oriented salespeople do follow-up, but due to the nature of the pressure needed to close during the first visit, many of the prospects they talk to never will come back no matter how many times you call. Realistically, if you drop the price trying to force a sale during the first visit and the potential client doesn't buy and leaves, what legitimate reason would you have to ever call him back? You just told him that this offer was for today and today only, and if he walks, you have to lie to him to get him back by giving him the same discount or even a bigger one if he now joins. He can simply wait another few weeks and hope you offer yet a bigger deal.

Trial memberships are weighted more toward a consistent follow-up and toward looking for that point where the member is comfortable with the club and staff and ready to commit to a membership. When you use trials, you have a legitimate reason to email, text, or call the person to check on progress and to answer questions or even to schedule him for a special event or programming.

Another key point for trial memberships is that you need to offer it to everyone who comes into the club. There will be a temptation to not tell a prospect who walks in off the street about the trial memberships until after you try to close them with the conventional methods. Tell the guest up front about your trial offer and then rely on the additional first-visit incentives and the power and image of the trial memberships to close the person anyway. When you use trials, you will get more sales, but these sales just might not always happen during the first visit.

Getting the Word Out

Discussing ways to market is always difficult because methods of delivery change so quickly. It is guaranteed that between the time you start this book and finish it, there will be at least three new social media companies that become important and two others that used to be big and are now gone and the old reliable ways to get the word to people will crumble.

Marketing is and always will be difficult in that you are constantly trying to throw a brick at a chipmunk. Most owners consider marketing as something done quickly at the desk with the media salesperson sitting in front them. The salesperson presents a badly done ad, you check for the right address and phone number, verify your deal of the week, and then let it rip.

Marketing done correctly for the financially driven owner is one of the hardest and most time-consuming parts of your business. Throwing a brick at a chipmunk means that the rules of marketing change so quickly that you have to intensely focus every ounce of your concentration before you toss that brick at the very fast and inconsistent target. Marketing for today's heavily competitive market is something that will take you much more time than we have ever allowed in the past. The first rule of marketing that you have to get into your head is this:

> You have to spend at least six hours
> per week building your brand.

Your brand is the combination of your public image spread through the visuals and in your marketing, the frequency of your marketing and consistency of your image, the word of mouth that is spread by your membership, control of your social media, mastery of mainstream media (such as websites and blogs), and your contribution to and participation in your community. All these done well will lead to increased potential member traffic into your business. If these are ignored or if you just depend on one to get the job done, you will most likely not reach the true revenue potential for your business. Dedicating six hours a week or hiring a specialist that can do this for you is what it takes to build a recognized brand that ultimately attracts sufficient traffic to your business.

Due to the changing nature of the avenues you could take with marketing, we will spend more time in this section talking about the concepts you need to master, such as the components of a good ad, rather than specific media. If you understand what it takes to build an image, you will do a better job getting the word out over time.

The next rule of marketing you need to master is the rule of consistency:

> You have to market your business every day
> for as long as you own that business.

The rule of consistency has two parts. The first part is frequency, meaning you have to create a marketing plan that is based on having a presence in the marketplace 52 weeks a year. The second part is consistency of image, meaning you have to settle on a projected visual image for all your branding that stays consistent year after year.

Frequency is consistency in motion. You have to have something new hitting the market—either through traditional retro marketing or through your social media—every single day for as long as you own the business. Consistency of image states that you adapt a look for your brand and then you stick with it over time. The combination of frequency and consistency of image leads to the next rule:

> Your goal is to build a recognition factor
> through your total branding effort.

There are probably not many people on the planet who couldn't connect certain symbols with certain brands. For example, who doesn't get the yellow arches, the big green circle with the mermaids, or the little doughy guy who giggles? If you can't figure out McDonald's®, Starbucks, and Pillsbury®, then you have been living under a rock, in a cave, or at the bottom of the sea. You know these brands because little about their public image has changed since the inception of these companies. For example, have you ever seen a Pillsbury ad without the doughboy? It is doubtful that almost anyone on the planet has ever seen one without the trademarked character.

All these companies use consistent components in their advertising and this consistency leads to a powerful recognition factor, which is the goal of your branding efforts. The issue for most gym owners is that they fall prey to whoever is in front of them at the time and most of these same owners have never spent the time or money to develop an image they can live with over time. If you take all the marketing most of these gyms have offered to the public during that last five years and laid them all on a table, it would most likely look like marketing from a dozen different businesses. The colors, images, logos, and methods would all vary based on whoever was selling something new to that owner that day.

You have to understand that if you are selling advertising or if you are consulting on a website, you don't make money by stating: "Yeah, what you are already doing is perfect and I wouldn't change a thing." You aren't going to make money as a salesperson if you agree with what the previous guy did. You only make money by saying: "Yeah, I can see the reason you are getting killed here. Whoever designed your stuff was horrible. If you let me take a chance at this I can certainly increase your traffic, but we need to completely redesign your entire image" (for extra money of course).

Before we go further, we need to understand that there are two different ways to market your brand. First of all, we use retro marketing, which is usually defined as marketing where you pay to play, such as newspaper ads, radio, or TV. The other way to market is by using electronic media, such as websites, blogs, and social media. Most of these methods don't cost much beyond initial design or preparation. For example, once you spend the money to get a website up and running, you really don't have to pay a lot each month to keep it fresh.

This leads us to the next major rule:

> You have to always equally cover retro and
> electronic marketing in most markets.

The sad thing is that this rule may be outdated by the time this sentence is finished. Retro marketing is now very situational in most markets, and in some major metro markets, such as New York and San Francisco, it is almost impossible to run any kind of consistent retro marketing that is restricted to just your part of the market. Electronic marketing is the rising star, but as of now, most owners can still benefit from a consistent retro marketing approach in their city.

Perhaps the biggest mistake many owners make is that they refuse to spend enough to buy that recognition factor in their market. If you want to be in business, you have to spend enough to stay in business. This number includes all retro and monthly electronic marketing expenses. Which brings us to the next basic rule of marketing:

> You have to spend at least 10 percent each month
> of your base operating expense on marketing.

For example, if you have a gym and it costs you $80,000 per month to cover all the bills, including debt service, payroll, utilities, and the rest, you should then budget about $8,000 per month on your marketing. That is $8,000 per month every month, you cheap people, and not $8,000 per year.

Training gyms have a different issue. Most owners of these facilities don't really believe they need to market at all, especially when it comes to doing retro marketing. Gym owners in this class—the ones who are usually about 7,500 square feet or less—often exist under the delusion that "If I build it, they will come," which is why so many of them struggle for so many years. There is also a rule for the training gyms:

> You have to spend a minimum of $3,500 per
> month if you want to stay in business.

We forget that marketing really has two purposes. The first purpose is offensive in that you market to create interest in your brand and eventually attract new potential business. The failure here for too many owners is that they run ads today and expect their businesses to be packed tomorrow. If it were that simple to make happen, the ad companies would be charging a lot more for their services than they currently do. Advertising and brand-building are slow processes. It takes months and years to create a good brand, not days and weeks. Which brings up another rule of marketing:

The longer you market a consistent image,
the better the response will be.

Owners often forget the second purpose of marketing—if it was ever known at all. The second purpose of marketing is defensive, meaning to market every day, every week, every month, and every year to keep the competitors away from your business. For example, if you budget $6,000 per month and spend it every month for 10 years in your market building your brand, how hard would it be for a competitor to come into town and immediately affect your business. Assuming that you have done all the right things as an owner, such as keep the place competitive, keep the physical plant updated, treat the members with respect, charge fairly, and hire a customer service-driven staff, then it would be extremely difficult for a new gym to get traction in your market.

The issue is that when we run an ad or do something on the radio, which is a dying method of marketing, we are so focused on our own process that we forget we are just another ad among many. We plan our ad, work with the salesperson or ad agency, book the space, and then the ad hits and we can't understand why 100 new people didn't come in today and carry it in their hand.

For example, let's say you ran a direct mail postcard piece that day—another somewhat hard tool to get to work without a great ad agency behind you—and that ad hits everyone's mailbox on Tuesday. First of all, in most of the world, anything in a mailbox is so retro that few of your under-40-year-old potential clients would most likely even see the piece. Secondly, let's say that on that day, all the major retailers in your town that still send out the big special offer mailers drop on the same day, meaning the mailbox is stuffed with a thick wad of advertising that most people simply take out of the box, walk to the garbage can, and toss it—unless you are that few who are looking for a new lawn mower or a discount on milk.

If you want effective marketing, you have to wear down the marketplace. In the case of the direct mail piece, you might try again next week and by pure chance be the only thing in the mailbox and you are finally seen. Marketing takes time to work and great brands are built over years, not weeks. If you are thinking you just can't handle this financially, you would be better off to fire a staff person or two, sell your car, or cut some other expense then you would be to stop marketing.

Think of marketing and the potential members that ultimately come through the door in response to a long-term brand campaign as food for your hungry business. If you are hungry, you get something to eat or eventually you starve to death. If your business is hungry (for those new leads), then you either feed it every week or it dies. Marketing is the last thing you should cut—never the first thing when times get tough.

Marketing and branding work best when you change up the delivery system. For example, if you run a flyer insert, which is an 8 x 11 glossy ad with your copy on both sides stuffed in the local newspaper once a week, for 52 consecutive weeks, it will completely stop working because you simply wore out the readership of that paper. If this paper has 30,000 subscribers and you run your insert for a year, everyone who reads that paper has seen your message. Even if you change the price special, which you should never run anyway, anyone who wanted to join your gym did so early in the ad campaign. If the newspaper adds a lot of new subscribers each month, you get more mileage out of the ads, but in reality, the paper can't add new readers as fast as your burn them up. Which brings us to another rule of marketing:

The delivery system will fail before the message dies.

Effective marketing requires that you change the angle of attack often. Changing the angle of attack means you mix up the delivery system in your retro marketing every 90 days. If you run a direct mail campaign for 90 days, you might then follow that segment with 90 days of flyer inserts and then revert back to direct mail again in a slightly different area of the market. There are exceptions to this rule. For example, if you live in a market that has a glossy city magazine that is published monthly, then you might want to commit to a full-page ad for a year. Magazines such as those have a longer shelf life and end up being kept, read again, or passed on to a friend. Again, this is why marketing is becoming so difficult because for every rule there is an exception to that rule.

It is easier to build a more consistent brand if you have a stronger knowledge of the components that should be part of all your marketing in the fitness business. The ones listed here can be changed often, but you still can use the same components over and over again. This is called *track marketing*, which is defined as always keeping the same theme but changing the components within that them each month. You probably see this often in most of the ad campaigns you have become familiar with through the years, but you may not recognize the concept. For example, if you see a Budweiser® beer ad, the ads themselves always change, but the basic components are always the same. You know there will be the horses, a tie back to their past with the beer wagon, the same logo the company has used for more than a century, and almost always the dog that rode on the wagon. Pillsbury does the same thing when it regularly changes the individual ads, but each one always has the same family feel and the same little dough guy. This brings us to another rule of marketing:

Always different but always the same

The following sections discuss the components necessary to build a service business brand. Keep in mind that we are selling future service, and to do that, you have to build trust in the brand over time. We are not selling a tangible object (such as tires), which often requires a totally different approach to selling, including price slashing or sales. When you sell a service, you sell based on the trust established between two parties: the buyer, who is taking a risk with his money and time when he believes you can solve his problem, and the seller, who wants to attract clients who will stay with him for long periods of time, but to gain that client, he must first create the belief that he can be trusted with your money and, in the case of fitness, with your health and well-being.

These are the four components that are designed to create a brand built on trust. All these should be part of all your marketing including all retro and all electronic:

The vehicle

Testimonials should be part of every ad you ever run in the fitness business. Fitness is a scary thing to people who have little experience with our product or who have tried and failed somewhere else, so running a testimonial of a real person who has gone ahead of this potential client kills much of the perceived risk in joining your business.

Keep the testimonials reasonable. Featuring the outliers in your ads, such as the person who has lost an extreme amount of weight or who competes in an extreme sport, doesn't really help you attract regular people to your business. The most common mistake an owner makes here is always featuring the person who has lost 100 pounds. This person is a success story, but few people can identify with him and running his picture and talking about his success is often more of a barrier than it is an attracting factor for your business.

The same is true of an owner who has lost an extreme amount of weight and who now wants to be in all her own ads. This same owner is also the one who just has to tell every prospective member how she got it done but then can't figure out why sales are horrible. We always have to remember that it is about the potential client sitting in front of you and his story and his issues, not about you and your journey. Testimonies should be from average people who have lost average weight and who give you and your team credit for getting it done.

This is also a good way to attack the weaknesses of the other competitors in town. For example, if your person in the testimonial ad tells you she was a member at another gym and hated the experience, then make sure that gets into her story—without, of course, the actual name of the other gym. You should compensate the members who appear in your ads by giving them at least a month's membership and you must always have every member sign a model's release, which can be easily printed off samples you will find online.

The tool

The tool is the offer you have attached to the ad. The only tool most service-based businesses should use is the paid trial membership—in this case, the 30 days for $39 option, which is adjusted for your gym by the rules listed earlier in this chapter. The belief system behind using a trial is this: I really do believe I have the best gym in town, but talk is cheap. Come see my gym, try it with no risk for 30 days for only $39, meet our staff, spend time with our coaching staff, and meet the other members, and at the end of 30 days, if I haven't earned your business, then I don't deserve to have you as a client.

The emotional cue

People usually make a decision based on one of two different ways. You can try to figure out intellectually if the decision makes sense or you respond emotionally and let your emotions take precedent over the brain. Deciding to join a gym, get in shape, and change your life are all about emotion and all your marketing has to be aimed at that target. Marketing fitness targeted at the intellectual decision-making process might be one of the bigger wastes of time in your business life.

Taking off your shirt for the first time in front of someone new you are dating, divorce, being in a wedding, going to the beach with your old high school friends, starting a new job, or just being disgusted with yourself because your new fat pants already don't button anymore are all trigger mechanisms that emotionally drive you to join a gym.

Everyone knows that if you practice health and fitness, you will live longer, live better, and look better and it is the good thing to do for you. We all know these things and we all spend a lot of time eating pizza and drinking beer discussing them, but nothing happens until the emotional cues drive us. Tell any middle-aged woman that she is going to be in a summer wedding with a sleeveless dress and she is immediately—not later—interested in getting in shape. Tell a guy who just got divorced after 20 years of marriage that he now has to date again and he is also interested in fitness now—not later but immediately, if not sooner. Triggers drive response and you have to fire these triggers by using an emotional cue in each ad. Perhaps one of the most powerful cues ever written that can be used in all fitness ads for any gym is:

We change lives.

This simple statement speaks to the heart and emotion of every potential member. Get up in the morning and those latest fat pants refuse to button. It is guaranteed that this person doesn't care about health, overall fitness, or living longer. He only cares about getting help today. If he has seen your ads for years—all using the same emotional cues over and over and over again—he is now your biggest fan and future client because you get him and are selling what he needs: a life change.

Use this slogan as needed in all your ads, put it on the back of your shirts, paint it on the wall, and make it your gym's cultural base that you use year after year. Speak to the emotion in all that you do and build this theme into your actual business plan and operation.

The positioning letter

Positioning letters are a more sophisticated approach to marketing in that you are now using a tool that begins to differentiate you from all your other competitors. If you are looking from the outside, all gyms look alike to the inexperienced potential member. However, if you are experienced, you can really tell the difference between the players and the pretenders. Positioning letters are tools that allow you to highlight the differences between who you are and who everyone else is, but most importantly, these letters allow you to build a more personal identity for your business. Which brings us to another rule of marketing:

You have to always personalize and localize your business.

Gyms don't do big online sales all around the world. Gyms don't have many people willing to drive hours on a weekend just to shop there. By the need of the member to use them every day, gyms have to be convenient in someone's life. Therefore, about 85 percent of your members live within about three miles of your business.

Your potential clients don't just want a membership, which can be purchased at any of your competitors. They want to support someone who has a face and a family and who is part of the community. Positioning letters place you and your business into the community and should be a part of all your marketing. This theme should also be woven into your website, social media, and member handouts. Who you are and what you believe is just as important to the potential member as the price. The following is a sample that illustrates how this is done:

To our friends in the community,

You live and die (sometimes too young) by the choices you make.

We have operated a business for more than 28 years that was created to nurture and support the women of Cape Cod. Operating this type of business for so long gives us a unique perspective about how women think about fitness and their bodies.

There is seldom an event, a party, or even a dinner where someone who finds out what we do for a living doesn't ask "So, what is the single best way to get into shape?" Everyone looks for the magic pill, that secret exercise, or that new wonder diet that will change her body forever. But after all these years, anyone who asks us that question is almost always disappointed by the answer.

Thousands of women have come through our doors in the last 28 years and we can unequivocally state that the difference between long-term fitness success for a woman, as defined by weight control, better health and energy, and a few dress sizes lost, is not a magic diet or pill. It is personal responsibility. Women who own the problem—be it weight gained or just plain out of shape and not exercising—are the ones who make changes and sustain those changes for years.

On the other hand are the women who blame the world, which includes such statements as "I just don't have the time" or "You don't know what it's like having kids" (which is a fairly absurd statement to make in a women-only gym owned by two women who have multiple children). These women start programs and then quit in a few months, blaming the universe and becoming angry with everyone around them because they failed yet again at taking control of their lives and making changes that might result in an immense rise in the quality of their daily lives.

Fitness is not easy, especially when compared to how easy it is to just ignore your health, not work out, eat badly, and then wake up 10 years later with medical issues and severe weight problems and be surrounded by stressful relationships. Fitness is not easy, but it is a choice and how you live and even how long you live will be determined by that choice.

Ask any woman who is in her 50s, suffers from myriad health issues, takes a handful of prescription pills a day, and who can't walk around the grocery store and has just been told by her doctor that her lifestyle is killing her what she would trade for just one healthy day? She will tell you she will trade just about anything—that is anything but the one thing that would change all this and that is committing to a fit lifestyle for whatever days she has left.

So, what does it take to enjoy the benefits of a fit life? It takes commitment to no one but yourself and the realization that the responsibility for your health, longevity, and quality of life is yours and yours alone. Commit to fit: Choose to live a full active life. Only you can make this choice.

Yours in fitness,
Sarah Smith and Kristen Jones

These letters would change in your marketing about every two months or so. The idea is to start a discussion and to get the potential clients in your market trained to look forward to the next installment. Most gym marketing fails because the ads are all the same and use the same tired tools that no longer work. Imagine a typical fitness ad that has a seminaked model, which is not a role model to the women in your market but the enemy, a bunch of bullet points listing all your equipment and services, and the price special of the week, such as half off the membership fee.

There is no emotional cue in this ad. There is no attempt to individual the business, personalize it, or separate it from the other competitors. Everything in this ad is all about the features in the gym and nothing about what is in it for the client.

The following is a second letter that would be part of the same series. Remember that these would be used with a trial membership offer and an emotional cue headline, such as "We change lives."

Has it really been 28 years already?

There probably aren't too many women around on the high side of 50 who haven't asked that question at least once in relation to a class reunion, anniversary, loss of a loved one, or perhaps fondly remembering a special trip. Time seems to accelerate as you get a little older and years start passing in weeks and decades fade faster than an hour free on a Saturday afternoon.

This year, we are celebrating our 28th year in the fitness business, and it seems that just yesterday, we were young, ambitious new club owners who were setting out to change the world of fitness for every woman on the Cape. When we started, there was only a handful of female owners in the country and women's fitness was nothing more than a few classes and chrome weights that wouldn't be caught dead in a coed gym. Today, there are more than 12,000 women's only facilities in the country and we are proud to have been pioneers through the years.

Our goal when we started was to make a difference. At that time, we had a difficult time actually defining what making a difference actually meant. We knew somewhere in my hearts that fitness should be an important part of every woman's life, but being young and having small children in tow, we never really had time or the experience to sit and define our grand plan for making change in the world.

We now know what we were seeking in those early days and we can define it clearly for all our members. This company was founded as perhaps the sole place in many women's lives where they could come and work on themselves in a nonthreatening and supportive environment and where they could commune with other women from all walks of life who are seeking to make themselves a little better every single day. Fitness is more than losing weight and a woman who moves a little every day, eats a little healthier, and finds that reason to get out of bed every day will be a happier and more fulfilled person.

We have had a chance to make a difference, and during our 28th year, we are taking the time to reflect on the opportunities and blessings we have been given. And looking back from our current position, we can unequivocally state that our companies have made a difference in women's lives and still do today. It is rare when we walk through the mall or sit in a restaurant that some woman doesn't come up and comment on being a member or former member of our clubs.

This comment is often so rewardingly connected to an additional note concerning how much weight she lost or how happy she feels just moving a little every day. In these small ways, we have made a change and we consider any woman who starts on the path of fitness and finds more happiness in her life a huge success story and a good reason for us to keep going to work every day.

We would like to make a difference in your life. Please come try our gym and find out why we are 1,500 women strong and still growing. You may try our gym for 30 days for only $39 and this includes a coach during every visit and a chance to try everything we offer in the gym. We are proud of our gym and what we do here. Please come meet our members and meet the staff and give us a chance to change your life too.

Yours in fitness,
Sarah Smith and Kristen Jones

Remember that the goal is always the same but always different. This letter tells a different story and should help potential members see a different side of the gym, but the goal is the same and that is to personalize and individualize the business. Join this gym and you just aren't getting a membership—you are joining a community of like-minded individuals all chasing the same goal.

Everything Electronic

Retro marketing built this industry, but electronic marketing will build its future. Websites, blogs, social media, and almost all other forms of electronic marketing change so fast that it would be impossible to keep up with them in a book. For example, the coupon sites were a rage for about a year or two and then died. Writing about how to design a coupon would have been an exercise in futility because that form of marketing came and went before the paragraph could be written.

Keeping that in mind, we are going to focus on the theories you need to master that can be applied to any form of social media or electronic marketing that might arise in your future. Understand the rules and any version of the game you play will be easier.

The most important lesson you can possibly learn about electronic marketing can be expressed in another basic rule:

> Hits, looks, likes, and the number of views
> mean nothing if you can't monetize them.

It is easy to get caught up in the grand game of social media if, for example, you sit in a bar and brag about the number of likes you have on your social media site. There can be great gamesmanship involved here, but these numbers mean nothing if you can't figure out a way to turn those likes into money. The ultimate goal of all marketing is to create interest, which attracts leads, who come to the gym, who become members, and who pay you money for the results you will help them get. If this sequence doesn't end with the getting-paid part, then it was inefficient marketing that proved to be a waste of your time.

The following is the entire theory of electronic marketing in one simple chart:

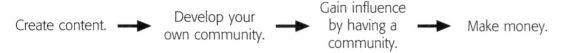

Create content. ➡ Develop your own community. ➡ Gain influence by having a community. ➡ Make money.

Creating Content

People love to learn, be challenged, be entertained, and, most importantly, hang out with a lot of like-minded folks interested in the same things. Electronic marketing—and especially social media—requires you to supply an endless stream of content. Posting content on almost a daily basis gets people to your sites and getting people to your sites regularly begins to build your community or, as the powerful writer Seth Godin refers to them, your tribe.

Content doesn't always have to stem from you. You can repost others' writings, find a tidbit in a magazine, recommend a book or video, and do a thousand other things that keep people coming to your sites each and every day. If you post a short informative tip on your blog three times a week, people become trained to go to your site during a break during their day. They will follow you because you are giving them information that somehow challenges their mind or entertains them, and if you do this consistently, you will eventually end up with a lot of people who care about what you say and now belong to your community. There is also a rule of marketing for this thought:

> You have to become the source on a specific topic.

You can become the weight loss expert, the sports performance for kids expert, the overall fitness expert in your small town, the body weight training guru, or just about any other niche you could imagine. You become the source or the filter that gathers information for his tribe and then posts the stuff daily that your tribe needs to see based on you being the master of that niche.

If you own a mainstream gym, your goal is to build a site for your business, but you as the owner should also have a site where you become the local expert on everything fitness. This gets you invited to speak at local groups or quoted in the newspaper as needed as a fitness source and this authority eventually drives people to your business because who knows fitness in this town better than you do—and that is proven by the last 300 posts you have made on your sites.

There are rules for content and the following are just a few:
- *You can challenge thought, but you should never insult, be mean, or put down someone by name.* If you disagree with someone, disagree with class and style and state both sides before making the position for your point.

- *Never post personal stuff.* This includes not posting pictures of your kids—unless it relates to your fitness mission—your dogs, your family vacation, you drunk on a beach in Mexico, you and the buds in a bar, or anything that might even vaguely distract the tribe from believing you are the source. It is hugely important to note that a decade from now, everyone who will ever consider hiring you or doing business with you will immediately pop your name into a search engine and also go to all the social media sites of the age. What do you want them to see? And remember that anything posted never, ever disappears from the web completely. Many younger people in the industry cry that this is unfair and their sites are their own private businesses. This is true, except for the fact that any person in any civilized country in the world can see whatever you post and nothing is truly private on the web. Post often, but post with the one thought that you are trying to improve your personal brand, not kill it.
- *Never repost without giving credit but always repost with a comment as to why you think this is important for your community.*
- *Post something fresh at least six days a week.*
- *Use pictures and videos several times a week.*
- *Remember that every post either enhances your brand or hurts your brand.* There is little in between.
- *Post and answer the comments as best you can each day.* If the community is working, you will start to see interaction and response to what you are writing. Don't wait a week to answer. If you post something controversial and expect comments, be there to answer and redirect the issue if needed.
- *Consider hiring someone to manage all your media.* This can be done for as little as a few hundred a month or as much as several thousand or more. The bigger you are and the bigger you want to be, the more you may need help posting daily and gathering the material for the posts.

The community

The content gathers the tribe. The community gathers around someone who pushes mental buttons and keeps everyone challenged. Content and community are in fact one big circle. You feed content and the community feeds back and around it goes again. The goal is to build a significantly sized group of people that follows what you do and what you write because you are the true source in whatever niche you choose to exploit.

The size of the community will vary from site to site and from niche to niche. One person might be a failure with 30,000 likes on his social media site, while another person might be wildly successful with 500 friends on his social media. Don't overestimate the need to build the largest community you can in your market. For example, a small training gym in a suburban area that has 500 followers on its site is doing quite well and that is enough to eventually start to turn that number into guests and memberships.

Building influence

Once you establish your community, you now have influence, but what to do with this new power? Think of influence as power to move the herd.

For example, you're a small country and you declare war on the neighboring country. You summon your army and five drunks show up with a few shovels and a club. This is going to be a short war and it will end badly for you and your army. But let's say you are a bigger country and you now want your loyal subjects to gather. You notice that you have 30,000 likes on your social media page and you want to sell your first e-book for $1.99 just to test the waters. Your community of 30,000 likes is far more likely to give you back sales versus the army of five. Put another way, when an army of like-minded individuals band together, whoever is leading that army has influence to make change—monetarily and through driving change in your industry or niche.

Making money

You have content in place that changes daily. You have built your community of followers. Your community represents a large enough segment in your niche where you can alter thought and drive change. You are now ready to monetize the process. There are rules to this of course. The following are a few tips when it comes to going after the money:

- *Do not—and this means DO NOT—try to sell anyone anything until you have at least provided content for six months.* Stated differently, build your community slowly without asking anything of them.
- *Once you starting asking for something, only do it once out of every 7 to 10 days.* Don't pound your tribe daily. Give, give, give for a week or so and then ask for that e-book sale. Give, give, give and then sell that trial membership. Build slowly and sell even more slowly.
- *Occasionally, give something away free just for being part of the tribe.* At least once a month, give everyone who follows you a free something, which is usually some short PDF tip sheet or an informational piece. Create one of these a month and recycle each one the following year. You want, you want, but you also need to give a little to your followers.

The following is an example of monetizing a social media site. This gym had 1,400 members at the time and also had about 900 followers on its social media site. This tribe of 900 was a mix of members in the gym, along with other people in the community who followed often due to the health and fitness tips that were posted daily, along with the videos that showed workouts you could do at home.

The gym's manager ran a post after about six months of gathering the tribe that said: "Post a video on this site in the next 30 minutes of you doing a burpee anywhere on the island, and if you are a member of the gym, you will receive 30 days of training valued at $300 for you and 30 days for your guest. Nonmembers, if you post, you will get 30 days free to the gym, which includes a full training package for you too."

The gym received 38 posts in 30 minutes. Out of the 38, 21 were members and the gym gave away 21 months of training and 21 guest months to the members to use with a friend. Remember the part from earlier where you need to reward the tribe with something free now and then. The other 17 posts were guests for a free trial month. In other words, this gym generated 38 guests in 30 minutes at no cost. Also, consider that this gym uses primarily group training and another body in the groups doesn't really cost the gym more money to service.

Another example from this gym was the use of the community and the influence with this community at generating revenue for the gym. The manager went to the local sporting goods store and asked the manager there if he would run a special just for the members of the gym, which is only about a half mile from the store.

The manager agreed because he had to do nothing. The sale was set for Friday from noon to 3 p.m. All members of the gym would get 30 percent off shoes if they presented their membership cards. On Thursday night, the gym's manager sent out a social media post stating: "Special flash sale just for our members. Go to Freddie's sporting goods from noon to 3 p.m. tomorrow and get 30 percent off any pair of shoes in the store just by presenting your membership card." The store sold 78 pairs of shoes. The gym's tribe was rewarded for their loyalty and support. Most importantly, the gym's manager could now ask for $500 to run the sale again because he had proven he has the influence to drive customers to the store. Everyone wins and the community grows because friends refer friends who don't want to be left out of these great special offers.

This formula applies to all electronic media because the basic progression is always going to be the same. Marketing electronically isn't hard if you have a plan and if you realize that everything has to lead to the ability to capitalize on your influence at the end of the day.

December 17, 2013
We are all different but are really all the same.

We all believe we exist as totally unique individuals, especially in the fitness professional field. However, the reality in business is that there are consistent and standardized rules that will work for everyone. Fitness professionals often stumble in business because they can't separate a personalized approach to fitness from doing business or even being an employee "their own way." When you own a business, there are proven rules that ensure you will be successful. When you are an employee, you work for someone else and have to master his rules to be successful. Knowing when to be you and when to follow the rules might be one of the hardest lessons in life.

December 20, 2013
What you do matters.

As the year ends, remember this: What you do matters and the people you touch have better lives because of who you are and what you do. Being in the people business can wear you down over time and it is easy to succumb to the beating and feel that what you do just doesn't matter. However, the reality is that you change lives. Clients can be rude, nasty, petty, and occasionally not worth the sweat they leave in the gym, but the other 99 percent who trust you with their health and well-being leave as better people after just spending a few months with even the average fitness pro. As this year winds down, never forget that fitness matters and professionals who patiently change people one day at time are doing important work that is seldom respected or acknowledged, but in your heart, you should know you made a difference, and as you sit quietly by yourself reflecting on the year that's just passed, that is all that matters.

15

Making the First Hour Count

You would think that after more than 60 years of sales training in this industry that we would be good at converting potential leads into new members, but the reality is that we are probably getting worse as time goes by.

The reversal of skills comes because how we sell and because the potential member's sophistication and expectations have changed over the last decade. In the olden days of the fitness industry, meaning just last week because we still insist on using technology that is outdated by five decades, we lived and died in this business by the pressure sale. Get a lead in the door, drop-close aggressively, and move on to the next lead.

Drop closing for you youngsters without psychotic experience in this business means you set a stupid price, such as $150, as your down payment and then leveraged the sale by dropping the number to $50 or so if the potential member signed that day. This still works if your client is as stupid as a pile of mud in the middle of the road, but for the most part, no one with an IQ over that of your average hamster believes anyone who ever signed up in this gym ever really paid the full $150. At best, this system is ineffective. At worst, it is insulting to the potential member.

This degrading system is failing in most of the chains and in the older-style mainstream fitness businesses and the industry as a whole is in a transitional period right now that is quickly forcing many owners to adjust their practices to more ethical and more effective methods. We still have to convert leads into members and that will never change if you own and operate a fitness business, but how we accomplish this is rapidly changing due to the more sales-experienced member and the amount of competition a typical club now has to face in its competitive ring.

The gold standard of sales analysis is do you have the ability to convert at least 60 percent of your qualified leads into real members? The answer based on national averages, which hovers below 40 percent, is we can't convert enough leads monthly to support most of the gyms in the market. Put another way, most clubs do get enough leads through the door each month—if they can accurately control and count the leads—to make that club profitable over time, but the owner simply doesn't have the skills to develop a staff that can effectively close those same leads.

This failure to close puts pressure on the entire club business system. If you can't close more than 40 percent of your leads, then you have to spend more on marketing to buy a greater number of leads or misses if you are holding at the 38 percent national average and just keep walking those prospects to the door, which most clubs just can't afford to do. If you can't close, something else usually has to give and that is almost always customer service because all your money goes into salespeople who can't get the job done, leaving very little left for hiring decent service staff.

However, you can rebuild if you are tired of living at the bottom of the fitness food chain. The following sections detail a few ideas that any club owner could implement immediately in his business that would make a big difference in a very short period of time. These are not those brilliant "write it down on a napkin at the bar" ideas, but most good business is really nothing more than mastering the basic skills anyway.

Get Control of your Leads

How many qualified leads do you get through the door each month, on an average Monday, on Saturday morning, or on any day of the week? Most owners can't honestly answer that question. However, ask any McDonald's manager what his average ticket sale is and he can answer that in about three seconds.

There are fundamental numbers every successful owner has to know and how many leads through the door during the month and during the primetimes are some of the most important. Use a basic inquiry sheet if you don't yet have a computer-generated tracking system, but start with the basic premise that if you want to fix your sales effort, you have to know how many leads you are getting through the door. If you don't know how many leads you have, then you can't determine your true closing rate, which means you can't tell how effective your sales effort is over time.

Do Sales Training Daily

Even if you are the only employee in your club, sit down at least once a day and read and study about how to properly present your business to a prospective client. Keep in mind that in today's market, sales are defined as the simple skill of helping someone get what he came in for when he walked through that door. We don't have to pressure or hurt people to be effective at sales, but we do have to learn how to help people take the first step on their fitness journey and that often means we have to spend a lot of time practicing how we present the club and its services. If you have a larger staff, go back to a 30-minute sales meeting every day to focus on numbers and short training efforts. Train every single day on how you can be more effective on helping your clients get involved in your business.

Hire Adults for the Job

Stop hiring young, stupid, male salespeople. The trend has always been to hire the stereotypical salesperson from the chain clubs. He is young, a killer at the drop-close, and knows every Tom Hopkins sales pitch in the book. He is also disruptive to your system, high maintenance, dates all your members, and can't be coached because he only knows one way to sell, which is far too dated and aggressive for today's market. Hire adults and usually look for that 30-plus female who has customer service experience. Her communication skills are better, she presents a better first image, and she can relate to a wider range of people, but most importantly, she will sell from a position of helping rather than forcing the pressure sale and she will often stay longer in your business.

Start a Basic Follow-Up System You Can Maintain Over Time

Phone calls are not follow-up. Phone calls are what you do when you don't train your staff on how to properly follow up a sales lead because no one answers his phone anymore. Use emails, try texting, go retro and use handwritten thank-you notes, and leave encouraging messages to get involved, but do not depend on harassing clients on the phone until they give up and join. You should have at least a three-step follow-up system in place and most clubs should have at least five steps over 30 days to be effective. Calling people at home and begging them to come back is not one of these steps.

Get a Dedicated Salesperson

You can't use multitaskers and expect to be effective. Get a dedicated salesperson whose sole job is new member acquisition and then pay that person well for the work. In most markets, you have to pay at least $12 to $15 per hour and commissions of at least $15 to $25 per sale to get anyone decent. Pay peanuts and get monkeys. Don't believe me? How did your staff of monkeys making $8 an hour do last month?

Owners also need to learn to sell. If you own only one club, then you should still do the majority of sales in your business each month. There is nothing more important than generating new memberships for your business. If you aren't any good at it yet, keep practicing because you can't teach it if you have never done it well.

Slow Down the First Hour

Fitness has changed during the last several years, but how we sell it commercially hasn't really evolved that much.

Today's potential clients walk through the door better read and more inspired than they have in the past. In the early days, they arrived seeking fitness but mostly having no idea of how to chase it, except for the guy who still wanted to do his high school weight routine because it worked so well for him about 20 years—and 30 pounds—ago.

Potential members today have resources past guests never had access to when they began their fitness pursuit. Type fitness, running, kettlebell, or any other industry-related term into any social media channel and you will pull up literally thousands of videos and clips.

Go online to Amazon and you can order Todd Durkin's bestseller *The IMPACT! Body Plan*, Rachel Cosgrove's masterpiece *The Female Body Breakthrough*, or Lou Schuler and Alwyn Cosgrove's *New Rules of Lifting* series. These books are so far superior to the old bodybuilding books we had access to in the past that it is like comparing a 1962 Volkswagen to a new Porsche. They might both be cars, but what's under the hood of one of them is mind boggling.

Not everyone coming through the door is well read and ready to rumble, of course, but even those who haven't been doing their research know that a couple workouts with a bored trainer and then starting a fitness routine based on a 1995 circuit is stupid and ineffective.

Why You Need an Assessor

Salespeople who are not trainers cannot sell training and it is laughable that anyone expects them to be effective at something they don't usually do and don't really understand. A trainer selling to his own client is sort of like asking a person who has chosen to do social work as his life's work to now become the president of a major financial company.

What attracted this person to the job in the first place is what defines him as a person, and as a person who loves people and loves helping them get results, he is not likely going to be someone who can sit and sell an expensive product. It is not that he doesn't have talent or is not smart. It's because advanced sales skills and being a compassionate trainer usually don't reside in the same person.

The old adage is that you can't sell a Ferrari if you have never driven a Ferrari has enough truth in it to apply to what we do in our businesses. Salespeople are seldom certified trainers, have never really problem solved with a client past typical sales pressure questions, and are not capable of projecting the client into the future based on chasing a series of fitness goals. Explaining the price of a training program mechanically across the sales desk is not anything like taking a client through an hour assessment and then placing that person into the training level that would most likely meet his needs and goals.

The unusual thing about training and fitness is that it is all future service based compared to selling a tangible object today. In other words, we are selling something that will happen to you in the future, such as changes in your body or happiness derived from getting into shape, versus selling someone a TV set they throw into the cart, drive it home, and watch it an hour from now. Selling future service is what training represents. Selling a TV is what a membership represents. These are two different products that need two entirely different sales approaches.

Because these salespeople are not trainers or don't truly understand the nature of training, the membership sale always comes down to such things as classes, equipment, or access or if we boiled all these down, most mainstream gyms sell nothing more than rental space on their equipment. There is always outrage about this comment when it is used around mainstream box owners, but the reality is that if only about 5 percent of the population of a typical box gym pays for traditional, old-style personal training, then that means that 95 percent of the membership is paying for do-it-yourself fitness and their monthly fee is for nothing but the rental of the equipment in that huge box.

Mainstream fitness facilities like the chains as well as YMCA, YWCA, and Jewish Community Centers should all target at least 40 percent of their membership as training clients using such tools as large group personal training and small group intensive coaching groups—all coupled with a small dose of one-on-one training. Doing this isn't that hard if the owners or managers are willing to break away from the traditional organization chart of a mainstream box club.

In the new world of fitness where the sale is based on getting the maximum results for the maximum number of clients, you can't use a sales-heavy staffing chart. This traditional method of sales has to be replaced with a dual approach using a lesser sales team that represents the front line of sales, such as drop-ins or buddy referrals, and then feeds those clients to the single most important person on your team, which is the assessor.

The assessor represents next generation staffing for today's model. This person should be a trainer who has experience and is not afraid of asking for money. This person does nothing but meet with as many potential members as possible and then place those clients somewhere into the training system. In other words, this person feeds all the rest of the trainers and generates the largest amount of monthly revenue for the gym.

This is the job of the future not only for the mainstream player but also for the training gym. Simply put, this is an acquisitions job that targets getting a larger percentage of clients into your training programs. As most of you have learned over the years, the last person who should ever be selling anyone anything is a trainer.

Trainers didn't get into the industry because they love to sell people things. They got in because they love to help people, which is a purely intrinsic motivation. This is why your assessor should be a trainer but also someone who is not afraid of asking for money and who is looking to move beyond the day-to-day routine of training clients.

The assessment tool itself is based on a simple premise: Time is the enemy of fitness. Most clients do not want to meet with a traditional trainer in a typical mainstream gym because they know that only two things will happen and neither one of those things are good. Either they will be asked (pressured) into one-on-one training or they will be given a circuit workout dating back to the 1980s and be made to feel like a lowlife because they couldn't/wouldn't pay for one-on-one training with this person.

Getting people to the assessor is as simple as stating to the client that time is the enemy of fitness and that our goal is to first find where you currently are on the path to fitness and then help you put together the shortest plan possible to help you reach your goals. Remember that you are not trying to work someone to death during this process but rather letting the person know that he can really do this workout thing, that you have a team of professionals that can guide him, and that you and your team are the most patient people on Earth.

The future of the industry is not selling memberships or renting equipment for the lowest price in the market but rather learning to get the maximum results for the maximum number of clients and charging fairly for that success.

How the Current System Works and Why It Fails

The current method of selling in commercial fitness is to start with a salesperson, who often doesn't know a lot about fitness beyond his own workout style, who then turns the client over to a trainer, who has no sales training, no interest in sales, and just wants to train clients, eat a lot, train more, and get a check.

The trainer takes one look at the person's car keys, sees cheap, and then loses interest because this client is obviously not a potential one-on-one victim. He sets the person up on a circuit, sets a few seats, counts backward from 10 a couple times, and then hands the client a big card with a workout on it that will fail the client in about six weeks.

The trainer then hands the client back to the salesperson, who now has to overcome the bad job and attitude the trainer brought to the process. This is stupid and inefficient and a leftover legacy from the 1990s, when you could get away with this nonsense due to lack of competition.

Nonprofits are even more inefficient. Most nonprofit fitness businesses are finding that the days where everyone just handed them money so they could waste it are gone and now there is the start of accountability within many of the organizations. These nonprofits do the right thing and their mission is the right thing to do for their communities. However, this group of facilities still uses the sales system based on fear of being thought of as a mainstream club.

Instead of helping potential members get some information that might help them make a qualified decision by using a trained sales team, the young counter staff at most nonprofits simply points toward the back of the facility and the guest gets a self-guided tour. The fear of the "sales" word makes the nonprofits and their friends a hard place to get help and guidance because no one wants to ask the guest to get started.

The last category is the trainer gym, where the staff wants to so impress the guests with their knowledge that they take the person through every test they can buy and then they spend an hour taking the person through a complicated and overdone routine that does indeed make the potential member come to a hard realization: Yes, I am fat, and yes, this is a crazy bastard because if this is the first workout for a deconditioned guy, I have no chance of surviving a regular workout.

The guy is there because he is fat and can't move well. You do not need to pull up his shirt, pinch a huge handful of fat, and call out a number nor do you need him to step over a string with a stick on his back to prove he has the moves of a 100-year-old meth addict. This is baseline stuff you use once he becomes a member, not something you do to try to impress a scared and nervous guy who knows he needs help.

The point of all this is that we can change the initial perception by using a different tool. The following are an overview:

- *Slow down.* You should spend at least an hour to an hour and a half with a person, teaching him how to work out. If he doesn't have his workout stuff, present the club during the first visit, but your best chance of getting new folks into your business is to get him working out using a positive experience. Sweat sells and a workout with a motivating coach who is actually teaching the "how" instead of "just do this" will increase your success.

- *Use two sales teams.* Use a regular salesperson and also use a second person who is a trainer who is not afraid of money. We call this person an assessor and his main job is to work with as many new or potential clients as he can and then place them where they belong in the system. The assessor/salesperson should try to upgrade the person into a training program and should feed the other trainers, who as I mentioned earlier are the last people on planet Earth who should be asking for money.

- *Use an annually structured assessment tool.* The sample format is described in the next few paragraphs.

- *Your goal during this first hour is to demonstrate expertise, professionalism, and a caring attitude.* Spend an hour teaching someone to work out, asking good questions about what he wants and what he is trying to accomplish and by basically doing everything that none of our competitors will do—and that is to spend quality time with someone interested in your business.

If you start the guest in the same format you use elsewhere for most of your training, he will fit into the system more quickly and can participate more easily in other club offerings, building up their confidence even more.

The format for the basic one-hour assessment is structured along the lines detailed in the following sections. Keep in mind that this is assuming that the client is dressed and ready to sweat. This is also assuming that the client either just purchased a trial membership or he is a new member and is starting on his free month of training.

All new members who join first visit and those who have not taken part in a trial program, such as a first-visit close referral from an existing member who brought a friend, should be given a VIP month of training with the thought that you will then get a chance to upgrade this person to a training membership once he experiences the full range of training products.

In other words, if the new guy comes in the gym as a friend of a current member and signs up today without using a trial, it will be very difficult to sign him up on any training program because he hasn't tried anything yet. The key is to get him started today on a simple access membership, meaning the basic membership to your gym, and then give him a full 30 days of training, during which he can experience all the training products the gym has to offer, with the goal that the assessor and sales team will follow up as he goes along and tries to rewrite this client into a higher membership later.

The meet and greet

All actual training should start with a one-minute meet and greet where every client in whatever group is going on at the time has a minute to meet all the other participants. The structure in the assessment follows the sale format but with a different goal. In the working assessment, the assessor should spend about 10 minutes at a table discussing three important issues with the client: What is your goal, what is your time frame, and what is your time commitment to getting in shape going to be each week? We can't help the client get what he wants if we don't know what he wants.

This 10-minute time period is important for a number of reasons. First of all, very few gyms will dedicate 10 minutes to get to know the client, his needs, and what he wants from your business. Almost every gym of any size—and the emphasis is on "every"—immediately moves into sales mode and attacks when the prospect walks through the door. The salespeople are so trained to go after the sale that practically no one will waste 10 minutes just talking to the guy casually about what he wants, where he has failed in the past, and what he is looking for in this gym. The salespeople have a story to tell and nothing—not even the potential client—is going to get in the way of that story.

Training gyms are not immune to this sales disease either. Training gym staff usually doesn't suffer from the sales disease, but it does suffer from the need to prove it has the world's best trainers, and instead of listening to the story, staffers want to prove their expertise so you will work out and you will work out hard and they will usually throw every technical term in the world at your head in the process.

There is an interesting phenomenon that happens in training: If a trainer progresses from a newbie who has to impress with an overly complicated workout to a true master trainer, his workouts and approach usually move from too complex to simple, which is often just what the client needs. In other words, the better you get, the simpler your approach to helping someone. This is the person who should be your assessor and should be the first experience for as many new and potential clients as he can handle.

Twelve-minute dynamic warm-up

This is the classic training approach these days and we vary this technique using a range of 3 to 12 minutes for the dynamic portion of the assessment because the condition of the client varies so dramatically from person to person.

The dynamic warm-up should be a graduated process, meaning start really slow and gradually increase the movement and intensity. The goal is to stop the client before he fails at a movement pattern. Remember that the goal of the assessment is to build up confidence in the potential client. He has most likely failed at fitness somewhere in the past, is most likely now overweight, and probably feels he might not be able to keep up or even do this at all. Slow down, spend time, and build confidence by having him successfully complete movements, not by pushing him into a movement where he is guaranteed to fail.

The 20-minute strength segment

The strength segment is fairly easy. It is designed to introduce the client to movements he most likely has never seen, giving the assessor a chance to be patient, coach professionally, and build confidence. These are also the fundamental movement patterns he will encounter in all the training he sees and does in the gym, so getting him started early understanding the method behind the madness is a good way to get him started. It is also recommended that you use these exercises exactly in this order for the strength session. By using a set format, you can use different assessor/salespeople and gauge their individual effectiveness because each one will be doing exactly the same sequence and you can then compare results.

The strength portion looks like this:
- Kettlebell swing
- Push movement overhead, even if it is a one-pound medicine ball
- Goblet squat
- Pull movement, preferably with a kettlebell
- Lunge movement
- Dead lift movement

This sequence allows the trainer/salesperson to demonstrate a high level of coaching and professionalism. For example, the swing looks so easy but takes some time to build up any proficiency for the client and this can only be done through the teaching sequence. Remember that your competitors aren't doing this and are using some version of stupid, so by slowing down and spending time here teaching, you are changing the mind-set of the client.

It is important to note that you should not be doing any type of formal movement analysis at this stage, but you really are doing it. What this means is that the assessor should be an experienced trainer who has mastered using a movement screen and who can spot dysfunction as he sees it.

More sophisticated assessors are using software designed for movement analysis, such as apps created for analyzing golfers, on their iPads and then videotaping a movement, such as the goblet squat, and showing the client what is happening in his hips or legs. Most of these apps are cheap and easy to use and find and give the assessor a major boost of professionalism with little effort.

Again, is your competition doing any of this? Your goal as a fitness business owner is to do everything you can to differentiate and separate yourself from the other pretenders in the market, and by using economical tools, such as a movement app, you can gain a nice edge over everyone else.

The 30-second to five-minute big finish

Finish big and put a smile on his face. He might only last for 20 seconds, but let him experience that small rush at the end of his workout based on pushing it just a little. The 50-foot rope is the perfect tool for this task because so few people coming back to the gym after years of being absence have ever used one. Make it fun and just a little challenging, but get the person breathing a little and a little damp to finish him off properly with a smile.

Taking the potential member back to the table and coaching cardio

There will be a large number of your potential clients who are not strength training experienced, and no matter what you tell them or show them during this hour, they secretly believe they will dedicate themselves to coming to the gym six days a week and walk on the treadmill for an hour, resulting in the weight just washing away quickly.

It is important that you intervene in this thought process. Coach cardio with the thought that in this gym, there is no cardio without intensity and then lay out a sample high-intensity interval-training program. Cardio will make a difference for the client, but modern theory suggests that the client will get better results more quickly if he strength-trains at least two days a week and adds cardio to that routine.

There are exceptions to this suggested course of training. If the client can't lift for some reason or is training for a triathlon, then obviously he needs a program that has running/cardio built into the routine, but for most newbies fresh out of fitness retirement, this should work. It is also assumed that you are doing some type of movement screen on the client to make sure he can do anything at all when he starts.

The following is a sample program that is easy to coach and, most importantly, easy to present during the assessment. This program is based on a 20-minute session and it is used to start a conversation on overall training for the potential client and to take away the nonsense in his head that walking slowly on a tread for an hour while watching sports will work for him to meet his goals. This is designed for a new person completely out of shape. You can talk him through the progressions to make it harder as you present the information to him:

- Walk slowly for four minutes.
- Walk fast for one minute/walk very fast/jog/run/run like a bear is chasing you and trying to bite you in the butt (the interval intensity is determined by his conditioning).
- Walk slowly for two minutes.
- Walk fast for one minute/walk very fast/jog/run/run like a bear is chasing you and trying to bite you in the butt.
- Walk slowly for two minutes.
- Walk fast for one minute/walk very fast/jog/run/run like a bear is chasing you and trying to bite you in the butt.
- Walk slowly for two minutes.
- Walk fast for one minute/walk very fast/jog/run/run like a bear is chasing you and trying to bite you in the butt.
- Walk slowly for two minutes.
- Walk fast for one minute/walk very fast/jog/run/run like a bear is chasing you and trying to bite you in the butt.
- Walk slowly for three minutes and you are done.

Once you explain the gym's approach to cardio, you can now move on to presenting the prices and closing. If this is the client's first visit into the gym and he has just signed up for a trial membership, you should present the prices, but don't expect him to close today. He will have to experience the gym first and that is what you want him to do. You eventually want him to be concerned about which type of training he wants, not about price issues concerning something he hasn't tried or seen. It just sounds expensive to him, so he will fight you with no frame of reference.

Presenting the prices

Always present the prices with your five to seven options listed with the lowest price on the bottom of the page and the highest price at the top. Remember, it is recommended that you include everything below the level the new member chooses, so it is logical to present your price options as a reverse pyramid. Before you ask the guest to decide which program is best for him, you have one more step.

The final question to ask the guest before he chooses his level is:

> "Are you the type of person who prefers working with a
> personal coach or are you the type that would rather be
> part of a group and share the cost of the trainer?"

This question allows the person to place himself into the type of activity he prefers, but it also allows him to place himself financially into a level he can afford without being embarrassed that he can't afford expensive one-on-one training.

The last step is to listen to the client's answer to this question and then suggest the level that meets his needs, his interests, and his finances. Do not always place him into one-on-one training or the most expensive program on the sheet. If he is under age 40 and loves the group dynamic, then suggest that he take that training program even though it is less expensive.

For example: "Joe, based on everything you told me about your goals and time commitment and the fact that you prefer to work out in a group, I suggest you start here at the team training level. It has everything you need to get to your goal and it is at a price you can afford. Let's get you signed up today and get you going."

Don't hesitate, suggest strongly, and make a recommendation. The client is looking to the assessor for guidance. You have already spent an hour with him, and if he has gone through some of the training first, you can strongly ask for the sale.

If the assessor presents the prices today but the client hasn't tried anything yet, the assessor will wait for a week or so and then catch Joe coming out of a workout and say: "Joe, you seem to really like team training. While you are here tonight, let's get you signed up as a full member and get the paperwork out of the way while I have you here." Joe says: "I still have several weeks left on my trial and I don't want to waste that time. I will sign up later." The assessor comes back: "Joe, if you want team training, I will give you an extra month free at the end of your membership and buy back those last few weeks. In the case of the team training, which is $129 a month, I will give you $129 as an incentive to get you going now. Let's get you signed up tonight and I will buy back those last few weeks."

This process is probably the most important thing in the book and will have the biggest impact on your business in the shortest period of time. Simply slowing down and spending time teaching and educating instead of merely getting the person started on a set routine will change your numbers.

If the person is truly deconditioned, you can offer what we call *fundamentals*, which is group training offered through your best coach four to six times a week, where the person repeats the same sequence and can learn the basic movements before moving on in the club.

January 3, 2014
Winners are willing to do what losers refuse to do.

"Winners are willing to do what losers refuse to do." This was a sentence written in an old notebook dating back years ago, but it has been a guiding principle in my life for most of my career. This simple sentence means you stay and make one more call, you get up a little earlier than other people, you help one more person before going home, and you turn off that TV and read one more story to your kids that night. Being successful is not some huge secret process that just happens to you one day. Being successful—personally and financially—is nothing more than a series of small actions you do that lazy-ass, unsuccessful people refuse to do. Any time I get tired and get lazy, I always remember that old saying and realize the difference between success in my life and failure in someone else's is just a willingness to suck it up, do a little extra work, and get it done. Somewhere out there, someone quit too soon and wasn't willing to do the work it takes to be somebody, but it won't be you and it won't be today and you have to promise yourself you will never let it happen in your life or career.

January 22, 2014
Working in the fitness business used to be something you did until you moved on and found a real job.

Working in fitness used to be something you did until you moved on and got a real job. The average fit pro usually lasted fewer than eight years and was gone. But that is changing. People now realize fitness can be your life's work and that you can spend the rest of your working career doing what you love. The day you declare to yourself and everyone in your life that this is it, this is my choice, and this is what I am going to do until you pry that last kettlebell out of my cold dead fingers will be the best day of your life. The challenge is to keep moving forward and up so there will be enough money to pay for family and your life. Increasing your business skill set, advancing your knowledge, and trying different aspects of the fitness world all combine to keep you funded and mentally growing, which is vital to stay alive in this field. Many people waste their entire lives searching for their perfect place in life, but maybe you have already found yours and you just haven't yet told the world that you are exactly where the universe thinks you should be. Knowing what you want, who you are, and where you are going makes for a very happy person in life and I hope that is you living a life in fitness.

Section 5

LEARNING HOW NOT TO HATE YOUR STAFF

16

Learning to Live With a Stranger in Your Business

If you're seeking growth and stabilization in your current business or if you dream of adding a second or third unit, then hiring and developing a second-in-command may be the most important decision you make concerning the future of your business. If you're that owner who has raised his gym from a small baby business, it may be time to consider letting a stranger come push the baby carriage for a while.

By adding a number two, which may be a manager, assistant manager, or just a strong administrative person, you free yourself to work on your business, not in it. Hiring a strong second gives you the freedom to expand your business beyond what you can accomplish yourself. One of the most important rules you will ever learn about small business is that you can manage more than you can do yourself. These means that by letting go, you can often accomplish more and manage more in your business.

In today's small business world and especially as it relates to the gym business, one person can't do it all. You have to shift the burden away from yourself and start relying on other people who are capable of taking responsibility to ensure the future success of your business. Even if you are that dedicated person willing to work until he drops, there are still only so many hours in the week when you can mentally function at a level needed to make good decisions and only so many hours you can physically work before you, super human being, need an extended nap. Perhaps the biggest breakthrough you will ever have is when you learn the power of leveraging other people's time and realizing the exponential power of a team compared to the short-lived manic energy produced by a single person.

Hiring a strong number two person also provides additional stability in an industry that typically has a higher-than-average employee turnover. According to the Bureau of National Affairs, the national average for employee turnover is 1.9 percent monthly or about 23 percent on an annual basis.

Our numbers in the fitness business often exceed 30 percent annually and usually reach as high as 40 percent, which is more than most financial institutions, which are recognized as areas of extremely high turnover with entry-level employees. Financial institutions encounter the same problems we do with young, low-paid, overworked entry-level employees, which ultimately leads to a high turnover at the lower levels. Giving the senior management team depth and stability with the addition of a number two should help your employee loss numbers drop. Adding more trained management people can provide more training and individual attention—two prime reasons that cause entry-level people to leave when these things are missing from their jobs.

While every owner dreams about having a strong number two who handles day-to-day operations, takes responsibility, and runs the place when you're out of town and does so in an honest, high-integrity manner, these people seldom just drop in and ask for a job in real life. If they do, they seldom last very long because they are talented enough to move to better-paying and higher-image real-life jobs. This means the only way you're going to get a second leadership person is to find and develop your own.

With your number two, you are like the Lone Ranger and Tonto, Picard and Riker, or Yogi and Boo-Boo. In other words, you are seeking to build a team that is stronger than either person is alone.

Before we go any further, let's first define what's meant by a number two or a second-in-command. The number two person in the business organization should be the owner's counterpart. He should cover the owner's weaknesses and bring other skills to the business that help to grow the facility beyond the owner's ability to do it on his own. In other words, there should be some type of synergistic effect where one plus one equals something greater than two. If the magic is right, the owner and the number two person should be able to combine forces and be more effective than both people working separately.

There are many reasons owners cite for never developing a strong management team or for losing that person when you do find him, but most of the time, it comes down to just a few key errors by the owners.

First of all, employees usually can't follow us or perform on their own because we don't develop systems. Most fitness businesses depend on the owner's on-the-spot decision-making capabilities to survive. If the owner isn't on the spot, then he is calling in every few hours to check the numbers and to make those instant decisions no one else can make. This happens because there are no set systems to follow by the employees that could be substituted for the owner's presence.

There are hundreds of examples of situations where owners make instant and inconsistent decisions that drive the staff crazy. For example, a salesperson is touring the brother of a long-term member. The owner just happens to walk by as the salesperson is explaining the prices to Joe, who is the guest, and to Bob, who is the member and who is sitting in on the presentation with his brother. Bob says to the salesperson: "Hey, can you give my brother the family deal? I know that Sue the owner is here. How about asking her if she'll give us some type of discount?" The salesperson asks Sue, who says: "Sure. Bob is a great member. Go ahead and give his brother the family deal."

The gym policy that the salesperson was trained on states that family deals are only for married couples. The owner made an on-the-spot, subjective, situational decision for the employee. What does the employee do the next time a friend of the owner, a good member, or anyone else asking for a deal comes into the gym?

How does the employee make a decision to act when the club has a policy the owner ignores depending on the member and the situation? The next time, will the employee follow the policy or will he make a judgment decision, meaning a special deal in this case, based on who he is talking to at the time?

The owner certainly has the right to give deals in her own club, but making these deals on a random basis in front of the staff destroys her ability to build a team of competent employees. Training employees to follow set procedures is relatively simple. Training them to interpret the procedures so they know when to make deals and when not to is almost impossible on a staff-wide basis.

This type of situation is why employees keep coming up to you all the time for answers instead of making their own decisions. This happens because the owners of the club don't establish and follow consistent guidelines. In this example, the employee should have known not to even ask the owner. He should have already known from the training he had received that there wasn't a deal possible because these two brothers didn't qualify for the family plan, but because the owner has a history of making deals, the employee had to ask to see what the deal of the day was going to be.

The second issue when it comes to developing a number two in your business is that employees go through stages of growth that often contrast with where you are today as an owner. We seldom find employees good enough to become key people because we are always comparing the employee's current stage of development against our own current stage of knowledge and experience.

The side issue here is that the longer an employee works for us, the better we get to know him. The better we get to know him, the more visible his weaknesses become over time. It's sort of like marriage. After a certain amount of time, we're more willing to hire someone outside our organization because that person is fresh, new, and without visible flaws. This is why we're usually overcritical of employees (or spouses) who have been with us for a while and who have given us time to see their strengths and weaknesses.

For example, a promising employee has two years of experience working in the same gym. The employee has gone through several seminars, has taken minor responsibility (the owner won't give up any major responsibility), and has worked in several jobs in the gym after starting at the bottom as an entry-level person.

The owner has eight years of experience in the business and is looking for a strong number two person to take on some of the management load and to help grow the business to the next level. However, the owner says that this promising employee just won't work in the new position because she doesn't yet have the skills or experience to take a leadership role in the business.

What's happened here is that the owner is comparing the employee's current level of skill and experience against his own eight years of experience acquired one day at a time by getting his ass beat in small business ownership and the employee just doesn't stack up with her current level of expertise. The owner is also comparing the employee against his own current state of business understanding, which has taken eight years of on-the-job training and trial and error to develop.

The questions that should be asked about her potential instead are: Where is the employee today? What is she capable of doing in the future? What responsibility is she able to handle now and in the future after additional training? We know that in this industry, the majority of our employees are undertrained and very few of our developing people could ever live up to the high and often unrealistic standards we set for them.

Most owners forget the price they paid to get the knowledge they now have after years of experience. In this example, eight years of daily decision making—right or wrong—has led to an experienced and capable gym owner. Two years of working for someone as a trainer or salesperson does not develop the decision-making process nor does it prepare the person to take responsibility. Only taking responsibility prepares someone for more responsibility.

Most employees never have a chance to learn responsibility because they never have a chance to fail on their own, which is the way most owners learned the business in the first place. If we only give them minor-level responsibility, their failures will be of no consequence and they won't learn anything from the experience, but we won't give them any real responsibility because we're afraid they'll make major business-threatening mistakes.

If it has taken a specific number of years for you to learn the business, how long would it take you to teach someone else? How much time do we really spend on education? The following is an example of a two-year employee who has worked up to manager.

This employee started his career at this gym by spending six months as a front counter person. His training for this entry-level job included:
- Two 8-hour days of orientation, or about 16 hours
- One staff meeting a week for 26 weeks, for a total of 26 hours
- One 2-day weekend training session, for about 16 hours
- Sixteen hours of general staff training, or about 16 hours total

Total training for this employee during his first six months is 74 hours.

The employee is then promoted to assistant manager—a job he holds for one year. His training for his new role in the business included:
- Two hours a month for special training, or about 24 hours during his first year on the job
- One-hour staff meetings for the year, or about 50 hours

- Attendance at one industry show, where he attended six seminars, totaling about 6 hours
- Two 2-day seminars, for a total of about 32 hours

Total training for the year for this employee at his new level is about 112 hours.

The employee is then promoted to manager—a job he holds for six months. The training he receives at this level included:
- One-hour staff meetings, for a total of 26 hours
- One 2-day seminar, for a total of 16 hours

Total training he receives in his new role over six months is about 42 hours.

The employee has received a total of approximately 228 hours, or about four weeks, of training over two years of employment. This number would normally be high for almost any typical gym, especially when it comes to time spent and paid for outside the gym in educational events. This owner has had this business for eight years. Eight years equals 416 weeks of ownership. Stated more clearly, he has had full-time responsibility for the business every day it's been opened for the last eight years.

As noted, the training for this employee is probably exaggerated for most fitness businesses. But we still feel that because this person has been there for two years, he should know the business simply by absorbing information while he is on the job. In reality, the only way to learn most jobs is to do them and to learn from your mistakes as they happen.

Another problem to consider when looking for a number two is that we often hire people who are too much like ourselves. Even if they aren't at first, most owners slowly mold the person into their own likeness. Ever notice that dogs and their owners start to look alike after they've been together for years? It's the same in gyms. Most owners have strong personalities and many of our new hires try to emulate them as their role models. After a while, the employee acquires your strengths, but most importantly, he also acquires your weaknesses.

One of the biggest mistakes in the hiring process is failing to hire people who are smarter than we are. The opposite of this, of course, is probably truer in that we constantly hire people who are dumber than we, so we always get to stay the big dog in our little dog minds. It's like the intelligent woman who always dates dumb guys because they make her look so much smarter in a crowd. She may never have great conversation, but she also doesn't have to worry about looking bad either. Some owners are like this. They don't ever want to be shown up or challenged, so they hire people with less talent. This leaves the owner with a loyal bunch of pleasantly dumb employees who are not capable of running the business to its fullest potential.

In the gym business, egos often dictate avoiding people who challenge us. For example, the number two person in many gyms (owned by young males) is either an attractive, very young, and usually very attentive female with little experience or education or a young male who is a workout guy like the owner but still without education or experience needed to grow the business. Neither one of these hires challenges the owner's opinion of himself, but neither one will ever offer a fresh new idea.

Even in the bigger fitness businesses, the number two is often the loyal salesperson who has no real experience in actually running a gym as a business but who has been promoted because he can make numbers happen in the sales department. This person is usually loyal and nonthreatening but never develops into the kind of person who could be trusted running the business if you were gone for a month. Good salespeople are often instinctual, and while a few can grow and lead, most can't. For example, look in the ski industry, where some of the best instructors are not always the best skiers, while the best, most talented skiers often make lousy instructors because skiing came so natural to them that they just can't grasp why everyone can't get it as fast as they did. Your number two should be someone who will make you think, someone who can challenge the decisions you make out of habit, and someone who can stimulate new ideas from the rest of your staff.

When you try to build a strong organization, consider hiring a person who is a complete opposite of yourself. If you're strong on people skills but weak on organization, then look for someone with adequate people skills but who can get you and the gym organized and ready for the next level of business. Most owners are good with people but not good with details and organization. What many owners need is someone who can get them organized and structured enough to move to that next level.

Hiring someone just like you can also slow down the progress of your business. For example, a 28-year-old single male owner in the northeast has two licensed gyms. He's a serious workout guy and is in excellent shape. His management team is made up of all males—all about 25 to 30 years old and all workout guys who are also single. They work together, party together, and chase women together on the weekends.

What kind of male-to-female mix do you think these clubs would have over time? The desired average is 55 percent female to 45 percent male in most mainstream coed gyms. In this example, these gyms are about 70 percent male. If the management team had to make major decisions, wouldn't its solutions all be somewhat alike due to the lack of diversity on the team?

For example, the club needed some new equipment on the workout floor and on the cardio deck. As young males and serious workout guys, most of the money was spent on advanced weight-training machines and very little on cardio. A different perspective might have sought more balance or at least equipment that would have attracted and supported a broader clientele.

There would also be issues of the club's atmosphere, colors and finish, music, uniforms, and member service. All these areas would end up with the same solution and same perspective—that of a single white male who lifts a lot of weights. Women, older males, and other gym populations would be ignored in this environment.

Before you can hire a number two person who can perform, you have to take time to analyze yourself as a boss and as a person. What are your strengths and weaknesses and what will you need from your second-in-command?

The following are some starting points to help you understand yourself better and what you want from your chief assistant.

Stay in Touch With Your Experience

You were the one who made the gym happen in the first place. For example, as an owner, you were good in sales, but now that you're the boss, you feel you should be actively doing something boss-like, such as paperwork.

Sometimes, it's good to go with your strengths and find someone else to take care of your weaknesses.

In this case, once you understand and master the numbers and the back shop part of the business, you can still sell and handle production for the company and hire a number two who takes over the paperwork, budgets, payroll, and other management necessities, but you always keep control of your business by being able to manage the person who manages the numbers that you mastered by spending time doing them yourself. By doing it this way, you're still improving the business with the addition of the number two, but you are also working within your strengths to grow to the next level.

You Can Manage More Than You Can Do Yourself

Streamline the business by farming out as much as you can. You could probably learn to do your own books and collect your own memberships, but why would you when these tasks add nothing to the gym's revenue stream? Remember the concept that your job in your small business is to create fresh revenue every day and that 95 percent of what we do is to generate more sales and money. Anything that gets in the way of this production has to get farmed out. You don't lose control by using a third-party financial service company to handle your memberships. You gain control because they do the work and you manage the results, which is must less costly in time and, ultimately, in money.

Many owners consider giving up parts of the business as losing control. It's hard to understand intellectually, especially if you are a born doer, but the more you give up and then manage, the more control you'll have in the end.

Also, streamline your business by creating set systems and procedures. Training a number two will be easier if you are teaching him how to follow a system rather than how to freestyle the management decisions. Put another way, systems are easier than teaching instincts. Good systems allows for someone's instincts to become sharper because the right way and the wrong way are clearly delineated from the beginning.

Provide Real Education

Here is a classic owner quote: "It would take me five hours to teach this task to someone or five minutes to do it myself, so why wouldn't I just do it myself and get it done?" This quote is the justification we use for still trying to do everything ourselves. The five hours of education, which we all know is a hyperexaggeration, could save you hundreds of dollars and many, many hours of labor in the long run. Your people will be more loyal and become better performers if you spend the time and money to educate them.

Lead by Example

If you don't do it and live it, then neither will your employees. For example, if you're 15 minutes late for an appointment with an employee, stop to consider the statement you have made about acceptable behavior in the business. Tomorrow, that same employee has an appointment with a member for training. What happens if the employee is late for that appointment? Whose fault is it? Could you fault an employee who learned from you that being late is the correct behavior?

Set Clear Objectives

People work better when they know what's expected of them. If an employee thinks he is doing a great job and his boss thinks he is not, you are already in a no-win situation. This situation arises because the employee is left to do his job without any feedback until he does something dramatically wrong and then the boss hits the fan. Managing by ignoring the employee is fairly common practice, especially in businesses that have varied shifts where employees can come and go without every running into a real supervisor.

The employee shows up every morning, leaves at the end of his shift, and does whatever tasks are written out for him, but his boss, who hasn't been in the gym at 5 a.m. for several years, thinks those morning sales and profit center numbers should be higher. The real problem is that no one from the management team has ever pointed this out to the morning guy. This becomes a problem, though, when the employee is now brought into the system in such events as a potential annual review, where both sides argue their stance is correct.

Ultimately, the boss is to blame for not setting performance standards so the employee knows how he is doing as he progresses throughout the year. If he is told that he has to do three sales per week and $1,000 through the register and he does that each week, then he has a set standard to compare his performance against without the need of having a supervisor, who has expectations but who has never shared them with this team members, having to intercede.

Praise and Recognize

As bosses, we too often fail to say thanks or to recognize an employee who is getting the job done. Because we are paying them anyway, we expect them to do a good job. Therefore, we only get involved if they are not doing such a great job, but because so few people do good jobs for the money they receive, we need to recognize effort that is ultimately on our behalf.

As owners, we too often reward the heroes and ignore the steady, dependable folks who are the heart of the business. For example, salespeople are always the stars, get the greatest pay, and have the best perks. We then ignore those steady, always-there employees who get the job done every day but aren't in the glamour positions. For example, that cleaning guy who hasn't missed a day's work in a year and keeps the gym ready for business is often overlooked—if ever recognized at all—by anyone on the management team. He gets it done but without producing obvious revenue through sales.

The steady producers who understand other aspects of the gym besides sales often make good number two people. This type of person needs to learn the role of sales in the business and should be able to do enough membership and training sales to lead by example, but he doesn't always have to be the top sales producer in the business.

Treat Employees as Individuals

No two employees are alike. The management techniques you use on one may not work on another. We need to develop techniques that can be adapted to individual employees. For example, a young employee who is chronically late may respond better to a stern warning that is written up and put in the file, along with a serious parent-to-child talk. However, older employees with the same problem might respond better to a sit-down talk about their role in the gym and how their behavior lets down the rest of the team.

Once you understand what it takes to be a good boss (and for many people, this process takes years of self-review and awareness), you then become ready to hire and start developing a good number two person.

Your number two person has a unique position in the company when it comes to his relationship with the other staff and with the owner. Most people in the world either like to give orders or they are more comfortable taking direction and working under a strong leader. The number two in most fitness facilities has to do both—take charge when you're off the property and defer to your authority when you're on-site. This means that the person has to have a certain degree of maturity to be functional in your organization.

The search for the perfect number two in your organization begins with avoiding the biggest mistake you can make, which is to hire too young. Hiring the youngest and, therefore, the cheapest employees we can find has forever been a tradition in the industry. But this practice is especially counterproductive when you're trying to develop your business by adding a strong assistant who must have working leadership characteristics. The following are a few reasons not to hire too young:

- *It takes more work to keep an employee who's too young.* Many of our young employees have not yet developed a real work ethic or have enough experience in other businesses to carry over to ours.

- *They are almost always less dependable than more established workers.* This means they're often still searching for the perfect job, they're likely still living at home, and vacating a job without notice doesn't really bother that person too much.

- *They have lifestyles that can be met by the pay offered at most any job.* Considering what we pay entry-level workers, their average lifestyle is pretty basic and can be replaced with almost any other entry-level job, meaning you don't have any leverage on this person. If something goes wrong for them or if they don't feel like working today, they are gone.

- *Most of our younger employees are undertrained and underexperienced in work that relates to making money in the fitness industry, such as customer service or sales.* Having a few months of customer service experience at the mall is one thing. Working through a six-month period, including the holidays, is something else entirely.

- *Weak communication skills are common among the younger workers.* It usually takes a number of years in the workplace to develop competent communication skills, especially when it comes to dealing with a wide variety of clients.

- *As a group, they may be young and not properly prepared, but most employees in this younger age group want responsibility quickly.* As owners, being aware of their age, we confuse more responsibility with the assignment of menial tasks. For example, we have a front counter person who's assigned to stocking the coolers—not an exciting job but one that has to be done. An owner might consider this responsibility, but the employee considers it a low-level task. To challenge the employee, we still might assign the task of stocking, but that person is also on the drink team for drink sales and is responsible for one drink promotion per week—under supervision of course. The difference is in the perception of what responsibility is and who has it: The owner, who usually sets up all drink specials, or now the staff person, whose first responsibility in the gym is running a weekly profit center promotion.

Guidelines for Hiring and Developing a Second-in-Command

Make sure you are ready to delegate authority.

Many owners never develop a number two because all they are really looking for is someone to do grunt work and menial tasks. To be effective and grow the business in tandem with the owner, number two people have to have the responsibility and authority to make real decisions, especially when you're not in the business.

For example, you're at a seminar in Las Vegas for the weekend. You either call the gym three to four times a day and end up handling the same problems you would have while you're at home or you relax and enjoy the pool, knowing that the club is in good hands and you can review the paperwork when you return.

If you're more likely to be running your club from the road, then your business won't grow because you aren't comfortable giving up partial control while you're there and still need total control when you're not. Remember that your job is to grow the business, and to do so, you have to pass along some of the responsibility so others can help you.

Make sure you have a clear idea of the traits and skills you desire in a number two.

Your number two should complement you, not be a clone. Analyze your own strengths and weaknesses first and then create a description of someone who is the opposite and adds to the mix instead of adding to the weaknesses that already exist. Hire to your weakness, not to your strength.

Ask yourself what it is you really want this person to do in your business.

Before you hire a chief assistant, write a job description that describes specific responsibilities and the authority the person would need to do the job. Include the duties you see this person handling for you as you continue to grow. For example, your second-in-command might handle one or more of the following responsibilities:

- Take over the entire staffing function, including staffing, staff training, monthly goal setting and teams (discussed in a later section), staff disciplinary action and files, and scheduling. This might allow the owner to concentrate on the marketing and sales function of the business.
- Take over the development and promotion of the multiple profit centers, including the daily promotions, monthly analysis of each center, teams and incentives, and ordering and stocking. Your second-in-command could also be your lead trainer who has the talent to still manage that department but who is interested in expanding his work into management.
- Take over the marketing, including the direct mail campaigns, newspapers, and public relations, handle the club charity, and set up and promote club events and programming. It also goes without saying in this day and age that whoever you hire has to have a full awareness and skill set to work with the gym's social media tools, websites, and any other electronic marketing you are engaged in at the time.
- Take over the sales and training functions, including training all the salespeople, training the assessor and other trainers to work in conjunction with sales, developing and stocking sales materials, and working with the head trainer, head nutrition tech, and lead salespeople to develop a consistent team sales approach.

- Develop and implement a procedure manual and staff training program, including all staff meetings, new-hire training, and the coordination of outside training events.
- Manage the gym's third-party collection effort, including all financial reporting.

These are not all the possibilities, but in most fitness businesses, the owner is currently doing all this stuff and more by herself. You're better off to follow the old adage of doing fewer things but doing them better and giving some of these tasks to your new number two.

Conduct an efficient search.

Once you have a working job description, where would you find this person? We often make the mistake of hiring someone we already know just because we are familiar with that person. This is opposite of not hiring someone because we know them too well and already know their quirks. The important part to remember is that the best person for the job may not be in your organization.

The common mistake is limiting your search to someone already in the fitness business. You should always look first for a fitness enthusiast with business experience, with a customer service background, or who has managed a number of people successfully over time. Again, look for the traits and not necessarily the skills we value in the fitness industry, such as training or sales experience. If the traits exist, then business experience or real-life service experience is more important, but we can teach the fitness functions later if the person brings the right traits to the table.

Pay equals performance.

If you want to keep a key person, you need to learn to break his lifestyle pattern in order to move him ahead in his career. Many of our key people become too comfortable in their jobs because we have let them become too comfortable in their lifestyles. This means we have trouble moving these people up because it's too easy to go back to their old comfort level they have been getting by on for years.

Here's another real-life gym story that illustrates this point. One owner was going to open a second unit in a town about an hour from his first business. He wanted to promote a female in her mid-20s—who had been with him for about two years—to manager of the existing facility. The manager would be responsible for all the day-to-day transactions in the gym, hiring and firing, and meeting goals. The owner was most concerned that he would train this person, start the second unit, and then she would quit for some reason.

The owner's original plan was to give her a raise and put her on probation for 90 days to see if she could do the job. He was going to train her for about 60 days on the daily operations and procedures she hadn't had experience with yet before he left for the other project.

This woman was ideal for the job and had been a loyal employee for a long time, working at most of the various jobs in the gym. She also had many of the skills necessary in business, such as organizational skills, that the owner didn't have. However, this hiring plan didn't meet the situation and might actually cause the new manager to leave because the changes only affected her job and not her lifestyle.

In other words, there was no risk for her to try because she could always go back to her other job or find an equivalent somewhere else in town. Her current compensation paid enough to cover her bills, pay for a nice little older-model car, and let her live fairly comfortably for someone her age by sharing expenses with one other roommate.

The revised hiring plan was to change her lifestyle in conjunction with her new job. Upon interviewing the woman, it was found that her personal goals were to have her own place and to get a new car. She was also concerned that even a management job at the gym was no guarantee of a long-term career.

The final hiring plan, which she participated in, gave her a small raise, a small loan for a deposit on her own place, and a new company car, which only cost the club $149 a month on a lease. Also, if she managed the gym successfully for one year, meeting goals and growing the business, she would be vested with 5 percent of the gym's stock in an equity-only position, with an option to buy 5 percent more if she wanted.

The revised plan changed her lifestyle, making it hard for her to go back to what she had done in the past after she had gotten into the new job. There were no other jobs in town that would give her those perks and future, so it would be unlikely for her to want to jump to something else.

If the owner had left her in her old lifestyle, meaning just a raise and the same old car and apartment, he would have created a situation where failure would not have been costly to the new manager. In her situation, failure means giving up an awful lot compared to where she had been in the past.

She was still hired under the 90-day probation for the new job and received more training than she anticipated, including business schools and a trip to a national trade convention, which made her feel ready to accept the responsibility to take on the new job.

It may often take two.

We sometimes need more than one number two. High-volume clubs or multiple units may need more than one number two. Two people may be needed to keep control of a large gym and staff, but they may have completely different job descriptions and have different functions in the business.

An example of this would be the training-centric staff structure mentioned elsewhere in this book. Reviewing that structure here, you would have a manager, a lead salesperson, an assessor whose job is to place clients into training, and a lead trainer, although the assessor and lead trainer can be the same person in certain gyms. In this model, the owner/manager would train the lead salesperson and the assessor as his senior leaders in the gym. Each has a separate area of responsibility, but each could handle other key areas, such as social media or marketing.

Create a systems-dependent business, not a people-dependent business.

Every procedure you have in your business should be documented so any employee faced with that situation can look it up. All new staff should be trained the same each and every time through their initial stages. For example, you hire a new employee—someone you think may fit well into your system.

During his training, could you show him:
- A set procedure manual for every basic function in the gym, such as cleaning and maintaining equipment?
- Working samples of every piece of paper and computer-generated form in the business?
- Procedures for every phase of the business, such as opening, closing, and handling renewals, personnel policies, and daily business reporting?
- Policies to handle common situations in the gym, such as cancellations, problems, and complaints?

Many businesses could not produce all these things in written form in manuals or electronically in your gym's computer system that are easily accessible to the staff. Most owners would have to talk the person through everything because nothing is in writing and everything they do in the business is situational, which means every problem that arises is handled individually as it occurs. In other words, do you limit or leave open operating discretion for your people? The more open the discretion, the more mistakes and less money you will make over time.

This lack of real working information is partially why we lose key people. They are eventually given responsibility toward making the business work, but they never really gain an understanding of our business on the backside. Your second person will do a better job if he has enough information to relate the task at hand to the bottom line and then is able to share that information with the staff.

The concept of sharing information with your people is new to most owners who grew up in systems and worked under owners who tried very hard to conceal every number. The basic idea of sharing information is to make sure everyone on the team understands why his job is important with regard to the bottom line of the company. If he is asked to do something, even something that seems menial at the time, he has an understanding that this job affects the bottom line in some particular way.

For example, if you or your number two are working with the staff on the importance of walking through each locker room every 30 minutes and shutting doors, replacing toilet paper, wiping off the sinks, and generally doing some basic cleaning, how would you make this job seem important enough to do without question?

One way might be to show the staff the revenue generated by the sales team. Then, relate these numbers to the overall financial picture of the club. From here, it would be a short walk to the payroll section. If sales go down because potential members see a dirty locker room, revenues go down, and eventually, the payroll would have to be decreased to compensate. Even the lowest-level counter person will do a better job if he knows why he is doing certain things.

Keep the pay competitive for your area or even higher than the market would dictate.

Another major consideration in keeping your number two is to find out if the salary you're paying is competitive for the area but not restricted just to other fitness facilities. It's helpful to find out what equivalent jobs, such as retail shop managers, get paid in your market. When comparing, include all the perks, such as health insurance, days of paid vacation, and other benefits we can offer to make the job more valuable. Buying talent costs money and you should often offer a higher wage than average in the area in order to attract the talented people looking to move up from other careers.

Even the smallest business can usually improve with the addition of a strong teammate for the owner—someone who can carry more responsibility and increase the workload beyond what one person can handle. An easy summary for creating a number two spot and for staffing in general can be simplified in some straightforward points:

• Avoid drastic overstaffing and understaffing.
• Clearly spell out (in writing) what you expect from your number two.
• Delegate major, not just minor, responsibilities.
• Encourage ideas, even if they are different from your own.
• Visualize, using visual management techniques, every staff member's goals, including your number two's and your own contributions.
• Visualize your team's goals so everyone has the same basic information about the business.
• Promote from within if possible.
• Set a realistic leadership example.
• Rotate job responsibilities with your number two on the really ugly jobs. You know, she fires one and then you fire one.
• Use positive incentives, goals, and performance standards to motivate.
• Accept mistakes. If there aren't mistakes, then no one is trying anything new and your business will die from stagnation.
• Give the low-level folks challenging assignments.
• Be liberal with praise, even on the little things you expect done correctly anyway.
• Criticize with tact. "Bonehead" or "You pork chop" are not acceptable staff names.
• Tell the truth, even when it makes you or the business look bad.
• Say "No" tactfully and only for good cause.
• Set up long-term incentive programs for your senior people.
• The more training and education, the better. You can't overtrain a staff person.
• Don't downplay bad assignments.

- Don't work with idiots. Don't expect your number two to do so either. If you hire badly, correct quickly and move on.
- Teach everyone time management—if you can find the time.
- Meet with and exchange information often with the entire team.
- Be consistent in your treatment of your number two and the entire staff.
- Show personal interest in your management team. Be aware of the issues in your life that affect them and, ultimately, you.
- Learn from the employees who quit. When good employees quit, they are telling you something.

Things to think about as you read this material

- Project your business three years into the future. Where do you want to be? How successful do you want your business to have become by that time? Now figure out what type of person—with what skills and knowledge—you need to reach those goals.
- Build a model of the pay, incentives, and job description before you begin your search for a number two.
- Build a systems-based business that does not depend on any one person to succeed. If your business is truly a systems business, you should be able to interchange staff without seeing a decline.
- Hire a number two who has practical business skills instead of fitness experience.
- Review the incentives you are currently using with your staff. Could you improve performance by changing incentives? Keep in mind that it's not always money that motivates people. Start with recognition as your prime motivator. Remember that the trend is moving away from using incentives to drive performance and toward a system that pays a higher base, therefore attracting a stronger person for the job. Incentives are only used as rewards for this person and not as motivators.
- Protect the key people you already have in your business. Learning to change their lifestyle to match their position makes it hard to leave you for another job that may not have all the great extras.
- Study and analyze your own work style. Most owners and managers are doers. Remember that you can manage much more than you can physically do yourself.

January 9, 2014
You are a role model—whether you want to be one or not.

If you have clients of any type or friends or even kids, you are a role model. Overweight trainers—whether it's fair or not—suffer from a credibility issue. Fit pros that are always late, badly dressed, hungover, or in constantly bad moods also have issues. There is also the weird side of being too extreme. Unless you train elite athletes, most of your people are just normal, everyday, real-life folks who struggle to get to the gym twice a week. Preaching hardcore extremism drives them away just as quickly as being the guy who doesn't work out much but thinks he is the master trainer. What you say, how you dress, how you live, and the standards you adhere to in your life all combine to establish your credibility and image. You may have never set out to be someone's role model, but you have to deal with the fact that you are—and who you are is just as important as what you know when it comes to long-term success.

February 12, 2014
True core strength

There are two types of core strength. The obvious one comes from quality training and reflects hours spent in your gym, but the other type of core strength is defined as who you are and how you live your life. True internal core strength is reflected in all the values that combine to make you who you are, such as integrity, professionalism, compassion, patience, empathy for those who struggle, and perseverance. When someone who is deconditioned starts a workout program, no sane coach would load a bar beyond the person's ability to handle it, but we often make that mistake in our own lives. You see this in people who go to some type of motivational workshop, get really inspired, and then lose that energy in a few weeks. This happens because the change was superficial and was easily lost due to the person's true core strength being weak. In other words, there is no change unless the core belief system changes to match the desired motivational change. True core strength can be built but can never be completed and will be a lifetime project. If you want permanent change in your life, look internally first and make sure your true core is strong because if it is weak, nothing you seek in life will be accomplished. You are who you are because of your core values and everything good in life stems from that center.

17

Why Is Your Employee Just Standing There Staring at You?

Ever wonder why that employee is just standing there looking at you like you're an alien or, even worse, one of their parents? It's because you may have hired wrong in the first place. Our traditional system of finding and paying employees has led you to hire a person who is too young for the job, never worked before in his life, and can only communicate with Beavis and Butthead, SpongeBob, or any of this year's nationally known slackers in life. In other words, you are suffering from the same staffing malady all your fellow owners and operators are suffering from: the "they're all boneheads" syndrome.

Staffing is one of those issues that raise a vast swing in emotions from a fitness facility owner. We can't live without staff, but we often lay awake at night wondering if we could get away with just killing a few chosen employees. Of course, this assumes that the employee in question is actually among the living and is not just doing a zombie impression at the front desk for low pay.

You understand the ones who really make us crazy, such as the counter guy who forgets to shave and always seems to have the wrong uniform top on when he comes to work. Nothing really serious here, but after a while, he simply needs to be killed. But even our plans to kill them won't work because just when we set the trap, the employee doesn't show up to work due to a massive hangover or because of a "significant other of the week" problem.

Typical owners in today's hypercompetitive markets will have to deal with almost a mind-boggling array of important issues in the near future in the fitness industry: raising capital, increased operational costs, the endlessly stupid low pricing from the big chains, and how to move toward a higher return per client and away from chasing volume. But two of most business threatening concerns you will face in the immediate future will be staffing and retention. These two key issues directly depend on each other because a weak staff prohibits any type of member service and weak member service leads directly to poor member retention.

The Traditional Fitness Staffing Model Doesn't Work Anymore

For our businesses to grow in the coming years, we need to re-evaluate how we find, develop, and motivate our employees. The reason staffing is such an issue for the typical fitness owner is that our traditional model of how we hire and pay employees no longer works. The fitness business has prospered over the years by depending on two distinct levels of staff: an elite high-paid sales staff and a very low-level, undertrained, and very expendable support staff.

But this system—a holdover from the days of chasing endless volume—is no longer effective in a generation of businesses that depend on getting the maximum results for the maximum number of members over time. The current membership supporting today's gyms come in two distinct categories. You either have members demanding more service and more guidance and who are educated enough to understand what more sophisticated training looks like and who support gyms that offer this service or you have clients who are literally searching for the cheapest price and who are willing to trade walking on a treadmill for $10 a month for no help whatsoever. The model mentioned that is based on a heavy emphasis on salespeople and a string of low-paid expendable counter staff now fails due to heavy competition that is forcing gyms to move toward the higher service model or offer none at all, but you can't survive in the middle any longer as a club that hammers sales without servicing its membership well.

As many of the big chains have proven over the past several decades, slick salesmanship is no longer the answer to the "thriving in business" question, especially because you now have markets crammed with dozens of fitness facilities all offering the same services, running the same price specials, and fighting for the same potential members. The big change is that these gyms now have to actually produce a solid product after the sale to stay competitive. You might get a new member, but he won't stay long in today's market because he most likely drove past four other gyms on his way to work out and any of them will be more attractive than yours if your service is horrible enough to make him seek a change.

Low Pay Buys Low Service

The old model of good employees for $5 to $6 per hour is no longer valid in most parts of the country. These old-style types of clubs can generate new business, but they can't keep this business because the support staff represents the lowest common denominator when it comes to hiring and training. Employees willing to work for $8 or $10 per hour in today's economy usually are too young, have little previous real-life work experience, and have poor communication skills. These employees are not capable of delivering the kind of member service it takes to keep today's more sophisticated members happy and in the system.

Another way to look at it is that the clubs hire bodies and not talent. You should know you are in trouble when you find yourself looking for any warm body to fill that morning shift—with the emphasis on the word *fill*. You didn't phrase the question to yourself: "I need to find someone who can generate a lot of money during those morning hours. I wonder who that is?" The concern was to find someone to fill a slot so you won't have to get up at 3:30 a.m. to open your gym. We too often hire bodies to fill slots, but there isn't usually a whole lot of emphasis on finding talent for these jobs, especially because we are offering pay at the lower end of the pay scale.

As Many of the Big Chains Have Proven Over the Past Several Decades, Slick Salesmanship Is No Longer the Answer

Without a consistent well-trained staff, there can be no consistency in the delivery of member service. With competition developing at a near frantic pace, the only thing that will separate the good clubs from each other in the future will be delivery of the product, not the product itself. Being a training-centric business is a huge advantage in today's market, but that edge will disappear as more training gyms open and the chains and the old independent players start to realize they have to adapt or die.

We'll all have decent physical plants and great functional-based equipment in the future. The winner in the gym wars will be the gym businesses that understand that long-term service is replacing traditional high-pressure sales as the central operating strategy for our business plans and that we are quickly shifting from volume-based businesses to results-driven operations that depend on heavy service and support for all clients.

The major flaw in the theory of delivery of the product is that the owner doesn't have the final say in the matter. The owner may truly believe in customer service, but it's usually the lowest-paid and most undertrained employee on the staff, such as the front counter person, that the members most associate with the club and its service image.

This undertrained person is the one who really has the responsibility for delivering the perception of the service product and will do so according to the traits he brings to the job and the skills he possesses. The flaw is that employees we now attract don't have the traits necessary for the club to be successful. Pay peanuts and get monkeys. The staff members that traditional low pay attracts are either good people too young and undertrained or just weak employees not able to deliver service under any conditions.

Traits in our business are defined as things the employee already possesses and can't usually be taught. Things that can be taught and developed are skills, such as the ability to learn a sales pitch or a specific training routine. On the other hand, enthusiasm is something that can be inspired but seldom taught. You either love people and are born to help or you are one of those people who need a computer job running numbers in the back of an office where you never see anyone.

This caring, people-person attitude is an example of a trait and is also something that can't usually be taught. Running a front desk computer system is a skill, but keep in mind that skills can be taught to people who still shouldn't have a job in service in a gym. It is a little known fact, but there was even a monkey at the St. Louis Zoo who could run a cash register. The monkey was so good at this simple task that the zoo's management got him a job at the zoo gift shop. He was bad at customer service, though, and kept spitting at the customers, so they had to fire him, and eventually, he got a job running the front counter at a typical $10-a-month gym where getting spit on was just part of the $10 experience.

For example, a trait necessary for a front counter person would be the ability to communicate with a variety of people on a daily basis, which is not an ability most employees who work for $8 per hour usually possess. Hiring a quiet, fearful person because he is the only body that applied is the norm for most owners. We then throw this undertrained and socially incompetent person into the fracas at the front counter on a Monday night during primetime—after only three to four hours of training—and expect him to be competent performer. Of course, if it were a new salesperson we were discussing, we'd never let that person on the floor without *days* of training. We assume member service to be self-evident and anyone holding the job can deliver the service, but the sales skills have to be taught.

Before we discuss how to find an employee, we should first explore the traditional thinking concerning what we offer in the way of jobs. Owners think working in the gym business is one of the most desirable jobs any person could have. What could be better than working around a bunch of healthy, seminaked people while you get to wear funny clothes and work out?

However, the truth is that the potential employee no longer defines our jobs as all that desirable. Today's crop of potential hires have too many options in today's job market—many of which offer better training, benefits, and a better starting wage. Let's look at what we think is a good job and then look again from the employee's viewpoint.

The Issue of How We Pay

As owners, we want to pay the lowest wage for the best employees. We think the typical wages paid by the industry—usually a little above the local minimum—are enough and should allow us to get decent folks to work for us. It's the theory the business was built on, and theoretically, this concept should still work. But every business owner is thinking the same thing. Remember the biggest thing that has changed in our markets: Anything works when you have no competition, but in the age of intense competition, we have to question everything we have taken for granted for so many years.

All the owners in the market want to pay $8 per hour (adjust this per region/substitute your local minimum wage) and get a dedicated employee. We—meaning all small businesses—are fighting for the same entry-level employee, especially in the service businesses. For example, in an intensely crowded market, with 20 or more competitors in your market ring of about five miles, there are also hundreds of other retail and service businesses looking for the same people willing to work for entry-level pay.

What kind of employee will actually work for that much or that little money anymore and are there enough of them in your market to fill all these entry-level jobs? Potential employees who are answering ads for minimum wage are probably too dumb to work for you or are using the club as their first work experience—neither of which is good for your business. Anybody who walks in and says "Hi, I'm Johnny and I'm here for that minimum wage job in the paper" is most likely not going to be the person who can deliver legendary member service. Why wasn't he going for those $10- to $12-an-hour jobs? Is it because he feels he is a minimum-wage type of guy and is really proud of the fact that minimum wage is the maximum he aspires to in his life?

Poor wages also means high turnover. Employees on the bottom rung of pay will quickly leave for a buck or two higher per hour once they gain practical work experience with you. If the employee has been somewhat trained and on the job for at least six months, it will cost you about 10 times the employee's monthly salary to replace him.

For example, a well-trained counter person would know how to recognize potential business in the pro shop, be able to make a shake, answer some basic membership questions, and be able to competently handle the phone. This trained counter person would also be able to recognize a potential member walking in the door and to promptly process that person. However, the new person hired to replace the exiting one who just left you for a few dollars an hour more wouldn't have the experience and training necessary to recognize that regular member standing at the counter waiting patiently for his smoothie. In fact, our new person wouldn't know the client's name or his favorite shake and wouldn't remember to thank him. This client has been paying you a membership for several years and this is the fifth new counter person he has to meet and break in, but after some point, the client gives up and realizes you can't keep staff and that after being a member of your business for a number of years that no one still knows or remembers his name.

The new counter person might also put too much of the basic ingredients in the shake, therefore lowering the profit margin, and might initially mess up a lot of phone calls—some from potential members—before they are comfortable. The business he loses or just doesn't see during his first six months could easily cost the club 10 times the monthly salary of the trained and capable person.

It would have made more sense to have paid a dollar or two more an hour to keep the first employee once he is trained and productive rather than constantly lose and replace employees, let alone figure the additional cost of hiring a new employee. In this example, the employee left you for a dollar or two more, which is still most likely top pay in the market. Meeting or exceeding that pay for a trained employee just makes business sense and it is bad business to lose a trained employee who shows any potential and work ethic in the job.

Another issue concerning pay relates to fishing. Lousy bait catches lousy fish—if any at all. The proper bait for the situation might get you the best fish. If we fish for employees with too low of an entry wage, we are only going to attract the most unskilled and weakest employees. By offering a better wage— usually a dollar or two over local minimum wage—we attract a better employee in the first place. If we properly train and develop our people, the employee is worth the extra salary anyway. Just be sure to hire all employees on a 90-day probationary period so any mistakes can be rectified in a manner that won't hurt the gym.

Local minimum wage is defined as what it takes to attract a front counter person. In northern states, that is usually several dollars higher than the federally or state-mandated federal wage. In southern states, flat minimum wage might be all it takes to fill that counter job. Paying $1 to $3 an hour higher than the local minimum wage is usually the difference between attracting a warm body to fill that slot and attracting someone with talent who can produce revenue for you in that position.

Poor Working Conditions

We think working in a gym is heaven on Earth. Many of us have had real jobs and most agree that ties, offices, and the other trappings of the real business world are undesirable things that have to be avoided at all costs. But to our employees, the gym business offers less than ideal working conditions.

Long shifts, no breaks, and usually no place to sit and enjoy lunch, along with constant stress from handling endless member service problems and inconsistent leadership, are just a few of the things employees have to deal with as part of their jobs in the fitness industry. Throw in a lack of meaningful compensation and work, petty tasks, and a cluttered, poorly lit workspace—all for $8 to $10 per hour pay none of us would even think of living on in our own lives—and we end up with a frustrated, short-term job holder.

Imagine working in an environment where you stand behind a counter on a carpet over concrete floor without even a place to sit down between customers. Throw in a few pieces of broken equipment the members have to deal with, flooded toilets, no parking, a lack of training to handle complaints, and a shortage of support staff during the busiest times. Don't forget to include a frustrating (if it's operating at all) computer system and you have an exciting and glamorous front counter job in the gym business.

We think of gyms as a sort of glamour job, but working long hours on our feet for low pay and doing repetitive tasks can lead to a quick decision to change jobs. We should be thinking in terms of what it would take to keep the people we invest in at the counter through training and consider consistent breaks—say, 15 minutes for every four hours worked—a regular lunch hour off premises, a break room with a locker, and a decent wage for the work performed or at least for the work expected. All employees are investments and every hour of training you put into that new hire represents a cost to you that you will have to repeat for yet another person you burn up in that low-end job.

Poor Training

In a recent survey among employees, we found that the majority of employees feel they are undertrained for the jobs they hold. On the other hand, the owners we surveyed felt they were giving adequate training for the employees and their jobs. This obviously leads to high expectations from the owners and managers and poor performance and job frustration from the staff.

The lower the level of the employee, the more training he requires. For example, front counter people probably need as many as four hours per week in training—in a combination of group and individual work. But it's usually the sales staff that gets the bulk of the training. These folks are sent to local sales seminars, role-play almost every day, and get spot help any time they need it from the sales managers, who are usually successful salespeople who have been doing the job for a long period of time.

Front counter folks, though, are usually taught once and thrown to our mad dog members—the regulars who enjoy working over the new front counter targets. Most of the training the counter people need to be effective in their jobs should be focused on the basics, such as phone work, handling complaints, member service training, and job essentials. The managers, senior employees, and owners should do the bulk of this training. Again, four hours per week every week would be about right for developing a good counter staff.

The material covered should be a mix of the basics and the introduction of new material. Employees should also be cross-trained to all other jobs in the business. A front counter person may never sell a membership, but he should have sales training to better understand the goals of the team and the role the sales staff plays. These counter people should also get team training for free as part of their job, attend group exercise regularly, and, in other words, experience and be able to discuss through personal experience everything the gym offers.

Lack of Structure

Most owners hate structure. They are entrepreneurial types, which means operating according to the disaster at hand. Owners expect to have good employees without setting a structure to ensure it happens.

On the other hand, employees love structure. They seek leadership and guidance in the parameters of being able to do their own thing. Teach me, train me, and then get the hell out of my way. But if I have a problem, I want someone to give me guidance and help me solve this problem and then get out of my way once more. Most employees also work better in a structured environment. Set rules, consistent follow-up, consistent enforcement of those rules, and an objective evaluation system all make for a better, more motivated employee.

A good way to create a sense of structure is to create a club procedure book. This is a master book kept at the front counter that has all the club's procedures documented in simple, easy-to-follow terms. For example, there might be a section on how to close the club that includes lights, heating and air, alarms, a final club walk-through, and even where the emergency key is hidden.

Other examples would be to show how to fill out a contract and include a sample, how to send in a contract to the financial company, policies and procedures on renewals, how to make change and figure tax, and how to do a proper information call. Don't assume anything. Every single procedure in the club—no matter how small—should have a separate page or section in the book. Start with the basics and add to them as needed. It may take a year or more to build a complete book that documents everything in the club. Be sure to keep a copy locked in the manager's office and another at home. You can do this online, but going retro here is just another way to keep the employee focused. It is usually much better to have an employee look something up in a book rather than go online and stay there for an extra hour.

A complete procedure book is also a great training tool. All the entry-level training for new employees can be done with the book. Another benefit of having a complete procedures manual is that you don't have to do all the training yourself from your head or by trying to reconstruct information from the daily tasks in the club. Anyone with any experience can show other employees how to do things by working though the procedure sheet for a job that's detailed in the book.

No Employee Benefits

We always hate it when a good employee comes in and says: "I have to quit. My mom says it's time to get a real job." Many gyms can't afford to put together a real benefits package, but every club should work toward a basic insurance and possibly a 401k package, meaning some type of personal investment package for anyone reading this outside the United States, for full-time employees as soon as the gym can afford it. We want long-term folks—ones we can count on to help the business grow—but we are usually not willing to make the job attractive enough for them to stay any length of time. In other words, if you pick the right employee and he gets better, then you have to get better and offer this person an opportunity to stay with you and improve his life at the same time.

Using Restrictive, Old-Style Management Principles

One of the biggest wastes in our payroll budgets is following the principles set down by our fathers. Everyone used to be a basic 9-to-5 worker glued to watching the clock all day. No one under 30 works like our fathers did in the 1950s and 1960s. Structured 40-hour workweek businesses offered in the 1950s in the United States are relics from a generation of employees that simply no longer exist.

We waste a big percentage of our payroll trying to give all our full-timers 40-hour workweeks. Go to just about any gym of any size on a weekday around 2 p.m. and you'll immediately feel payroll getting flushed down the toilet. There are always at least three people standing around the front desk just waiting for something to do and this group usually outnumbers the members in the gym at that time. This group of bored and nonproductive employees is there because we believed we had to give them 40 hours a week to keep them in the gym, and in today's market, we are often wrong about hiring this way.

Most of our next generation employees would be happy working a 32-hour workweek, with a higher base pay and light bonuses and commissions, which would be considered full time by most of them. This means an employee could work four 8-hour days and be considered full time by the owner. This would also mean one less person standing around on Friday at 2 p.m. burning up the payroll.

For example, most of us need our lead salesperson during primetime on Monday through Thursday. But we usually make that person come in on Friday because we need to give them full-time hours, meaning the traditional 40-hour workweek—hours that could easily be filled by a secondary and less costly employee.

An option would be to give the person four 8-hour days and have him there Monday through Thursday or give him four 10-hour days during the same time period and simply give him other tasks to do during slower afternoon hours. Either way, you save the cost of the clog on Friday afternoon. However, a note here is that if the employees want to work four 10-hour days, they must sign away their rights to overtime on a document to be kept in their employee files.

In this example, you could keep a good salesperson from burning out by only working the key hours and save wasted payroll on nonproductive days. Having a job where you can make decent money and still have time off is one of the most desirable job requirements for most of our under-30 employees.

The Kiss of Death in Member Service: Hiring Too Young

Another negative by-product of low wages is that it forces us to hire too young. Many of our front-line people, such as entry-level trainers, salespeople, and most of our counter people, are simply too young and inexperienced to do the work we expect of them. There is a rule of thumb here that holds true almost anywhere you could operate a gym: You never want to be anyone's first job. Your goal is to hire someone where you can teach the person what to do in that job, but you never want to hire someone where you also have to teach them how to work, how to show up for work, how to dress and groom, and how to say hello. Let someone else take the first job beating and concentrate on only hiring people who have some type of basic work experience.

The problem with an employee who is too young is the lack of communication skills. A big part of member service in any job in the gym is the ability to listen and understand what a disgruntled member is trying to get across to you. Once it's established what the member is trying to make us understand, the employee then has to rectify the situation or pacify the member until a solution can be found.

Often, simply listening well and then talking the member through the problem can settle the issue. Employees who are too young seldom have developed good communication skills. When you spend your life with your face buried in a personal device, you usually don't know how to listen well, you lack common ground with older members, and you can't really talk the member through the problem. "Hey, I'll text you" isn't always what a pissed-off member standing at the front counter and screaming about no toilet paper wants to hear from our new counter person.

We lose a lot of good members because they simply walk away frustrated over a problem that could have been simply handled by a sympathetic ear and a smile instead of a shrug of the shoulders and an "It's not my job" attitude or the "I'll talk to my boss when he comes in" put-off.

A prime example is the lead counter person. This is usually the person who is at the front counter during the busiest hours of the day until closing. This is the one person in the club who sees everything, is in contact with virtually every member who enters and leaves the club, and acts as the traffic cop for directing and leading the other staff members. In a gym based on member service and results for every client, this might be the most important job on the team, but it is often one of the youngest and least-trained people we have in the system.

A perfect person for this job would be someone with good communications skills, a strong presence, and the ability to work with a wide variety of members and who could give some guidance and direction in the gym to other staff as to what must happen at the moment.

The ideal person for this position would probably be a woman in her late 20s to whatever age, as long as she is a workout person and has had some type of customer service job in the past. This person should also be a people person who also can multitask, which is why we normally leave most young males out of this role in the gym. This type of person would probably have far better communication skills than your average 22-year-old male or female. Remember: "Yo, dude" is not a standard club welcoming statement.

Finding a staff in today's market is tough. Everyone who is any good is probably already working for someone else. Traditional sources of employees, such as help wanted ads, are useless. In today's market, if you want to work, you probably are working, which means you aren't home answering traditional and extremely dated ads in the paper.

Currently, you usually only have two choices to find help. Advertising on any form of electronic want ads is the place to start when you're looking for people in the age groups we want to hire in the gyms. These vary from country to country and could be offered as an extra through the town newspaper or through specialty websites that are based on a variety of lists, including jobs, things for sales, and other ways to put people in touch with other. This is always the first place to start searching for staff in any market.

There is also plan B—or the "steal everyone you need" plan. If you can't find good employees because they are already employed, then we need to strongly invite those employees to change jobs. This has been going on for years in the real business world, but we've always had qualms in the fitness industry about such a sensitive subject.

We don't necessarily have to steal from local competitors, although any club over a couple miles away is probably a fair target. However, that gym may have just as lousy employees as you do. We do need to learn to steal from other types of service businesses, though, because we are still looking for the traits the employees brings with them with the understanding that we can teach them the skill sets they need to get the job done. These traits are most likely already proven in any employee who has been surviving in any type of retail or service business for any length of time.

Remember, we are looking for the strong traits, such as naturally good customer service, the ability to talk and to look you in the eye, a good work ethic, and a professional appearance. If the person has these traits, we can usually teach him the skills he needs for their specific jobs in our businesses. If the person doesn't naturally have these traits, all the training in the world won't make him much of an employee.

The perfect example would be an employee of a national chain of clothing stores who helped me at the mall. She was personable, had a strong sales presence, a professional attitude and look, and was about 25 years old. She was also making about $10 an hour after commissions. How do you find this out? You ask. If you've ever had anyone praise your work, then you know how flattering it would be to have a complete stranger offer you an interview after a brief encounter. A simple "You're really good at your work—you're not looking for a different job, are you?" is all it takes.

This person had all the traits necessary for our type of work and was susceptible to a steal because of the type of work she was doing and the pay she was currently receiving. To steal this person, you would have had to offer at least $12 to $14 per hour, plus light bonuses and commissions, but she would be worth it because she could be productive at a higher level with less training.

It is important to note that in today's market and with today's employee, you are always better to pay a stronger base wage and then go with lighter commissions. This type of pay system allows you to attract a stronger employee drawn by the higher base pay. The old school thought, which has no basis whatsoever in research, is that high commissions drive performance. The reality is that if you pay enough to hire strong people in the first place, then you probably hired someone capable of doing the work anyway at a much higher level and the commissions wouldn't make any difference in total performance. This is true in any job in any gym: Pay more to buy quality and keep the commissions lower as rewards for good work but not incentives to drive the work.

The biggest plus in the woman in this example is that she knows how to work. You don't have to teach her how to show up, be on time, and have a good work ethic. She learned that on someone else's payroll. Many of our potential employees who arrive fresh from college programs have never held a job in their lives. They want $40,000 a year and a title and yet have never worked toward anything—ever. You not only have to teach these people the job, but you also have to teach them how to work too—something much more difficult than working with someone who has the basic traits.

However, many owners are afraid to steal employees because they're afraid someone will come back and steal theirs. If they steal yours, maybe it's because we aren't meeting the employees' needs, as we discussed earlier. If an employee is paid decently, works in a reasonable environment, and has consistent training and support, he will probably be pretty hard to steal. Happy, rewarded, and appreciated employees are hard to steal in the real world.

Hiring Right the First Time

It's been said thousands of times, but it's still true. Most employee problems occur because the owner or manager hired wrong in the first place. He simply put the wrong person in the wrong job and had to live with the results.

The first phase of your hiring process is to seek talent, which is something you're going to have to pay more than your competitors if you want to consistently hire the best talent in your market. Cheap employees may be a bargain for a week or two, but they shortly become more of a liability than an asset.

Offer base pay in your area high enough to get decent people to work for you. We also pay bonuses and commissions as part of the employee's incentive package. Every employee should have the chance to earn a little extra if he meets his goals for the month as a reward but not as a driver of performance. Often, commissions and bonuses are restricted solely for salespeople and managers. Every employee should have a chance to achieve an extra level of compensation no matter what position he holds in the gym. Goal setting and incentives are discussed in depth later in this chapter.

Your payroll may be slightly higher with this system but not always. Better employees usually get more work done and achieve more than weaker people and often cover the higher pay with increased production. In other words, you can get more performance out of fewer people if those people are motivated and willing to do the work.

For example, let's say you normally pay a front counter person $8 per hour with no additional bonuses. This time around, you start the new counter person—who is a little older, has more work experience, and needs less training—at $10.50 an hour plus small incentives from team bonuses. At 32 hours and $8 per hour ($8 x 32 x 4.2 weeks per typical month = $1,075), the first person would gross about $1,075 per month or just enough to slowly frustrate him enough to either get a second job or eventually leave you for a higher-paying one when he gets some experience. Just when you get this person trained and productive, he leaves you, burning up the training expense and forcing you to toss another rookie into a key production job.

At 32 hours per week and $10.50 per hour, the second person starts at about $1,400 per month ($10.50 x 32 x 4 weeks in a typical month). In this example, the second person would also have the opportunity to earn an additional $75 to $125 per month in team incentives from the multiple profit centers. Even if the second person hits all the team goals in the profit centers, he's only getting an extra $300 to $400 per month more than the first "bargain" employee.

The question you have to ask yourself as an owner is what type of person or employee did the $10.50 per hour draw in comparison to the $8? In most markets where $8 per hour is normal service pay, the $10.50 per hour is a huge difference and would attract a much more sophisticated worker and probably someone with a lot more talent and experience. If this person produces, he is worth the extra money. If he doesn't, he has to be let go at the end of the 90-day probationary period and the club is really not at much risk financially.

The $300 $400 is a big difference but only if all you want is a body to stand at the front desk and fill the slot. But this difference may not be such a big hit on your payroll if you are trying to attract an older and more qualified worker who can provide member service, produce revenue in the gym, and do extra work generating extra revenue, such as help with customer service calls and other retention work that has to be done in every gym of any type.

Profiling Our Employees

When you hire for traits, not skills, you need to start with a basic profile of what you really want in your employee. Each position in the gym should have a profile of the traits necessary to successfully do the job. If you already have a type of person in mind written down on paper, then you'll have a much better chance of recognizing the real thing when it comes through the door.

The following is a profile of an entry-level (counter person, basic trainer, and entry salesperson) position for the typical fitness facility. Use these points as a checklist for the hiring process—in addition to building a profile for the job itself.

The person should have and exhibit these traits:
- He is generally enthusiastic and outgoing in personality.
- He makes eye contact easily, smiles often, and is relaxed with other people.
- He is interested in personal fitness, as demonstrated by his personal workout program and interest in other sports. (Remember, this hire doesn't have to be in perfect shape, but he should be a work in process. If you have lost 20

pounds and still have 20 more to go, welcome to the gym, but if you need to lose 30 and haven't yet started, you may not understand what we do in these businesses.)

- He has held previous jobs that require customer service and he held these jobs for at least six months.
- He appears to be a "people person," as demonstrated by the activities he enjoys and jobs he has held. (For example, someone who says he prefers to run races on the weekends is most likely a better candidate than someone who prefers to hide from others and read by herself.)
- He demonstrates the traits of a self-starter and hard worker. (You can usually determine this by asking one simple question: How old were you when you had your first job?)
- He has a wide range of interests and accomplishments.
- He has held previous jobs that required being a self-starter (e.g., newspaper delivery person, cut lawns, or worked at a fast-food place while in school).

If a person has these traits, we could train him for most positions in a gym. Often, we overlook these traits for skills, which may or may not prove to be valuable in the actual performance of work in your system. For example, a person may have had sales experience in another fitness facility but has to be completely retrained because he doesn't fit with your current sales system. You bought skills, but now you must constantly fight the "Well, we did it this way at my other job," which is hard for many employees to get over.

Other jobs in the facility might require different traits. Managers need to be good with numbers. Salespeople need strong self-confidence and strong communication skills and trainers need to be patient and empathetic. By profiling each position, we concentrate on looking for the type of person we want in that job and then train him to the system he will work in at the club.

Interviewing

Interviewing is a lost art dating back to pre-Columbian pottery and the early Elvis days. Very few people are good at it anymore and even fewer care to learn. Most interviews in gyms consist of the owner begging the potential employee to please take that morning shift starting tomorrow so he doesn't have to open for the 20th time in a row.

Good interviewing for the gym business consists of three steps and a real understanding of the law. We'll talk about the three steps here, but you need to attend a good human resources workshop on the legality of hiring and firing in the state or country where you live and start understanding what you can and cannot ask potential employees legally during an interview. For example, you can't ask age in almost any country in the civilized world. You also can't ask any leading questions that try to determine age. You can ask how old a person was when he had his first job—one of the most effective interview questions. But you can't ask what year that was or who was president or any other trick questions that allow you to figure out his age.

Assuming you have read up on the legal aspects of interviewing, all interviews should be done in a three-step process.

Step one is an easy step and is simply a plus or minus on first impression and is a pre-screening for the next two steps. There is a sample hiring sheet at the end of this section that should be used during the first step, although as with any legal form, make sure it is legal to use in your state or where you live.

Normally, it's the manager or assistant manager who's in charge of the staffing and also the one who would do the initial screening. In the smaller clubs, meaning fewer than 600 members, the manager or owner might do the first interview, but even these gyms should have an assistant who has basic HR training who works with the staff—in addition to reporting to the manager.

The first impression is very important and is the key to the first step. If the person has grubby pants on, a hat on backward, huge snake tattoos on both arms, and hasn't shaved in several days, this is probably a person who won't fit your uniform code. Is it fair to judge a person on his first look? Is it fair for an owner to have to interview someone who doesn't even know how to apply for a job and who is not experienced enough or smart enough to shave and cover the tats at least during the interview process?

We're not talking ties and dress shoes as needed for the interview here. We're talking someone showing up for an interview with neat, clean clothes, a clean-shaven face, combed hair, and a limited number of pierced body parts that are exposed. You have a right to wear what you want and dress as you please. We as owners and operators have the right to not hire you to work in a million-dollar professional fitness organization if we think how you look will offend our clients and potential business.

For example, the first impression of your staff may be the deciding factor for a sale in the club. A potential member walks into several clubs in one day, looking for a place to work out. The gym with the staff that looks and acts professional and that can provide member service will most likely get that person as a member. Therefore, the staff needs to look and act professional and be able to communicate with a large number of people. It doesn't always come down to money for the client, as many inexperienced owners think. There are cheap clients looking only for the cheapest in the market, but there are so many more clients willing to pay more money to get away from those cheap low-end members in the other gyms and this group of people will base their decision on the perception of quality and service in the business they choose.

This is also a good time to discuss diversity. The best staffs are the ones that represent a wide range of cultures, colors, and looks and orientations. The worst staffs are usually the ones that all come out of the white bread mold of America. Many young owners tend to hire people who look just like themselves.

For example, a young single white male owner ends up hiring young single white guys to run the club. If there is a problem, the answer is always the one that a young single white male would come up with at the time. This type of owner isn't hiring to run a business. He is hiring to build a posse of drinking friends who all look, act, and talk just like he does. Diversity gives the club texture and feel and truly expands the member service and moneymaking potential of the business because a variety of unique people often combine to come up with a much wider range of solutions to the gym's problems than six identical clones could produce.

The same person who did the first interview (and the person who runs the department where the new hire will work) also performs the second step of the interview process.

Even in the smallest training gyms that have only six to seven employees, it's good to have a manager, a lead salesperson who handles the acquisition of leads, and an assessor, whose primary job is to work with every new or potential client and place that person where he belongs in the system. All these people should all receive the same type of management training because this way, you have back up if you lose the manager or if you're the manager/owner and eventually might even want to take a few days away from your business.

The second interview is more in depth and structured. Keep in mind that we're trying to hire people we can train to be productive and who can deliver outstanding member service. How this possible employee communicates in the second interview sets the tone for what he will do on the job. The second interview should also be based on a set series of questions that center on work history, personal interests, and customer service situations they have faced elsewhere.

Some sample second interview questions include:
- How old were you when you had your first job and what did you do?
- Describe the last time you received bad service as a customer. What would you have done differently if you had been the employee?
- What's your idea of a great personal workout?
- What do you like to do when you aren't working?
- Tell me how you delivered customer service at your last job.

There are many possibilities in an interview, but stay consistent and keep the questions limited. It's better to ask fewer questions and let the interviewee talk more about what he does and where he worked in the past.

The manager or the on-site owner who is acting as the manager always performs the third step in the interview process. This is the person ultimately responsible for the new hire and who should also have the final decision. The final step is more relaxed and is geared toward questions the potential hire may have about the company, the specific job, or the hiring process itself. If you're going to hire, always offer the job during the interview—unless you've lined up too many choices, which is unlikely if you've screened along the way.

We get into problems when we become desperate for help, so we hire the first warm body, put him at the front desk, and then suffer because we find out this new front counter person is shy and quiet and has never used a computer. Try to stay one entry-level person ahead at all times. It's worth the extra money to constantly stay slightly overstaffed and production doesn't stop if you lose someone suddenly, which is the way the business works.

Summary

Staffing will be the key issue in the coming years in the fitness industry. How you hire, train, motivate, and develop your employees will be what sets you apart from the competition and will ultimately become your competitive edge in the marketplace.

The old model of hiring and staffing doesn't work anymore in the fitness business. In the past, we've followed the fast-food model: Hire cheap, turn over often, and keep payroll and benefits costs at the lowest possible level. This doesn't work in a thriving economy. The good people in this category are already in the workforce, leaving pretty weak candidates for the money we are accustomed to offering in this industry.

To grow our businesses, we need to hire a higher caliber of worker—one we won't get unless we change our hiring and pay practices. The consumer expects a much higher level of member service for the money they pay and someone who can communicate and solve problems can deliver this level of service. This person is not the typical 19-year-old we traditionally place at the front desk that spends his time texting on his cell and staring at the clock, waiting to run madly for the door at the exact minute he is done with his shift.

The gyms are also switching to more multiple profit centers, such as putting an emphasis on training and recovery shake bars, and these also require a more sophisticated worker to make these businesses within a business more productive. The days are gone where someone merely stands behind the desk and checks people into the club. Today's worker needs to understand our product, be able to sell and promote profit centers, and be cross-trained to handle other jobs in the facility as the need demands. Member service means being able to provide service where and when the member wants it. That takes a more sophisticated team than we've hired in the past decades in the gym business.

One of the primary problems is the pay itself. Minimum pay gets minimum results and the people who work for the lowest pay need more training, more supervision, and a lot more skill development than the older and more experienced worker. Better pay attracts better, more qualified people who perform more efficiently earlier on in the job.

Another major issue is staff development. Most of our employees feel they are undertrained for the positions they hold. Training makes employees feel better about who they are, makes them perform better in their jobs, and makes them harder to steal from us in the long run. The prime trainer should be the manager, but you should also use a wide variety of outside educational sources each year to keep the staff fresh and growing.

A manager should devote about 50 percent of her time to staff training and driving production. If your manager spends most of his time on sales, then you don't really have a manager—you have a salesperson with a great title on his business card. Training makes the company more productive and this vital task should be delegated to someone as part of his job. How they train and the results they get should determine how that person is paid.

Hiring is getting tougher all the time. The traditional methods of ads in the paper don't bring in the qualified candidates they used to in the earlier days of the industry. The best people are probably already working somewhere else and these should be the ones we go after for our businesses. This is called stealing and it's perfectly legal and ethical in the business world.

When you hire, look for traits, which are the natural gifts someone brings to the table with them. An enthusiastic personality can't be taught. You either have it or you don't. Computer operation can be taught if the person has at least seen one or is interested in one. Hire for traits and then teach the person your business. The person will stay longer and be more productive in most cases.

A Few More Things to Think About When It Comes to Staffing Your Business

- *Hire the best people you can afford.* Research your market, determine what the local minimum wage is, and then go after people a level or two above that one.
- *Set up a recruitment system based on going after people who are already working.* Carry cards and actively go after people who impress you with their professional look, customer service, or just plain good attitude.
- *Set up a formal hiring system based on three interviews.* Learn the law and make sure your interviews are clean and legal. Involve other members of your team in the hiring process, but reserve the final decision for yourself or your manager.
- *Be creative in your hiring.* A housewife returning to the workforce would be a great lead counter person for 32 hours per week. A retiree might make a great club opener. What a concept! Why not hire a person who likes to get up at 4 a.m. instead of some young guy who usually gets in at 4 a.m. and then tries to make it to work.
- *It's almost impossible to overtrain someone.* Start training aggressively on the first day a new employee starts working and continue with a consistent and intense training program. Also, start the training at the bottom. Most clubs put their training into the higher-level employees, such as salespeople, and neglect the entry-level folks. Think of training as a pro football team would. Who would need the most intense work—a seasoned pro quarterback or the rookie just out of college? The old pro may need a few reminders or help with a specific problem, but the rookie needs the most help and not just with being a quarterback but how to adjust to the team's system. Your rookie employees are the same. They need job-specific training as well as cross-training in all areas of the club. They'll be better employees if they understand the entire system.
- *Set up a staff training schedule and make it mandatory for all full-time employees.* Staff development meetings should be set weekly (on the same day and at the same time) so employees can make this part of their regular schedule. Fridays at noon to 4 p.m. or the best hours to train staff in most gyms. Keep the meeting segments to an hour only and structure it on a positive note. Chewing butts every week wears out the staff and

decreases the team's moral. The following list is a sample of one-hour meetings focused on staff training:

✓ Answering the phone. This can be repeated every month for emphasis.

✓ Handling a complete phone inquiry

✓ Greeting members and providing member service at the front counter

✓ Efficient check-in procedures for the members and updating computer skills each month as needed

✓ Focusing on one profit center and how to promote it, such as talking about the benefits of your smoothies and how members can use them as recovery tools

✓ Working renewals in the club

✓ A 30-minute club walk-through (including a quick clean in the locker room, the cardio area, and the club's entryway)

✓ Education from a team leader, such as the nutrition tech, who educates the staff on a new product

✓ Greeting a potential member

✓ Developing a wait policy for potential or regular members who have to wait more than five minutes for a tour or appointment

✓ Using the trial membership cards as a focus tool for the staff

✓ Reviewing key procedures in the club, such as teaching everyone how to make a shake, handle a renewal, or do an information call

✓ Member service for the trial members

✓ How to handle member complaints and how to work the complaint card system

✓ How to sell special club events and programming

✓ Handling problem members

✓ Working with trial members as a team

These are just a few examples of one-hour training sessions. You should pay the staff to attend these meetings, even if they are not scheduled to be there at that time. Instead of their regular pay, give them training pay, which is usually minimum wage. All meeting times are posted 30 days in advance and are mandatory for full-time (over 32 hours per week) employees.

Figure 17-1 is a hiring sheet to be used for the first interview. It emphasizes the traits necessary to do the job and is designed for entry-level people in the company.

Be sure to look for a professional dress and attitude. We're not necessarily looking for a shirt and tie or dress, but neat, clean, and well groomed are important. If someone shows up for an interview in ragged clothes, he is going to bring that same attitude to work.

The person has or demonstrates the following traits:
- Enthusiastic and outgoing
- Makes eye contact often
- Has a fitness look, is interested in fitness, or is currently active in some type of program
- Has held some type of people job where customer service was part of his responsibility
- Has the trait of being a hard worker or self-starter
- Self-motivated (advanced in other jobs or took on more responsibility)
- Wide range of interests or accomplishments (Boy Scouts, active in church, and/or ski team or soccer team as a youth)
- Held previous jobs that would require being motivated or a self-starter (first job might have been as a paper delivery person at age nine)
- Has strong communication skills demonstrated by speech, language, and attitude
- Has the ability to relate to a large number of members and could provide member service in a patient and friendly manner

Sample interview questions:
- Tell me about the last time you worked with a large number of people supplying member service. What did and didn't you enjoy about the situation?
- How old were you when you had your first job?
- Describe the last time you received bad service as a customer. What would you have done differently if you had been the employee?
- What do you like to do when you don't work? What kind of workout or physical activity do you like to do on your off hours?

Figure 17-1. Hiring sheet

February 9, 2014
Seek quiet time.

Find at least an hour a week that is all about you. Walk in the woods, sit quietly and read, or just go to a coffee shop and read something that makes you smile but is meaningless. The intensity most of you live in your life will take its toll. You have to find time to recharge and heal, but most people who are trying to create lives that matter don't know when to back off for a few hours and let their minds and bodies recover from the stress and intensity. No gadgets and no contact—just you and a cup of tea and your thoughts for an hour a week. If you can, make it an hour a day every morning before the world finds you and proceeds to start your daily ass kicking. You spend your life taking care of others, but what are you doing this week to take care of yourself?

February 5, 2014
Discounting kills your true value

Discounting what you do for a living absolutely kills every shred of credibility you have worked for through the years. Once you establish a rate, stick to it no matter what. Do not discount if people try to prepay in any form. If your rate is $50 an hour, then charge $50 per hour and do not discount if someone prepays for 10 sessions with you. Your hourly rate is your credibility. If you discount to $40 (5 for $200 or 10 for $400), are you really a $50 per hour professional or a $40 per hour hack. Stop selling yourself short no matter what business you are in. All most of you have to sell is your time, and when you sell it, get what you're worth and avoid what a discounted cheaper rate reflects on you because someone flashed a credit card in front of your nose. Establish a rate and then establish one way to pay (such as "I am $50 per hour, but my services are sold at 5 for $250 to make it easier to pay"). Initial consultation should be for an hour and a half and that should be at a premium. In this example, you might charge $120 for the first hour. You have worked your entire career to master what you do. Don't discount your professionalism and hard work by selling yourself cheap when it most matters.

18

If Your Employees Were as Good as You Are, They Would Have Your Job

Many owners expect—and in fact demand—their employees to be as motivated and as skilled as they are at working in a fitness facility, but these same owners don't spend the effort to provide leadership and the training the employee needs to develop to his full potential.

Employees want to be led and will gravitate toward strong leadership. They want you to show them how to do the job. They want you to provide the training they need to be effective. And employees want the chance to fly and make mistakes on their own. They also want you to be there to guide and lead them, not just give them minimal training and then ignore them.

Employees want to be led by a person with vision and leadership skills, not beaten into submission with a 1950s militaristic style of leadership. Leadership styles have changed over the past 60 years in the fitness industry, but most owners haven't adapted to these changes. Today's owners think of themselves as entrepreneurs, which is a polite way of saying "Get out of my way—I'd rather do it myself" instead of learning to lead and develop others to do the job with them.

Most employees leave their jobs because the management failed them. There are always employees who we want to leave reflecting the concept that no matter what you do, you will still make hiring mistakes and need to correct that mistake as soon as you can, but there are many more employees who would have stayed and contributed to the business if only the owners and managers understood how to lead and guide their teams.

Expecting greatness and then becoming disappointed is humbling and depressing as an employee. I once worked for a person who I thought was truly inspirational—a man with whom I thought I'd like to spend a great many of my working years. Ten years after I started, I walked out of my office completely beaten down and carrying a small box full of junk from my desk. I started as someone who had confidence that I could learn and grow in that job, but I ended up a decade later as a person who had little faith in myself or in my ability to work in the real world.

This boss was raised in the old school style of management from the 1950s. People managed in that era by using fear and intimidation and by constantly making employees feel stupid. Years later, I realized that I'd let this happen and that buying into someone else's negativity was my responsibility, but as a young and impressionable employee, I didn't realize at the time what was happening and let myself slip further behind every year.

There are many valuable employees who want to be led—but not by people who manage out of their own insecurity and who work to keep the employees in their place by fear or by a constant barrage of beatdowns. Today's more sophisticated employees want to work for a person who can provide inspiration, motivation, and education and who can create a vision the team can follow through the fire pits of hell and back because the leader said "Go and do the job I trained you for over the years."

Bill Gates leads this way. Steve Jobs built a creative empire through micromanaging the details yet attracting and hiring the best employees in the industry. With his leadership skills and his vision and by inspiring an exciting company culture, Jobs created one of the most dynamic companies in recorded history.

Other great companies, such as Google™ in its early days or Nike®, are defined by their style of leadership and the company's vision. These companies aren't just good places to work. These are places where the employees belong to something big and important and management that can instill this belief in their employees is changing how things are done in the marketplace.

Fitness facilities could be the same way. These facilities are staffed with young gung-ho staffs that want to belong to something—to be part of an exciting business with direction. The driving force that makes this happen is the leadership style of the owner. The block wall that prevents this from happening in the gym is that most owners instinctively end up following the old, authoritarian approach to leadership and to their businesses.

A simple definition of the authoritarian style is that the boss makes all the decisions and manages the people in the organization through intimidation. There is no teambuilding. There is no discussion as to the way to do things. The manager makes the decision and the employee carries it out. The armed services are based on this system, with a very narrowly defined chain of command.

Being attracted to this style of management is one of the downsides of being an entrepreneur. You took the risk, you started your own business because you were probably tired of working for someone else—or thought you could do it better than someone else—and now that you're on your own, you're going to do it your way and you are going to make sure everyone who works for you is also going to do it your way.

The classic owner assumption under the authoritarian style is signified by how expendable the workers are. They don't make decisions and they don't have to think—they just do it the way you tell them and everything is fine. The trouble with this logic is that the employees of today are much more sophisticated, want to share in the decision-making process of the business, and seek more responsibility. In other words, good employees won't work under this type of leadership.

Old-Style Management Prevents Growth in Your Business

Signs that your facility may be suffering from authoritarian suppression are pretty easy to spot. For example, does the club have a high turnover of employees at the lower levels? Are the employees working for minimum wage? Does the gym offer benefits for full-time employees? Is the club understaffed during key hours, which leads to burnout for the employees you do have working? And are your producers working on commission only, high-pressure numbers, and unrealistic quotas?

These are all signs that the staff is working under adverse management conditions. If the club has no benefits, is understaffed, puts salespeople on a chase after unrealistic numbers, and has a high turnover at the front desk, then employees know they are expendable because everything in the gym's business system leads them to that truth.

People want to be led by inspiration, not by intimidation. In your business, maybe the followers aren't following because the leaders aren't leading. And the results you seek from your business may be elusive because the staff is not fully committed to your cause. Most importantly, many of today's employees want to participate in the business and do often have ideas to offer that can help a business prosper. These employees read about the tech companies and understand that other businesses allow their employees to learn, grow, and take part in what happens in that business and that their contributions often lead to better jobs and more money.

The Search for Good Faith Effort From Our Employees

When you impart an inspirational style of leadership, you get that extra effort from an employee that you can't force and you can't buy. This extra effort is called *good faith effort*. It means the employee has the faith and trust in you to give you what he would normally hold back in other jobs.

A weakness in most small businesses is employees who are not totally committed to what they are doing and who they are working for at the time. These are people who work for you, do their job, but never really give you their full potential. On this employee's best day with you, she might give you

80 percent of what she is capable of doing in her job, but she is not engaged and, therefore, will not give you that extra and perhaps most valuable effort.

For example, an employee at your front desk is on the clock and doing her job. A new member shows up at the front desk a little confused about her first visit to the club. The employee is courteous, tells the member where the locker room is, and tells the person that once she is dressed to come back to the front desk and she'll find her scheduled trainer waiting for her. Technically, the employee did the job we pay her for each week. She was friendly, helpful, and provided basic member service.

Our competitor's front desk team is faced with the same situation. Her employee walks the new member back to the locker room (of course there is always a backup to cover the desk while she is away), shows him how to find the right locker, and then finds the trainer and has her waiting for the new member when he comes out of the locker room. This club's staff gave better member service, made a new member happier, and opened the door wide for a member referral. Why? Because the staff gave more effort than was required—or good faith effort. You can't force it and you can't demand it, but it's what makes your business special and successful.

Many times, a fitness business will fail because the owners create an organization that undermines motivation and discourages good faith effort. These clubs fail because of burnout among the producers, mistrust, missed opportunities, and resistance to change. In other words, these organizations waste their most precious asset, which is the organization's human potential.

The Function of Leadership

It's easy to define the function of the leader. The leadership function is what the leader brings to the business that is beyond just keeping the business profitable and running, which represent tasks that are nothing more than part of the basic job description for any owner or manager. Many owners lose because they confuse management with leadership. The following are a few basic functions for a manager but not what it takes to define a leader:

- The management function includes building a proactive business plan based on projecting the business three years into the future.
- Develop a marketing plan that leads to the sale of new memberships.
- Create a training-centric business model that can generate revenue equal to or greater than the gym's monthly membership dues
- Develop a mature and motivated employee base through strong and inspirational leadership.
- Learn to satisfy members, which leads to repeat business in the form of renewals.
- Work toward long-term profits for the business.

The key to good leadership is to balance these points. If the owner doesn't balance and understand all six areas, then the business doesn't grow.

CHAPTER EIGHTEEN   *If Your Employees Were as Good as You Are, They Would Have Your Job*

Some examples of an unbalanced approach include the following:

- An owner who strongly believes in member service but who undertrains the staff and is never able to build a strong member service plan or have great member retention

- An owner who is too nice to the employees and makes everyone a friend, but then he doesn't have a strong business because there is no accountability from the employees. You often can't fire your new best friend.

- An owner who will do anything to get new sales and who then puts all the money into the sales and marketing effort but doesn't put any revenue into member service. This gym will sign up new people, but it won't keep any in the long run, putting even more stress on the sales effort.

Leadership Begins With the Core Attributes

Learning to be a good leader starts with understanding the basic attributes a leader might possess. These aren't all the attributes of good leadership, but these do represent the ones that affect how we do business in the fitness industry.

A leader should have deeply held values about other people.

There are basic core values a leader should have that help him rise above merely being a manager in his own business. Fairness, seeing a sense of worth in others, a belief in the equality of people, and a sense of right and wrong are all values necessary to lead a young staff into business battle. For example, would an owner who says he is fair and honest aggressively drop-close someone in a closed office with the purpose of pressuring a potential member to buy a membership today? Would a respected leader refuse to hire blacks or women in the gym? It's hard for a young staff to follow someone who says one thing and then does something totally different in the workplace. You are the person you are defined through your actions, not through your words.

A leader has respect for an employee's unique talents and quirkiness.

You come back from a trip and find one of your trainer/salespeople on the floor with a group of six women. You ask the manager what's going on and she tells you that this group of potential members is participating in a group tour and workout led by the trainer. Your policy is that every potential member must start one-on-one training with a salesperson so the gym can have the highest potential for getting that new sale. Out of the six women in the group, only two are actually members and they are the ones who referred the others. The trainer/salesperson finishes the group, signs up two more new members, and makes appointments for the other two to come back and work out again. Would you respect the employees' unique solutions or would you be upset and bring up the policy? Old school management would chastise this employee for breaking the rules, and in many chain clubs, he would most likely be fired. In new generation management, you have to ask yourself several questions: Did he take initiative? Did he do the right thing for the gym by organizing this group around the two members and their referrals? Was he successful at his

389

attempt? Did you as the owner learn something new by watching an employee take the lead? The trainer broke a rule, which probably needed to be broken, took some initiative, and ended up getting the job done, which would get him fired in most gyms.

A leader has respect for a person's contribution on his behalf.

Your front counter person calls off on short notice. Your other evening employees have a busy night with member visits, but they still manage to get four sales and they also do a respectable job in the multiple profit centers. You come in late in the evening and the first thing you see is how dirty the club is. Without knowing the situation, you immediately start chewing butt because the locker room is dirty, weights and dumbbells need to be put away, and the counter area is trashed. In this example, the owner showed poor leadership by not finding out the entire story and, most importantly, not respecting the job the remaining employees performed that night on his behalf. Bad managers shoot first and aim later, meaning they react without asking about the current situation. Good leaders step back, take a breath, assess the situation, and then deal with their current reality.

A leader has to be skilled at creating an environment that brings out excellence, accepts risk taking, supports creativity, and accepts mistakes from those who really are trying to do a good job.

Your young manager, who has been with you for several years and who does a good job, takes over the printing for your ad campaign. This is the first time she has handled the entire project by herself with the printer. She orders 25,000 pieces at a cost of $1,500.

She made one small mistake though. When she and the printer proofed the piece, they overlooked the fact that the gym's phone number wasn't on it. The manager signs off on the piece and you have 25,000 cards with no phone number. Do you now do all future projects yourself? Do you yell and scream and try to blame the printer? Or do you calmly find a solution, such as getting stickers printed and attached to each piece, and write it off as an experience for the manager that probably won't be repeated? Good leaders have to accept mistakes as part of the learning process. Mistakes that occur once are learning opportunities. The same mistake that occurs several times is a leadership and training opportunity, which forces you to assess the "how" and the "why" your team can repeat a mistake more than once. You will find that sometimes it is your choice of staff and perhaps you have someone in a job he simply can't do well. You will also find as an effective leader that the system itself is often flawed and needs to be fixed and that repeated mistakes, such as an outdated membership collection company that constantly makes billing mistakes for your members (who now blame your manager), is the real problem.

A leader has to be patient.

It took you many years to learn what you know about the business. Can you really pass this information along in just a few weeks of training? For example, you've been in the business for eight years, running the club yourself. You hire your first manager and set about teaching her the basics. Even if you taught her full time for two months, she is still about eight years short of having your experience and knowledge. There is no substitute for eight years of experience but eight years of experience.

Even with a dedicated, intensive training course during her first three months on the job, she still wouldn't have the most vital skill a manager needs, which is the experience from practicing and learning on the job from the decisions she makes. Until you make the big decisions, you don't really ever learn how to lead and manage. Being patient until a person has acquired some of this hands-on experience is very trying for an owner but important while learning to be a leader.

A leader must have integrity.

Let's say you hire an old sales dog with big-chain, high-pressure experience as your sales manager. As the owner, you have established a policy that the club and the sales team have to get a consistent membership fee, meaning no deals for anyone. However, the new guy will do anything to get a sale.

For example, he gives two women who come in together a two-for-one membership fee. The next guy in pays no membership fee in exchange for signing up today. The third guy in the gym today is unsuspecting and inexperienced in the business world and actually pays a full membership fee because he just wanted to join because his friend is already a member. This salesperson isn't following the club's rules, but he is selling a lot of memberships, so you hate to say anything. What has the rest of the sales staff learned about you, your leadership style, and your integrity? How do you now enforce other policies in the gym with the rest of the staff? Leaders always have to do the right thing—at least according to your own core values. If your policy is no deals and every new member pays the same rate, then you have to stick with this rule. If your policy is to get what you can, then that decision also reflects your core values. Your staff members always catch the disconnect, meaning they will immediately notice the difference between what you say you believe and how you act in your life and business.

A leader must have trust.

You hire a manager to start taking some responsibility in the club. After about six months of training, you feel somewhat comfortable with the person's progress, so you decide to take a short vacation. While you're away, you call twice a day to see how things are going. What concept did you teach the new manager? Is there trust in the relationship? Will the manager live up to the trust you have shown her, which is none, by not managing and waiting for you to make all her decisions?

Leadership goes beyond just getting the staff to do what you want. Good leadership inspires a staff to go beyond the base expectations you have set for each one of them. It inspires your team members to be a part of something special you create, and most importantly, good leadership allows you to reach levels of success very few people ever achieve in this industry.

On the other hand, the lack of leadership affects your business way beyond the performance of your staff. Every aspect of leadership—no matter how small—affects your future as a business, as part of the community, and as a moneymaking vehicle to enhance your life. Your staff and the members in your gym know who you are by how you lead and how you treat all of them. Weak leadership, questionable ethics, and owners who take everything they can without regard to the staff or members are rewarded for that work by the loss of all of them over time. Strong leadership can last for years, but bad leadership always results in a business that ultimately fails.

People like to be led, as was said earlier, but they like to be led by inspiration and not intimidation. If your staff is not giving you what you want, it's because you either made the wrong choice when hiring those people in the first place or it's because you haven't yet learned leadership skills.

Leadership can be learned. You don't have to be a born leader. The skills of effective leadership are there to learn in a thousand books and blogs, but it does take time and experience to learn these principles and make them yours through daily application. And it also takes extreme patience too. You should also keep in mind that leadership makes a statement as to the kind of person you are in the eyes of those you are trying to lead. What you are and what you believe in directly affect the type of leadership you will give.

The Common Leadership Failures and Mistakes

Mistake #1: Failure to improve yourself personally

Almost all business owners get to a point where they think they know everything there is to know about their chosen business. When the owner reaches this point, which is usually about three to five years into the experience chain, the business becomes stale due to a lack of new ideas and stimulation and it starts to decline. When you are not growing and developing personally, you run the risk that those around you might be moving forward and leaving you behind. It's hard to be a leader when you're more concerned about defending what you know than questioning what you don't know. To avoid this happening in your business, try to keep the following growth points in mind:

- *Be open to change:* We are in the business of change. Trends in equipment force change. The sophistication of the members forces change. The central body of knowledge in the industry expands and forces change. Business methods change over the years to reflect the current level of owners in the field, the changing nature of competition, and the evolution of fitness itself. Everything changes except the old entrenched gym operators who refuse to admit that what worked last year may not work this year. Good leaders seek change. Bad leaders ask "Has anyone else done this and been successful because I don't really want to go first?" Leadership is just that: leading by going first. You can be the 10 percent of the owners who are proactive and seek change and who are the ones that drive change in their market or you can be the other 90 percent who wait until they are forced to change in reaction to their competitors, their declining revenues, the loss of members, or even as something as simple as an aggressive ad campaign by a club down the street that forces you to advertise for the first time this year. You don't lead from the back. You lead from the front—and great leadership is proactive and drives the market where your business exists.

- *Don't avoid the numbers side of the business:* Businesspeople run fitness facilities better today than the old sales-driven owners from past decades. These new owners thrive on numbers and information. Many of the staff we hire today do a much better job when they understand what really happens in the business. The problem is that many of the old style of owners only know the sales side of the industry and don't learn the backside of the shop. Better leaders lead better when the troops have the right information. There are always key indicators in every business. In the fitness world, you need to master numbers, such as average payment per sale, closing rates for the sales team, conversion rates to training memberships, growth of the membership and training receivables bases, and average return per member. Numbers drive the business, and if you don't lead by mastering and reacting to your numbers, then you are leading by emotion, which is at best inconsistent and situational.

- *Seek out advanced training and education for yourself and your team:* The best businesspeople in the world don't know everything. However, they do ask the best questions. There is always education available—inside and outside the fitness industry—that can take you to the next level. If you want to be effective in the fitness business over time, you need to continually add to your business skills, along with mastery of what it takes to train today's clients. No one should own any type of fitness business who isn't a certified personal trainer and who doesn't understand how to train clients based on what we know today, not what we thought we knew about training in the 1980s. You have to be good at business, but if you want to compete successfully in the fitness business, you have to be even better at understanding current training philosophy and how it has to be applied in your business.

- *Cut down on time-wasters in the business:* Many owners waste their days by doing work that could be farmed out to lower-level employees. This busy work prevents them from working on their businesses. In other words, eliminate the unnecessary and learn to work on your business, not always just in it. The rule is this: 95 percent of what we do each day is create fresh revenue and the rest is management. Farm out anything that gets in the way of production. When you're in your gym, you only have one purpose: What can I do today to generate new revenue for this business? There is a difference between being busy and truly being effective in business. Busy is busy, but it is seldom being effective.

- *Learn and practice time management:* Simple time-management techniques, such as learning to make a work list and set priorities, could greatly improve an owner's or a manager's production during the day. More efficient use of time means more time for training and staff development. Never start a day without a plan to make money that day. Stop returning phone calls randomly. Set a time each day for an hour or two and return all your calls at once. Turn off your devices and actually get some work done. Unless you are expecting a vital call that is life changing or unless you are in the middle of a construction project, turn off your phone and go to work. The member in front of you is far more important than the voice on the other end of that call.

- *Set personal goals:* The perfect goal for most owners would be to write a 12-month self-improvement plan. For example, what five things could you learn in a short period of time that would improve your business? Once you achieve your basic goals, create a new list and move forward again. Keep yourself and your business constantly projected into the future.

Mistake #2: Limiting yourself to only one part—or a very narrow part—of the business

By limiting yourself to just the specific parts of the business where you are comfortable, you're setting yourself up for several costly mistakes. First of all, you make yourself vulnerable inside your business by letting someone else gain knowledge about your business you don't have, such as an owner who has a nutrition program but hasn't attended the school and doesn't really know how it works. If you create a new program, you and the entire management team should have a working understanding of the program and be able to maintain it at least at the minimum level.

It has also been stated a number of times in this book that we are in the business of fitness and of getting results for each and every client. You must get current and stay current in what is happening in the training world and not limit yourself to just selling memberships or pretend you are hiding on the business side. If you own a restaurant, you need to know how to cook or you will be held hostage forever by someone else in your business who has a skill set you don't and who could walk out at any time, leaving you unable to at least get through the day. It is the same in the fitness industry. You can't own any type of fitness business unless you are a certified trainer who stays current in theory each year. You don't have to train anyone. You just have to understand what we do for a living in this business.

Another example is if you start a new nutrition program, you should go through all the basic training for that new part of your business, as should your manager, assistant manager, and the person who will actually run the program on a daily basis. You can't lead if you don't understand what you own. Group exercise/aerobics is a good example of a program that faded rapidly in the early 1990s once the owners stopped taking classes and stopped supporting the education function connected to staying current in the field.

Secondly, by limiting yourself to just one part of the business, you are also setting yourself up for burnout. Doing the same thing year after year will lead to a decline in your performance, and eventually, you will be forced to start stepping away from the business more often, which will lead to even a further loss of control. The typical scenario in our industry is an owner who becomes burned out, owns a flat and unexciting business that is slowly declining, and then steps away to try to start another business. He hires a manager and then just leaves that person on her own so he can concentrate on the new project. For a while, that project is fun and exciting, but eventually, burnout sneaks in there too. To stay fresh, stay current in all aspects of the business and keep learning.

Mistake #3: Failure to accept responsibility for your own business

If your business is not as successful as you wish it would be, it's your fault and your responsibility. Leadership starts with accepting responsibility for your business, your staff, and the decisions you make. That old saying "What you are today is the result of all the decisions you made yesterday" is true. Some of the best excuses ever invented in the fitness business come from owners who refuse to start with themselves as the problem. For example:

- The gym could make more money if we could find good employees. This means you don't know how to hire, lead, or motivate employees. If they are truly rotten employees or, worse yet, truly rotten relative employees, who did the hiring and who is training these people—if they are being trained at all? If you can't find good help, who set the pay scale and did the looking? If there aren't any good people in your town, who chose to open there in the first place? Somewhere and at some time, it all comes down to you and the decisions you made—or didn't make—in the business.

- No one came in today because the weather was rotten. No one came into the gym yesterday because the weather was too good. You can't have it both ways. Maybe it's your marketing. Maybe it's the fact that the new training gym down the street is killing you because you are still in the membership at any price business.

- My competition is underpricing me out of business. Who set the focus and niche for your business? Who didn't establish more value in his product? Who hired lousy staff that brings you down to the competition's level? Who had six months notice that the low-priced guys were coming to down but who refused to acknowledge that fact and just waited to see if the business would really be affected.

- No one is in my group exercise classes and I hate child care people. Who has failed to change his business to meet the changing demands of the consumer? Who made the decision to run programs that are outdated in your business? Who is losing money every month in his business but refuses to deal with the issue? A good exercise for this area is to list the five most glaring weaknesses in your business and who is responsible for these areas. Then, list what needs to be done to improve these weaknesses and in what time frame. Even the simple step of writing down the problems and accepting responsibility for them helps you move to the next level.

Mistake #4: Letting yourself become too successful and thinking it will last forever

Some owners actually become too successful. They hit a long streak of endlessly successful business and then come to believe this success will last forever. This "once successful, always successful" thinking hurts their businesses because they become too slow to react when adverse conditions in the market and business negatively affect the strength they have come to rely on over the years. In many ways, it's harder to lead a staff in times of success than it is when the gym is in its lean and hungry years. The expenses slowly creep up, money is wasted, and the staff and owner forget what it took to achieve that success in the first place.

When you lead from a position of success, you need to establish working goals for the business that keep the team moving forward. Protecting a profit margin is not a workable business plan. If you're not growing your business, then it is already in a state of decay—the rot just hasn't caught up with you yet. There is only one speed in small business and that is full forward, and if there isn't growth, then there is death. Simply put: Grow or die in small business.

When you seek growth, start with the desired profit margin for the business. How much is enough and when will it be there? If you are already at the desired profit level, list five ways you can grow the business during one-year, three-year, and five-year periods. List five things you can do to protect the margin while you're growing the business to the next level. Always remember the difference between growing the business and merely sitting in a defensive position and trying to protect what everyone else wants to take away from you.

It is also important to learn that what drives revenues in your business will change from year to year. Tanning was big decades ago and now it is gone. Traditional aerobics were huge in the 1980s and drove memberships in every club in the country, but it also eventually failed. Training was a secondary income for years, but now it is the single most important revenue source in the industry, with the potential to rise way above membership income. Just because it worked in the past does not mean it will work in the future.

Mistake #5: Failure to make timely decisions

Fitness owners are notorious for putting off important decisions. They call all their friends in the business, see if anyone else is facing the same problem in his gym and what he is going to do about it, attend a seminar and look for solutions, call a consultant or two, and then this owner eventually just doesn't do anything and hopes the issue will go away on its own.

Most major decisions should actually be made months before the owners get around to making them. For example, you are standing at the front desk and you get complaints about the gym being short on cardio equipment. These comments are important because they are coming from a few of the regulars, and then on top of those comments, an employee notices a few aggravated members bitching about the gym to each other and you finally start looking into the problem.

A few weeks after that, you admit there is a problem. This leads to a few weeks of research and negotiations that end up with an order that now takes four weeks to arrive. Instead of anticipating the shortage by watching the influx of new members, the time of year, or the increased renewal rate in the gym, the owner waits until someone actually complains before doing anything. By then, it's too late. You've lost members, you've lost your credibility, and you are now vulnerable to any competitor that opens with enough new and shiny cardio toys. The theme in this chapter is to be proactive, not reactive, and part of being a strong leadership is anticipating an ass-kicking before the guy shows up with the bat. It is too late to take martial arts lessons after you were beaten up in the bar and it is too late to make decisions once your business has already suffered.

Mistake #6: Losing touch with the business

A common disease in the fitness business is the "I finally made it" malady that affects so many owners of all walks of life. Once they start making a little money, the disease hits hard. Most stop working and just start dropping by for a few hours a day. They walk in, pick up all the cash, shake a few hands, and then they are off for the golf course. In their mind, they have paid their dues and they are ready to take it easy. In reality, this is when the club needs the most leadership, not the least. The business will start a slow decline once the owners lose the day-to-day touch to stay profitable.

The problem with getting out of touch with the business is that you're out of the leadership loop. Guiding your staff and making the hard growth decisions are hard enough anyway and can worsen if you're not there enough to watch the details.

For example, one of the first things to go in the club is its atmosphere. If you were there, you'd quickly pick up that the music is on the wrong channel for that time of day, no one cleaned around the cardio area last night, and the shades in the front windows are still down long after the sun left. Leadership is often compared to feeling the pulse of the business. It takes time and a practiced eye to stay on top of a constantly changing business.

Mistake #7: Failure to control expenses

One definition of profits is wasted expenses we are able to cut from the business each month. Because of their experience growing up in sales-driven clubs, most owners only have a sales solution to the problems of the club. The only question they ask is: How can I generate more income through more sales volume?

Providing leadership in your business means growing your revenues but also watching and controlling the wasted expenses in the business. You grow through the sales effort and the multiple profit centers and you also grow by watching the expenses and keeping them in line.

Leading a staff requires the ability to do both. Just working on sales is a self-defeating business plan that eventually leads to a sales-driven environment short on member service and member retention.

Mistake #8: Failure to make sure any job assigned to any employee is understood, supervised, and completed

The problem with being a leader for most people is that they don't have the patience to turn around and tell the people who are following them where they are going and what their role is going to be.

People will do their best work for you when they know what their jobs are and when they know exactly how you want them to do that specific task. We often assume an employee has the same skills, cultural background, and work experience we've had in our lives. When we tell a staff person to do something, we assume that person is operating with the same basic wiring we have. They don't and often what we assume to be intuitive action for us is often the hidden "I have no idea what in the hell that man is talking about" response from the staff person standing there shaking his head up and down like he really understands.

The key to leadership is realizing that the people who work for you learn and gather information in different ways. Some do best when you show them what to do and they learn by watching. Some learn by having you explain in detail what you want them to accomplish. And some function best by doing the task while you watch and correct.

Failure to understand these different learning styles is a failure in leadership because the employee will have a difficult time accomplishing what you want done because he doesn't understand what you expect. Another way to state this is that you conveyed your wishes to get something done but the person didn't get the message—or in other words, he was open to reception but the information didn't connect with his style of processing.

For example, a person might learn primarily by reading and secondarily by doing and then having someone correct his efforts as he makes the attempt. If you are this person and your employee learns by watching and doing, he is already off to a bad start in dealing with you and your management style. You want a specific task accomplished, you put out a memo, and you expect the work to get done. The employee reads the memo and has no real idea how to complete the task. His heart is willing, but he simply doesn't learn how to do things the way you do.

Let's say you're trying to get the staff to start cleaning under the treadmills once a week and checking if the belts are loose. You spell out all the directions clearly in the email or memo you leave at the front desk. The staff person who learns by seeing the task demonstrated will have a hard time understanding the email or memo and will also have a difficult time successfully completing the task unless he first has someone take him through it once so he can watch. He then has to try it on his own with someone watching. Learning can only be accomplished in the mode one works best with in his own head.

This is a simplistic explanation of learning styles, but it does illustrate how a leader could fail because he simply doesn't understand that the followers don't understand what he wants done and are failing not because they don't care and don't want to do the work but because they simply don't understand what you want.

Unclear instructions, indecisiveness on your part, vagueness, and only partial information are often to blame for an employee's lack of performance and his failure to get the job done. It's up to you as an owner or manager to clearly tell your people what you expect and in a way that makes sense to them so they understand what you're trying to accomplish.

Because you may never really understand how an employee internally processes information, try to cover all the learning styles each time you teach the crew something new. An easy way to make sure they are getting what you're saying is to use a notebook system.

Each employee should have a notebook given to him when he starts work. The notebook is kept at the gym, except when he is traveling to special educational events. Every time you teach the employee something new, he is expected to write out the procedures in his notebook. You explain the new task, the staff person tries it once in front of you for correction, and then he writes down the process in his notebook to make sure he has it.

You're covering all three parts of the learning process by doing it this way and now you have something in writing that you can refer back to when you check later for understanding.

Checking for understanding simply means: Does the employee understand and is she able to do the task? If not, check back to her notebook and start again by telling, showing, and having her correct her notes. This system also allows the staff that has been with you for a while to start passing on information to more inexperienced staff members because now they have documented how things work and what you expect from each typically assigned task in the gym.

For example, let's say you're trying to teach the employee to fill out a membership agreement for a new member. She brings her notebook to the training session and you start by verbally explaining how to fill out a contract. You then have her fill out a sample on her own, with you looking over her shoulder and giving pointers. Finally, you have her write down the procedures in her notebook and staple the sample to her page.

When she is on her own, she has something to refer back to if she is having trouble. If she still has difficulty, verbally review her mistakes, have her fill out a new sample—concentrating on the parts she is having problems with—and have her update the notebook. This passes the burden of ownership of the material to her because she is responsible for adding it to her book.

Leadership of a young staff is not an easy task. Make sure you can communicate your needs before you expect your desired results.

Mistake #9: Wasting time doing work that should be delegated

First, master the task ad then delegate it. It's a simple premise of leadership. Much of the work that consumes a typical owner's day is work that does not grow the business. Collecting your own membership agreements, handwriting checks, paying bills every day instead of twice a month, personally giving workouts to your favorite members, and taking a desk shift to save a few dollars are all examples of working in the business, not on the business.

To be an effective leader, you need to know when to work and when to let others do the work for you. We often confuse being busy with doing the important work of growing the business. You work all day, come home exhausted at night, put your feet up on the couch, and wonder what in the hell you really got done that day that made a difference in your business. Part of leadership is learning to delegate and to do this you must learn to simplify most routine tasks in the gym.

The rule of thumb is to create a powerful image in your head as to what your time is really worth and where you should be spending the bulk of your day. Try this by imagining that you or your manager's time is worth $500 an hour. Keeping a number like this in your head forces you to ask yourself this question: What is the best use of your time at any one period in the day? Are you doing $500-an-hour work growing the business, which means working on the marketing, training staff, selling a membership, or working the profit centers? Or are you standing at the front counter filling a regular shift on the schedule that's worth $8 per hour? Before you do anything, always start with the concept of what the best use of your time is at this moment and whether that task is worth $8 an hour or $500 an hour?

Mistake #10: Failure to rethink your business

You've had trouble with employees for years. The ones you attract are always too young and they don't stay with your business after you invest time training them. Maybe it's not them. Maybe it's you. Are you still offering almost the same hourly wage you did several years ago? Maybe the wage is wrong for today's market in your area? Maybe your area has changed? Maybe you need to rethink your hiring and compensation methods to attract and keep good people?

This is like trying to fix your bicycle with the same broken wrench. You try and try and you just can't get that tire off the bike. You need to sit down and think about replacing that broken wrench with one that works.

In business, it's often the same in that we try to fix our problems with the same broken solutions we've used for years. We tell ourselves: "It can't be anything I am doing because what I am doing worked so well for so many years that it has to be the people who come in for a job."

Good leadership means supplying the team with the best solutions or tools for the job you expect. This means you have to sit down on a regular basis and analyze the tools you are using to accomplish the job at hand, which is to build a financially successful business. Pay is the perfect example of something that becomes routine for owners who have been in business for a number of years. Mentally, it's hard to realize that it takes $10 per hour now to hire for the same position you paid just $6 not too many years ago. Markets change, competition gets tougher, and wages rise, but many owners get stuck in the past and just can't make that next-level adjustment it takes to stay current.

Make every tool in your business system a suspect. Many of the things we do in this business are simply habits copied from other owners who stole that idea from someone else 20 or 30 years ago. Why do you charge the way you do and why do you still use the same pricing system you did 10 years ago? Why do you offer a set number of guided workouts for new members when common sense tells you only two or three workouts are not enough? Why do you pay, hire, and train the way you do when you still don't get the results you want in your business? If your business is stuck in a deep rut, maybe the reason is that 15 years ago, you became frozen in time and haven't learned a new thing or made a significant change since then.

Mistake #11: Failure to keep your word

This business problem is probably better known as trying to be liked instead of working toward being respected. When you try too hard to be liked by your staff and members, you'll tell the person in front of you whatever he wants to hear so he'll ultimately be pleased with you. Telling people what they want to hear is always easier than telling that person the truth, which may not make him happy at the time, although you do avoid any type of confrontation

Are you the type of person who does what you say you will do or are you the type of person who has a lot of excuses for not doing what you promised? Broken promises, such as "I'll drop the check in the mail today" and then you send it two days later or "I'll call you on Monday at 10 a.m." and then you get busy and call on Tuesday, really make people question your integrity and leadership ability.

Staff promises that are given as encouragement but have no real substance can destroy a developing staff person. "You're doing a great job managing this club. I'm going to open a second club for you to manage and give you some ownership as part of your incentive package. I should be able to get that done in the spring."

This promise may have been made with some sincere belief that it's going to happen. The owner may be thinking that this is a possibility in the future. But in the manager's mind, it's a promise. When you break this promise, even though there was no intent to do wrong, you are a leader who is no longer dependable or trustworthy.

People don't care why you didn't do what you said you were going to do. They only care that you didn't do what you promised. Once you break the faith with your staff (who follow your vision of what the business is going to be in the future on blind trust), it's almost impossible to get it back. They trusted you as a leader and you failed.

Again, the promises don't have to be big ones. In fact, it's often the little ones that do the most damage. "Good job. Let's talk about a raise at the end of the month" or "You're doing a good job as a trainer. If Bill ever leaves, it's your job if you keep working the way you are" are innocent comments meant to motivate, but in the staff member's head, these are things his leader promised would happen. If these promises don't happen, you've completely demotivated what might otherwise have been a good employee.

The development thought is to review your personal style. Do you promise everyone everything and are you trying to be liked or do you only promise what you can really deliver and then work to gain a person's respect instead? Also, reflect back on a typical workweek. Did you deliver on what you promised or did you have excuses for why all those simple and quick comments weren't fulfilled?

Mistake #12: Failure to set a personal example

As a leader, you want the young employees to look up to you and respect you, but you date the members (or, worse, your staff) and are a legendary all-night party person. You want everyone in the community to support your business, but you haven't given a dime's worth of time or money back to the community since you opened your gym 10 years ago. You give a sales tour to a potential member about the benefits of working out, but you're 15 pounds overweight. You want your employees to work hard for you, but they are undertrained, yelled at in public, given wages lower than you could hire trained monkeys for, and their boss (you) is a moody SOB with irregular work hours, a bad attitude, and no life outside the gym.

It seems we may have a leadership problem here. Leadership starts with the example you set for the staff. The old "Do what I say—don't do what I do" theory is not a form of leadership in a small business. If you can't live it yourself, it's hard to expect the staff to meet the standard. How you look, how you live, and how you treat the staff are the pillars of leadership in a fitness business. Make sure your personal example is at a level that can stand scrutiny before you attempt to lead.

Mistake #13: Failure to ask employees for their solutions and insights for club problems

Gym owners are generally entrepreneurial by nature, meaning they want everything done their way—whether they know anything about the situation or not. The problem is that most fitness businesses are too complicated for a single person to control and understand every single component every single day.

Your employees, meaning the ones who actually do the work each day, often see creative solutions for the problems you face during the normal course of business. But as entrepreneurs, we always have to look good, so we try to come up with all the solutions ourselves instead of including the people who probably understand the problem better than we do into the creative problem solving.

Employees like to be challenged in their jobs and to feel part of the decision-making process in the business. Everyone likes to believe he has good suggestions that could help solve a problem. Part of leadership is knowing when to let go of the need to feed your own ego and get your team involved in the business. The following are four steps to keeping employees challenged and involved in the creative problem-solving process:

- *Let the staff participate in some form of management:* Show your team how the numbers work, let them help decide on uniforms and profit center items, and let them have some level of responsibility in their jobs. In other words, let them be in charge of something even if it's small.

- *Let your team help make the rules concerning their work and how they do it:* You don't have to turn over your business or lose complete control, but staff members should participate in some of the rules that concern them in their jobs. For example, what happens if someone on the team comes in late? They are usually harder on themselves than you would be in an employee manual.

- *Let them take part in the decision-making process:* The gym needs new treadmills and your ready to consider other brands than the ones you now have. Let the staff try a few other models, let them work with the equipment reps, and let them have a vote in the final decision if possible.

- *Keep all your key players informed about the details of the business:* Employees work better when they know what's going on in the business. They also like to feel like insiders. Sharing information keeps them in the loop and keeps them more involved in the outcome of your business.

Here's an example that illustrates getting the team involved in a small but important way. The club's drink sales are flat. You've tried every idea you could come up with to sell more drinks, but nothing has worked. The problem is that the process usually stops there. You've tried everything you know, so there must not be any known solution to the problem.

Why not run a contest to see which employee can come up with the most innovative gimmick to sell drinks that month? The employee whose idea sells the most gets a $50 bonus or something he wants, such as new shoes, as a reward. The key to leadership in this example is that the owner sought and obtained involvement from the staff. Most owners complain that staffers just don't care about their businesses. Telling them to get involved doesn't work. Asking them to get involved by seeking their help immediately solves the problem.

Mistake #14: Making decisions for your employees instead of having set procedures or guidelines

Every time you make an arbitrary decision concerning a business situation in the gym, you have taught your employees to be ineffective. You must have systems that guide your employees to make their own decisions. Guidelines and procedures in the form of a procedure manual must be in place. These guidelines are where the employees look for guidance instead of coming to you or the manager for decisions concerning a situation that you handle differently each time depending on who's in front of you. Handling the same problem a different way every time is called *situational management* and this style of management is probably the least effective way there is in small business to train key staff.

For example, the policy in your manual states very clearly that any member who is 30 days past expiration must renew at the current rates and fees. An old member is standing at the counter trying to get back into the club. You walk by, greet the member, and then tell the staff person that she was a great member and let her in at her old rate and no additional membership fee.

What does that employee do the next time he is faced with a similar situation? Does the employee give a deal and break the policy because he saw you do it or does he follow the policy because he doesn't know if the former member standing in front of him was a "good" member or a not-so-good member?

What will probably really happen in this situation is that the employee just comes to you to make the decision for him because you just make things up as you go along anyway. By making the decision for the employee, you've taught him not to make any decisions for himself. When you ask yourself "Can't anyone make any decisions around here except for me?" the answer is "No, they can't" because you taught them not to decide anything important or even minor without you.

If an employee comes to you with a problem, learn to say "What is the procedure on that?" or "What have I taught you previously about handling that type of problem?" Don't say "Do it this way," which means "Don't worry about ever making a decision on your own. That's why I'm here—so I can teach you to bring everything to me and so I'll never get anything done except handling routine, mundane questions all day that should be covered by my staff."

Mistake #15: Failure to develop a second-in-command

You're hurt in a car accident and you're going to be out of the gym for six weeks. Who is trained to run the business when you're not there every day? One-man shows are a sign of poor leadership. If the gym would suffer in its day-to-day business because you're not there for only a day or two, then you have signs of an immature leader who thinks giving up power and information undermines his leadership position.

If you've put off finding a second-in-command for years, maybe it's because when it comes down to it, you won't give up the real power and authority to get the job done. Some people like having people come to them for every decision, but great businesses aren't built that way. You might be willing to give up the small, petty things you hate to do in the job, but you cling to the important things that would allow someone to run the show when you're not there.

Good employees will follow a strong leader—one who can make work seem important, fun, and exciting all at the same time. Leadership can be learned and can be sifted down to a few key points:

- *Leaders must have vision and the ability to set goals.* Leaders must see the whole picture. If leaders have unclear goals and incomplete vision of what is going to come to pass and no plans in place, how can you lead if you don't know where you are going?

- *Leaders must be trustworthy.* Are you a trustworthy person? Is your word good? Do you deliver what you promise? Do you work to earn the respect of your employees or do you try too hard to be liked?
- *Leaders inspire participation.* Poor leaders can get people to work for a short period of time through intimidation. Good leaders can get people to rise beyond their basic job. That is where employee satisfaction begins and profits grow.
- *Good leaders practice diversity.* Good leaders are diverse in their personal interests, are well rounded in life, and have an outside life beyond their businesses. Poor leaders are narrow in scope and usually hire other people who are usually mirror images of their selves. Practice diversity in your own life and in your hiring of the people who work for you. Think rainbow and hire a wide cast of characters of all shapes, colors, and orientations, and while you are in a completely crazy mood, actually read something every week that has nothing to do with what you do for a living.
- *Leaders are big-picture people.* Good leaders spend a great deal of time working on their businesses, not in them. Good leaders expect their people to have creative solutions and support that creativity even if it isn't right all the time.
- *Leaders are high-integrity people.* Good ethics is good business. Promise less and deliver on every promise you ever make.
- *Leaders making learning a lifetime passion.* When you think you know it all is when you really don't know anything anymore. The business changes, the consumer changes, and times change—and so should you.
- *Good leaders have a sense of community.* We support the community and then the community supports us. You want, you want, you want from everyone in your market, but what have you given back to anyone in your community since you opened your business?

The following are a few things you can do to help yourself master this material:

- *Start with you.* Are you the leader you should be? Write out your five strongest gifts as a leader and your five biggest weaknesses you need to work on in the next six months.
- *Review your systems.* Are your employee systems, such as pay, hours, and incentives, relics from some age-old club or are they vital and current? Can an employee grow and thrive in the environment you've created in the business?
- *Review your hiring systems.* If you're not attracting the type of people you need to grow your business, this is the place to start. Remember that most owners that have been in business any length of time almost always refuse to pay enough to attract higher-level employees. The market they work in changed, but they simply didn't.
- *Review your training strategy.* Most owners don't understand the learning process. Institute the notebook system and slow down. Make sure your people truly understand their tasks and what you expect from them on a daily basis. Most employees like to do a good job—if they know what a good job is.
- *Assess your leadership ability.* Leadership can be learned. Write out all the things that you need to change before you can become the leader you want to be. Also, write down the top 10 leadership mistakes you have made with your staff in the past and how you should have handled those situations.

- *Improve your staff training process.* Training is everything. Write out a 30-day training program for all key positions in the business (see Figure 18-1).
- *Learn to delegate.* Create a list of at least 10 things you do that could be delegated to someone. These items should free up more of your time and give the employees a sense of participation in the business.

- Outline what the employee should anticipate—the good and the bad in whatever job he will fill in the gym.
- Explain how you will measure performance.
- Explain how you will recognize and reward good work.
- Start with member service on the first day.
- Create a detailed job description.
- Assign another employee as a big buddy.
- Spend at least two hours a day on the basics of working in a gym, such as phones, member service, and basic sales information.
- Build working examples of member service situations that have occurred in the club and let the employee work through the solutions. Build at least 10 different examples.
- Let the person follow a variety of employees around the gym. He will have more of a sense of teamwork and understanding of what everyone else does each day.
- Let the person try or tour every profit center and get started training, spinning, and doing whatever other activities you offer.
- Review the employee manual in depth.
- Train from the procedure manual. The employee doesn't need to memorize every procedure. He just needs to know where to find them.
- Try to not let the employee work alone during the first two weeks.
- During the third and fourth weeks, end each workday for the employee with a 30-minute training and review session of his work.
- Include a formal review at the end of the 30-day period.

Figure 18-1. 30-day staff training program

February 4, 2014
Have you ever wondered … ?

Have you ever wondered why, knowing that 70 percent of the diseases of aging are self-inflicted, people still continue to sit on their asses and eat until they die early? Why smoking is the known path to early death and disease and people still choose death and continue that nasty habit? Why, when just walking an hour a day can change someone's life so dramatically, you see so few walking? Why the lie continues that healthy food is more expensive than junk? It's not, but we still use this tired story as an excuse to justify a 34 percent obesity rate. Why the average person who is 40 pounds overweight doesn't at least die trying to get healthy rather than just dying? Why people get into working with a trainer and then lie to the trainer about food and workouts? Most importantly, why do really overweight women wear tights that look like monkeys are wrestling in the back of their pants when they walk and why do fat guys insist on wearing really short running shorts from the 1980s and then insist on doing bench presses? Why, people, why?

February 3, 2014
We become trapped by our pasts.

Many people become trapped by their pasts. The anger and emotion left from failed relationships, bad partnerships, and lost businesses often eat away at people to the point that they can't function in the lives they lead today. People seeking help often like to live in the past and if left alone would spend hours telling you how they got to this point in their life. The harsh reality is that no one, not even skilled professionals, can change how you got here. Where you were in the past is the least important thing in your life, but where you are going in the future should be the single most important thing you focus on. You also have to replace the negative emotion and need to constantly rehash the past or blame events that happened years ago for where you are today. It does not matter where you came from in life. It doesn't really matter much how many mistakes you made or how badly you screwed up yesterday. It *does* matter who you are going to be tomorrow. Living in the present is a wonderful thing, and given a chance, most of you will find that today is simply a beautiful day and tomorrow can be the time of your dreams if you let go of what doesn't matter anymore.

19

Hiding From Your Members Isn't Usually Considered a Good Form of Member Service

Somewhere at some time, someone is going to figure out that the most important part of getting enough customers to keep a business viable over time is learning to keep the clients we already have using the business. In other words, we should be in the business of repeat business.

In every market, the new sales cycle will start to deteriorate at some point. The gym may run hot for a year or two, but then new client business settles into a level of new sales that becomes steady from that point forward and eventually almost every market then throws a 5 to 10 percent decrease at the owner, lowering the previous established sales norm. There are always a few months that are records or over the norm, but the year-to-year average usually doesn't change beyond a few points either way for an extended period of time and then it reaches a point where the gym's numbers decline slightly, establishing a new but lower ceiling.

There has been a lot of energy, money, and effort spent trying to disprove this theory. For example, the low-priced players who offer memberships in the $9 to $19 level always claimed that their type of operating system was immune to the sales ceiling and that even if a plateau were reached that the number representing the total net membership revenue would never decline. However, time worked against their plan and low-priced providers found that same law of decline hit them too, but in fairness to that type of system, the ceiling and eventual decline didn't happen until the fifth year or so.

There Are Several Factors That Create a Ceiling

This eventual decline of new sales illustrates the necessity that renewals are important to the future growth of the business. The following chart illustrates how member service and renewals are related in the business:

Member service = renewals

Renewals = lower operating costs for the business and an increase in membership at a lower cost

Lower costs and increased membership = higher overall efficiency in the operation

More efficiency = less vulnerability in the market due to competition

The opposite of this formula is what happens to clubs that ignore the internal and just focus on the external aspect of the business, which is called frontloading, or the total focus on nothing but new sales. The following formula illustrates how this could also negatively affect your business. Remember that a club may run hot for a one to three years, but then it settles into a level of new sales that becomes pretty steady from that point forward. However, low-priced clubs run hot for four to five years and then average sales begin to decline due to everyone in the market who was motivated by price being drained. At this point, sales decline and will do so continually unless there is a large influx of new candidates into the market.

Low/poor member service = low renewals

Low renewals = demand for new sales to replace lost members

Demand for new sales = increased sales and operating costs in the form of more advertising, increased commissions, and higher employee-related costs

Dependency on high volume of new sales = high vulnerability to competition and other fluctuating market conditions

Member service is key but is also one of those subjects that is so subjective in nature that everyone who talks about member service is an expert because no one else knows what the hell he is talking about either. Another way to look at typical customer service is that you can often read an entire customer service book and walk away with no concrete methods or techniques that you can apply to your business. For example, what do you do in your business when the advice was have your staff smile, hire only nice people, be polite, dress nicely, and learn how to use the phone? In the real business world, it is much easier to talk about member service than it is to implement a truly outstanding program because there has been so little definitive advice available.

In the fitness industry, there is usually a large gap between understanding the importance of member service and implementing a member-focused quality program or, more simply put, learning how to understand and meet the needs of the members.

One of the hardest things to understand in the business is why reasonably competent owners who are honest and hardworking people with nice gyms in good markets still fail. Some folks believe that gyms fail because they are traditionally undercapitalized, while others believe that compared to most other types of small businesses, gyms cost too much to start and attract owners who are not businesspeople but are merely passionate about their chosen lifestyle and rely on that passion over learning even the most basic business skills.

The real reason why many fitness businesses crash is related to lack of balance in the daily operational plan. Good balance comes from understanding the relationship between getting new members and fighting just as hard—if not harder—to keep the ones already in the system.

New sales are easy to understand and most owners can figure out how to work that side of the formula at a basic level of play that allows the business to survive over time. The more advanced play where the owner moves beyond simple sales and starts to seek a higher return per member/client is now the separation point that defines a good owner and a great owner and many owners never really get to that level, but what it takes to rise to that point is defined elsewhere in this book. However, mastering service is something any owner of any type of business can achieve and is one of the fundamental rules of survival in a tough and competitive market.

Member service sounds easy, but in reality, it is a difficult concept to master and very few owners ever really understand or will do the necessary work and investment to keep the members who have already bought once. It is just plain easier to chase new clients than it is to keep the ones they have, which was a working business plan in 1995, but in today's market, it is a sure way to fail in just a few years.

The challenging question is how many members did your gym lose last year to poor member service? How many members bought, believed in you, and then left the gym or failed to renew because of the indifference showed toward them by you and your staff? Every owner believes his teams are nice to the clients, but few owners have a set plan that is measurable in place and that can be taught directly to new staff.

Before we discuss how to implement a member service program, let's first discuss what member service isn't. Owners define member service in many strange and wonderful ways but seldom in specific acts that actually benefit members and make them want to remain long-term members.

Most owners lose their way because much of the member's perception about the business just doesn't make sense to the average owner. A guy joins the gym, pays each month, and then expects service for that money. When the member has the nerve to stand at the front counter complaining about something minor—minor from the owner's viewpoint—the owner becomes stressed because all the crazy members do is moan about the perfect gym the owner has spent his life and money creating.

What the owner has to learn is that the member paid for the right to moan and most members aren't shy about exercising that right. If the member believes he didn't receive value for money spent, he will get even—often in a negative manner by withholding his financial referral support from the club.

Members expect and seek equity in their relationship with your business. The gym's staff has to understand the member's need for equity to provide a higher level of member service. Equity is achieved when the member is satisfied that he received equal or greater value for money spent. Staff members also have to understand that unless they learn to exceed a member's base expectations of the business, they'll never be able to reap the benefits of this equity relationship.

Everyone in the fitness business talks about giving good member service. Everyone who owns a gym believes that he gives the best member service of any of the competitors in the area. The sad point is there is a huge difference between wanting to give great member service and actually delivering the product. We've all heard "We have the best gym in town" or "We provide the best workouts." But the real management challenge is to translate these slogans into actions that the member will understand and that separate you from the competition.

To start this translation process and to understand the equity relationship, begin with a common premise: The number one purpose of you, your employees, and the services and amenities you offer is to attract, satisfy, and preserve customers. You are not there to provide a great well-equipped gym, the best workout in town (which is not enough and usually not what the member is looking for from his purchase anyway), or a staff that smiles the most.

You are there to satisfy customers. Satisfied members are those who purchase and receive value from the service you offer and then continue to support the business over time through continued business or through referrals. It's not what you want that satisfies the member. It's giving the member what he wants. If he doesn't like what you offer or the way you offer it, he can go elsewhere. But when he does walk, taking his money and friends with him, you and your organization suffer. Satisfied members create profits in your business. Dissatisfied members still spend the same amount of money. They simply spend it at one of your competitors.

The average gym will lose between 40 to 60 percent of its current member base by the end of next year. For example, if you have 1,000 members currently working out in the club, 12 months from now, there will only be between 400 and 600 of them left. This represents the industry average. The majority will leave because of their personal perception that the equity relationship was in your favor or that you were receiving more from the relationship than they were as paying members.

Member satisfaction is like an election that is held every day in your gym. In this case, the members will vote on the member service they receive. If they believe it's poor, they vote with their feet by walking out the door. The destructive thing is you may never know why they left your business. Often, they simply disappear and are quickly forgotten about in the search for a replacement member represented by this month's sales numbers.

For the gym business, member service needs to be defined as equaling renewals. Renewals will be the most important issue clubs have to face in the coming years. We are in an age of severe competition. Learning to satisfy and preserve the member base you fought so hard for in the first place is the key to your future business success.

But before you can jump in and start working on the equity position of your members, you need to first understand why they do what they do. Why do members behave in certain ways and why do they sometimes choose to renew or sometimes simply disappear and end up elsewhere?

Understanding Why Members Do What They Do

Members are motivated to act in particular ways because their actions will either result in a gain (reward) or will avoid a loss (punishment). Members are rational people. If their experience in the gym is positive, they will probably come back. If it is negative, they will stop coming and disappear altogether, along with that much needed monthly payment.

Members first come to the gym with base expectations that need to be met at the very first level. Base expectations are the basic services and needs that the member expects to be met as part of doing business with you.

Owners and their staffs are traditional— if nothing else—but the following items define what service isn't more than what it is in today's more competitive market. Remember, these items once defined service and were enough in 1995 to grow a business, but today, these items are mere base expectations by the client that need to be surpassed each and every day you are in business:

- You consider your gym clean.
- Your training system is to give the member three or four workouts and then expect him to solo (do-it-yourself fitness) if the client fails to sign up for traditional one-on-one training.
- You have new generation equipment, such as suspension training tools and kettlebells, but you keep them locked up for the trainers only.
- You let the staff take all the good parking places in front of the gym because you have plenty of parking still available.
- You offer training and coaching, but it is only for the elite few who can pay for a bunch of sessions all at once and who only want one-on-one training.
- You offer monthly payments but refuse to offer a weekly alternative.
- You set the date each month for the EFT draft, but it is only one day and you then prorate the member's first payment.

- You carefully selected four different types of leg extension machines at the last trade show.
- You have group exercise instructors shouting into a microphone when there are only four students in class.
- You pride yourself on giving a good tour and a free workout if someone wants to try the club.
- You control the front desk by forcing members to show their cards every time they come in to work out.

All these perceived methods of member service have one thing in common. They're all good for the club and the staff and none of them are really aimed at finding out about what the members need or want. And none of these actions actually benefit the member beyond what's expected from a normal business open to the public.

A clean gym is not member service. It is a basic expectation you have to fulfill just to get into the game. Trainers who are available to help the member set up a program and who are around to help them with the mechanics and necessary changes is not member service. It is the very least a member expects from the club for the money he spent with you.

As noted earlier, members expect clean locker rooms, enough equipment so they don't have to wait an unreasonable amount of time, a friendly and well-groomed staff, usually towels, and enough help to be able to participate in a basic program. However, this is where the trouble occurs because many gym owners confuse meeting these basic expectations with providing true member service.

The following chart explains how base expectations relate to member service.

Base Expectations	Not met	Met	Exceeded
Member Attitude	Indifference	Passive feelings	Committed to the gym

For a member to renew, spend money in the profit centers, and bring in guests, he has to be emotionally moved beyond having his base expectations being met (the passive feelings area) into the area of commitment by having his base expectations exceeded. In other words, you don't get his referrals and trust unless you make this guy really happy over time about his choice to support your business.

In the chart, even if a member's base expectations are met, the member is still in the area where he feels passive about the gym. It's okay and meets his base needs, but if something better came along, he'd give it a try.

Meeting base expectations is no big deal. He expected that in the first place. The only way you impress the member is to move beyond base expectations being met to the expectations being exceeded.

We make our biggest mistake in member service by thinking we are providing great member service by meeting a member's base expectations.

That still leaves a member in the area of indifference or at best passive, where he has no commitment to the gym in the long run.

To really understand how the member thinks, we have to also take a look at the equity theory. The equity theory is just a fancy way of saying that as human beings, we work very hard to keep everything in balance in our lives. If you invite me to dinner, then I feel obligated to repay that kindness by inviting you to my house for dinner. If I don't reciprocate the gesture, there is no balance or equity in our relationship and one of us feels slighted.

This theory is really the base for what happens to members in the gym. If the member joins, he feels he has already done you a favor by picking your gym. He had choices in the community and in fact drove past four competitors just to get to you, but he picked you. Therefore, he feels you owe him and it's up to you to balance. In other words, now it's your turn to pay back because he made the first gesture and commitment.

If the member doesn't feel you evened the score early, then the situation gets worse once he starts making payments. Eventually, the member will seek equity, meaning he will even the score on a negative point rather than a positive one.

For example, the member at this point feels there is an inequity on his part. He put more in than he received. Once he feels this, he will either start ignoring you (stop coming or stop payment), demand attention (love me now or lose me forever), retaliate (bad word of mouth to everyone that will listen), or withdraw from the situation altogether by cutting off all support, money, and friends.

You can benefit from this theory though. If you exceed the member's expectations, meaning the member perceives he is getting more from the gym than he is paying for in his membership, he will also seek balance because he now feels he owes you something for all the extra benefit he is receiving for what he pays to be a member. This feeling results in a positive imbalance and it has to be corrected in the member's mind. The member wants to pay you back by buying a product at a premium price, bringing in a friend, or, most importantly, renewing when it is time. The ultimate goal for member service, then, is to work toward creating positive imbalances by exceeding member expectations.

But again, the hardest part of member service is taking the concept and translating it so members perceive you are exceeding their base expectations. Even if the owner makes a commitment to getting a real member service program started, the breakdown in delivery occurs with the people in the gym who actually have to deliver service on a day-to-day basis.

You may build a $5,000,000 gym, but it's your lowest-paid front counter person and trainers who will often determine your financial success by how they deliver member service over time to potential clients and existing customers. At Starbucks, it's not the president who demonstrates the service standard. It's the young barista standing behind the counter who smiled, showed courtesy, and tried to get you to buy a pastry with that drink. Starbucks is known for its service as a result of the training the company puts into its most inexperienced staff who represent the business to the public each day.

To members, the front-line people are the business. These are the people who the members come into contact every day—the ones who they perceive as the real gym. Therefore, the front-line people need to be the best-trained and most service-oriented people you can put into the field. But what happens if they are not the best trained? How can a weak front-line person really affect you?

The following is a typical story from a gym member. We call the member Joe Smith in the story and he is definitely in a negative equity position with the club:

Joe Smith has been a member of the gym for two years. His dues are $40 per month. He's been on the same routine for a year because no one at the gym has offered to review him and update his workout and because he found the gym's elite one-on-one training program simply too expensive for him. He currently trains four days a week, has gone through the gym's nutrition program, and buys a drink every time he's in the club.

During his last visit to the club, he stopped at the juice counter, but the gym was out of his favorite drink. He also stopped in the pro shop to make a purchase of a ball cap for his brother-in-law's birthday, priced under $20.

The new counter person, who had been there about three months and who was about the tenth new counter person Joe has seen since he has been a member, didn't recognize him, so she asked him for an ID when he tried to pay by check. None of the staff said hello when he came in and no one thanked him for his purchase at the counter.

Joe just received his renewal notice in the mail but decided to lay it aside on his desk and just try a few other gyms before he sent it back. He was a little upset with the notice, especially after his last visit to the gym, because it began "Dear Valued Member."

Joe's thoughts were that after two years as a member, if they don't know me or care about me, then it's time to shop the other gyms in the area. In other words, Joe doesn't think he is getting $40 worth of value a month from his relationship with the gym, let alone the extra money he spends there every visit.

Was the situation that bad from the gym's viewpoint? After all, the gym was simply out of a drink and the counter person was only following procedure by asking for an ID. The club was open and clean and all he had to do was ask and a trainer would have helped him with a program—for a fee he couldn't afford of course. To the gym, member service was there and the owner thought he did a good job.

However, the important point is Joe's perception of what happened. In his mind, he was rudely treated when he was asked for an ID. He's been a member for two years, paid each month as promised, and was supporting the club by buying $20 worth of merchandise.

In his perception, the front counter people are the club and they treated him badly. Even his base expectations—getting a drink, being able to write a check, and being served by friendly considerate people—were not met, let alone exceeded. And this gym owner was also out of touch because there was no group training, workshops, or other lower-cost methods for a member to get training information. The owner only has two products to sell here: a basic membership to the gym and elite training, which leaves out the majority of the membership.

What does this improperly trained front-line person really cost the club if he loses Joe?

Joe pays $40 a month or $480 per year. Joe is a resident of the area and enjoyed the gym. If he was a member for five years—and yes, we need to start thinking of members in the long term—he would be worth $480 x 5 or $2,400.

Studies also show that an upset member tells, on average, 11 other people about an unhappy experience. A very damaging number that we usually ignore altogether is who these 11 people that Joe complained to now tell.

This is called secondhand word of mouth or "No, I've never really been in that gym, but a friend of mine said ..." These 11 will tell five others each. So, who is really unhappy and how far does the story go?

Joe Smith starts out the bad word of mouth = 1 person

This one person tells 11 = 11 new people
in the word-of-mouth loop

These 11 people each tell 5 others = 55 new people now
have a negative image of the club

We have the potential here for 67 people to have a negative image of this gym. Why? Because an underpaid, undertrained counter person didn't correctly handle your most valuable asset: your long-term member.

Even if only 5 of the 67 didn't come in, quit if they were members, or drove off others, you still have a huge loss. Five times $2,400 is $12,000. Again, the $2,400 is from one member staying five years. This doesn't count other money he might have spent in the gym.

Don't believe this sequence? Look at any social media site, such as Yelp (I am hesitant to mention specific names here because you never know how long an Internet company might last, but this one is a social site where you can post complaints about local businesses), and view the complaints and people who jump into debates over a business that never actually had direct contact with that business. You can also see negative reviews on Amazon of books the person never read but heard from a friend or just didn't like the author from his last book. You don't have to be a direct recipient of bad service to jump in and be part of the negativity loop. You just have to have a friend who had a bad experience.

An important number here is that it costs the gym six times as much to attract a new member than it does to keep one already in the system. The cost of advertising, commissions, staffing costs to get the new member in the system, and administrative costs are all more expensive than the service it would have taken to keep this guy around the gym. If the counter person really cost the gym that much money, would it have been worth it to hire slightly better people at a slightly higher rate and then put more training into them?

One front counter person in a bad mood, with bad breath or bad hair, or undertrained can do serious financial damage to the gym. What should this counter person have done if he would have been properly trained?

What he could have done to deliver better service is simple. For example, if you were out of a drink you normally carry, you could have given the member a discount toward another drink. Or you could have given a rain check discount toward the next purchase when you have the drink back in stock. You could have bought the member a drink if the owner or senior manager was present. You could have done any number of things except say "No," which is the last word to ever use in a customer service dispute. It was not being out of the drink that was the problem. It was how staff handled the situation that hurt the business.

It's the member's perception that you don't care about his experience in the club, you didn't care about his two years of support, and you didn't treat him as an individual. And you certainly should have taken his check. By simply changing the gym's current policy to asking only nonmembers for IDs for checks could have made a negative situation positive for our long-paying but now upset client.

Implementing a member service program is extremely hard, and in some ways, it's also very simple. The hard part comes from trying to get past the thought that we are already doing great customer service in the gyms, when in reality, what we are doing doesn't really qualify as member service at all.

The simple part is that it's easy to get started on the right program. We can do it by simply listening. Learn to listen and to understand what the members want. Fitness owners should define member service as paying attention to your members by listening to, understanding and meeting your members' and employees' wants and needs.

Member service can also be defined as asking a member what he wants and needs, listening to the answer, and then responding the best way we can. Any good business can tell you that customer service is simply asking the customer what it takes to get and keep his business.

But most owners are afraid to listen to their members and employees because they fear they will want them to change things in the business and because a lot of what members and employees tell them goes against the owner's preconceived notions of what the business should be. It's hard to dream about opening a business for three years and finally get it open and then when you talk to the first five members about what they want, you find they don't really like what you've created.

In reality, most gyms that open are already outdated by several years, reflecting what fitness used to be, not what it is in today's market. The perfect example is the box club that opens with rows of free weight equipment, including all the plate-loaded equipment and bench presses it could buy. Yes, you have a fully equipped gym, but it is equipped for business in 1995 and the bodybuilders, not the more active, full-body type of workouts the trainers and up-to-date owners are embracing today.

There is also the problem of "old-timers disease." This happens to owners who were fresh and innovative when they opened, but one year later, it's hard for them to make change because "That's the way we've always done it here."

What is the main reason for this resistance? It's simply that the known is preferred to the unknown. Until the discomfort level forces change or until pressure from the members becomes too great or until the new idea is proven (often by your friends or competitors) to be significantly better, change won't occur. When most owners change their business plans, assuming they have a business plan, it's usually because they are forced to change their operational plan by outside forces, and by then, it's usually too late.

The truly great owners learn to make major changes in their businesses to keep them growing before it's necessary and before their competitors catch up and copy what they are currently doing. Perhaps one of the best quotes ever said by a successful gym operator was "I can stay current and upgrade my gym faster than all my competitors can copy me, which gives me a huge edge in this market." A successful owner learns—often from his members—to anticipate trends and changes that will affect the future of his business.

Gyms that are in financial trouble or are not as profitable as the owner would hope or are just plain flat have everything they need to know to grow their businesses to the next level right in front of them. But to do this, you have to ask the members, listen hard to the answers they give, and be willing to change.

If you ask and then listen, the members will help you answer the following questions:
- What's wrong with my club?
- Why don't they refer their friends to the club?
- Who are your best staff members for delivering real member service?
- What could you do to make more money in the gym?
- What would they buy if you sold it?
- What do you sell that they won't buy?
- Who are your competitors and why do people buy from them?
- What attracted them to the gym in the first place and how can you use this information to attract other potential members?
- What would it take for them to keep paying you in the coming years?

- What's broken and what needs to be fixed in the facility?
- What kind of equipment do you need to buy in the next few years? Often, their answers about equipment are completely inconsistent with an owner's buying equipment to fulfill his own personal equipment fantasies.
- Is there anything else of value you might need to know to save your business?

Understanding members is right there for the asking, but few owners ask. We don't ask because we always seem to be too busy, it's too time consuming, or—and this is the worst blunder—we believe we already know what every member in the gym is already thinking. We always have enough time to sign up a new member, but we never seem to have enough time to ask current members what it would take to get them to stay for a while.

Perhaps the ultimate question to ask the members was proposed by Fred Reichheld in an article in the December 2003 Harvard Business Review titled "The One Number You Need to Grow." Reichheld is credited with creating the Net Promoter Score®, which is a simple way to find out if your business is indeed on the right track and what to do about it if it is not heading in the right direction.

The author grouped people into three categories: customers who were promoters of your business, customers who were passive, and customers who are working against your business, known as distractors. The system he proposed simply subtracted the percentage of distractors from the percentage of promoters, with good being defined as a positive score. For example, you could have a -100 percent score if every customer is a distractor who hates your business, and yes, this is possible in the fitness business. On the other hand, you could have a +100 percent score if everyone loves you—something a few training gyms can achieve due to low numbers of clients and loyalty. In reality, any score that is a positive score is a good score.

The question that is asked that sets all this in motion is: "Would you be likely to recommend my business to a friend?" This question is then followed by: "If not, why?" There are companies that specialize in this type of information gathering and most of this is done electronically now to keep old-fashioned phone time down. The key is, of course, what do I do with this information now that I have it?

Let's say an owner has a survey done on 100 of his members. The survey finds that 40 percent are promoters who would most likely refer the gym to their friends, 30 percent are passive, and 30 percent are distractors. This would give the owner a net promoter score of +10 percent, which isn't great but still positive (NPS = promoter percentage − distractor percentage).

However, the key for great customer service is the second question that is asked of distractors: "If you wouldn't recommend this business to a friend, why?" In this example, let's say that the clients in this category almost all state that the gym's parking lot is horrible and there is never enough parking during prime times, which is a common complaint about gyms everywhere.

The owner reads this and then goes proactive. He arranges for his staff to park off-site, has a local company repave and line the lot, opening up additional spaces, and adds 10 new slots by eliminating some unneeded landscaping. He then posts these changes on his website, social media avenues, signs in the club, and emails. His goal, of course, is to turn as many of the distractors as he can into promoters. He is in essence telling his membership: "I asked, I listened, and then I acted according to your wishes."

The perfect world goal would be to then repeat this survey quarterly and then chase those clients who are currently residing in the distractor category at the time. What most owners find in the real world is that there is no perfect and that there will always be distractors in your business, but most importantly, he will learn that the membership responds to an owner who is constantly listening and responding to the ever-changing needs and wants of the members.

A hard lesson to learn by all inexperienced owners is that someone else may pay attention to a member, ask him what he likes and wants, and then do everything they can to make this member happy. It's too bad when it's our competition that is doing the asking and the listening— and we are not taking the time to create a responsive business.

Implementing a member service program can be easily broken down into a few basic steps. These steps should be followed in exact order to be effective. The further you get in the steps, the more successful your member service program will be.

Remember that member service in our gyms is our future because good member service means good word of mouth. Good word of mouth means more renewals and more sales, the staff is happier and more motivated when the members are happy, the multiple profit centers are more productive because they are designed to the member's needs and wants, and overall profits increase.

A final point here is that you may have already instituted some member service concepts in your gym. In fact, you may already be on the right track when it comes to listening to the members, but as famous American humorist Will Rogers once said: "Even if you're on the right track, you'll get run over if you just sit there."

Step One: Understand What You Are Trying to Accomplish

It is easy to fail at customer service if you don't have a conceptual basis to build on. In other words, what is the core belief that represents what you are trying to accomplish within your business?

The easiest one to grasp for most owners and then use this basis to make it easy for the staff to understand is to equate the business with something everyone can relate to in his personal life. Perhaps the strongest analogy to use is also the simplest to understand:

My house, my guests

If the business represented your house and the clients represent guest who are coming over to your house for a party, what would you do differently each day to increase your customer service? "My house, my guests" is a strong reference point that gives you guidance in handling almost any customer service issue.

For example, if guests were coming to your house for an important event, such as an anniversary or a family gathering (avoid the image of 30 drunks coming on Sunday to watch football), how would you treat these guests and how would you plan the day?

First of all, how would you dress for these guests? Probably at least decent pants and a nice shirt or an appropriate dress would at least be the minimum attire? Equating that scenario to the gym, if the business represented your house and the clients your guests, how would you dress your staff for business each day? Would you put everyone in a cheap T-shirt and jeans or would you dress for the guests who are coming to the house today?

The same holds true for every aspect of the business. If a true guest of the house spent money on a smoothie, would you slide the change back and say "There you go"? If you believe this analogy, you would also thank every training client after each visit, thank each group exercise student after he leaves each class, send birthday cards, offer nice soaps and extras in the locker room depending on the club, and keep the gym as nice as you would prepare your house to have your family spend the day. In other words, we dress for the guests of our house, we are polite to guests of our house, and we are always on time and courteous to each and every guest that trusts us with his money. "Our house, our guests"—and you will respect the guests of this house.

We also forget three important things in customer service, and by losing sight of these three points, it is almost impossible to deliver any type of real customer service:

- If you take someone's money, you as an owner have an obligation to provide extraordinary service. Being in a service business is much like being a superhero: If you wear the suit, then you have to answer the call for distress. You can't be a super guy and then sit home watching TV while the city burns. In our businesses, if you accept money from someone who trusts you, reflected by that person handing over his hard-earned cash, then you now have an obligation to live up to that commitment. You took the cash, so now you are obligated to live up to that trust and provide the service that was implied by the transaction.

- Coming to the gym is a job to us, but to a member/client, it is the best part of his day. The client is paying for his time on his terms and expects everything to be perfect every time. Yes, this is impossible to achieve, but nevertheless, that is his goal and it should be ours. The client comes to escape business, family, and stress, with the main goal of establishing his time and his space. He also might accidently get into shape while there, but that is not always the prime reason a person commits to a gym, even in the training world. Making sure this daily mini-vacation for the member is always right is the only thing that really counts in service.

- In the client's head, what he pays is always worth more than you receive. The owner says "He is only paying $39 a month and I give him everything and he still moans and bitches." The client says "I pay that loser $39 a month and can't even park here, and after six months, no one still knows my name." We need to remember that value is established by perception of service and not by the actual money paid. In the client's world, $39 may be a lot of money and he picked you out of a crowded market to give his very hard-earned money to each month. Where we lose perspective is when we think what we are providing for that money is always enough, when in fact, it can never be enough. Service is about exceeding value for price and not about providing minimum service for a set dollar.

Step Two: Create a Simple Message That Conveys How You Feel About Service

Here is a sample mission statement from a club that will make money in the coming years:

We change lives!

If the owners don't believe in member service and taking the commitment to the next level, then they won't successfully implement a higher level of service. If the owner believes in member service but the manager doesn't, then it won't work. If the senior management of the club believes in member service but can't get the staff to buy in, then it won't work. Everyone on the staff—from the owner to the babysitters and janitors—has to be on a mission to make the club the number one fitness business in the country when it comes to member service.

Your goal—your vision of building a business we'd all want to own and work out in and one that all the members want to belong to—is a gym that does the following:

- Commits to providing legendary member service in the club industry and refuses to be anything but number one in everything it does
- Values its members and employees above all else
- Works harder every day to become better in its delivery of true member service

Your vision as an owner or senior manager has to be the driving force in member service and it always has to come from the top down. A motivated employee can make a difference for a while, but she only has to hear "Sure, we believe in member service, but you still have to tell the members that there are 20-minute limits on the treadmills on busy nights. That's our policy" from her boss and then she knows that the member is not really number one.

This is also the point where she realizes that what's convenient for the club is always going to take first place over the member's needs and wants. It's a sad fact, but most gyms are still internally oriented, meaning they're focused on what's best or most convenient for them and not what will ultimately please the member enough to stay longer and pay longer, which should be the goal of any fitness business.

But keep in mind that the member is not always right. That's not what's being said here. The person who wrote that the customer is always right died a very impoverished death, working at a fast-food restaurant somewhere. A better way to think about it is that the member is always right—up until the time bad business begins.

For example, a member might request the owner add a neck machine to the club's equipment list. Neck machines are brutally dangerous and only an insane owner—or one who owned her own insurance company—would ever put a neck machine in the gym.

Sometimes, the member is not right. But if a member complains that he has to wait for 30 minutes to get on a treadmill and that the time limit is unfair to someone who pays $40 a month to work out here, then he is right. The gym needs more treads and the time limit is not good member service. It's an owner's poor attempt at disguising poor member service.

The mission statement cited earlier—"We change lives!"—is the only one most any fitness business would ever need. But those words are also deceptively simple and don't refer just to getting someone in shape.

In a competitive world, the gym has to become more than just a place to rent a treadmill. Owners who want to stay in front of the growing competitive curve in the coming decades will have to move past providing just simple fitness and start to understand that the gym is becoming more of a communal part of the member's life and that he has more expectations than just basic working out.

For example, a more sophisticated client wants more education than clients in the past. In the old days, just doing a guided workout was enough for most clients, but today, the client wants coaching, but he also wants more of the "how" and the "why" and less of the "Just do what I tell you." This means the gym now needs to offer everything from a video library online of all the common exercises and movements to daily eating tips on the social network sites. The gym would also need to offer online nutritional support and education as well as free or low-priced special events, such as kettlebell workshops or planned but limited intense training experiences for the clients who want more. The client has changed and that means how we service the client also needs to change.

The communal experience is also better served in the group experience—something the aerobics people have know for decades but that the trainers are just starting to realize in most markets. Being part of a group working toward a common goal is a special part of the human experience and that concept has built most of the big companies in America, such as Apple, Facebook, and Starbucks.

The gym has to become not just a place to go to where fitness is done, but it has to become imbedded into a member's life. Always remember that you need to change how you think about the member. In today's market, the member/client is no longer replaceable. If you believe this, you will create systems that provide more total support to the members with the thought that if the client gets more help and support, he will stay longer and pay longer, which is what retention is really all about.

Mastering the Listening Game

The following is a basic training guide for the staff that covers the rules of interaction between a staff person and a member who is not happy at the moment. This process would be one of the first things a person learns when starting work in a fitness facility and it should be reinforced on a regular basis. Members who complain are important to your business plan, but over time, complaining members can wear down any owner no matter how motivated he might be. Implementing a process keeps the interaction more professional and leads to less wear and tear on owners and staff.

Free styling or, worse, allowing yourself to become emotional and overreact to a disgruntled member will cost you money and eventually your sanity. Train all new staff early in their stay with you on how to listen, respond, and respect the client who is paying you each month but at the moment might not be our favorite person. In this scenario, there is a disgruntled member standing in front of a staff person. What do you do and how do you handle the situation?

Stop what you're doing and listen.

Acknowledge the member in a sincere way even though the member may be worked up at the time because of the negative experience he just had. Nothing appears ruder to the member than the staff person trying to do three things at once—one of which is barely listening to someone who is mad and needs attention. Stop all the things you're doing, look up, and give the member your full attention. It doesn't matter if you have heard the story before and this guy is the 10th that is complaining about the treadmill being broken. While he may be the 10th, this is the first time he has told the story and he needs to be respected and heard.

Never argue with a member about the complaint he is trying to make.

Members need to vent. The problem obviously upset them enough to complain. Arguing, defending the club, or blaming someone else just irritates them more. However, most young employees feel the need to defend the gym and end up arguing with the member, which just makes the problem worse. Don't argue—learn to listen. The venting process is the relief the member needs. Being heard in full is a powerful way to drain someone's anger and letting him tell the story and complain is often enough for the member and most likely solves his problem. Remember, most customer service issues are nothing more than someone being momentarily inconvenienced. There is usually nothing really wrong here except this member came in exactly at the same time he does every day and went to treadmill #3, only to find it had an out of order sign on it. His routine was interrupted, he needs to express that irritation, and then life will return to normal for him and the gym.

Don't let a member get you mad.

It's not the complaining member that's the problem. It's the problem that's the problem. Young inexperienced staff members often take a complaining member personally and then get mad. Teach the team to ignore the mannerisms of the messenger and get to the message, which is the problem we need to hear and fix. Staffers need to learn that an angry member is not personally attacking the staff person—just using him to yell at because he was the unlucky guy standing at the desk at the time. If the member does make it personal, a manager needs to step in, take the client off the floor and away from other members, and correct the situation. Personal attacks (unless warranted)—such as sexual harassment or other inappropriate behavior by a staff person—are unacceptable, but it is up to the owner or manager to handle the situation.

Listen patiently until the member describes the entire problem.

Most complaints are not new or original. The staff has heard them before and therefore wants to step in and finish the story once the member gets started. Resist the urge and let the member finish his own story at his own pace and time. If the member was inconvenienced by the problem, venting the story often helps to alleviate the problem for the member. There was one legendary member, though, who got his tie stuck in the urinal-flushing-handle machinery. This complaint was a fresh and welcome change for the staff from the common run-of-the-mill treadmill or missing weight stack pin complaints. Learn not to interrupt, except where you need to guide a member to the end of the story. "What happened then?" or "How can we make this right for you today while you're here?" are sample ways to keep a member on track with the story.

Let the member know that we are on his side and that our job is to listen and then do everything we can to fix the problem.

Simple comments, such as "Yes, I understand how you could be upset," are an easy way to let the member know we are on his side and that it's our job to help him solve his problem the best we can. Try to understand that his inconvenience is our inconvenience and that if he leaves the desk satisfied and maybe happy, we have created a customer that believes we exist for his benefit. Perhaps the most important thing to remember about customer service is that there will always be customer service problems and that there will never be a day in any business that depends on daily customer traffic to survive that will be without at least one service issue to resolve. Knowing this, you can then understand that it isn't the problem that drives customers crazy. It is how you respond to their problems and how quickly you are willing to solve them that builds loyal customers for life.

Get them to fill out a member complaint card.

No matter how big or how small the problem is in reality—and remember that to him, the problem is always big and to us it is always routine—if it's important enough for the member to complain, then it's important enough for us to get a card filled out. Be sure to get it filled out now while the member is standing there ready to get it out of his system. Filling out a card is just another form of venting and also a written guide for problem solving for the management team. See Figure 19-1 for a sample member complaint card. Refrain from giving these cards a cute name, such as "A new challenge," and deal with the reality of what is really going on here. The member is complaining now in front of a staff person, so give him a complaint card so he knows we are listening and not sugarcoating his concerns by trying to go cute.

If you can fix the problem, then do it immediately while the member is still in the club.

If the problem can't be fixed immediately, then tell the member what you plan to do to get some action started. For example, if the member is upset because there is no soap in the showers, then immediately go put some soap in the shower. If it's a problem we can't fix that easily, tell the member we will take the card and immediately turn it over to the manager for attention. But if the staff can fix the situation or if the manager needs to immediately jump into the game, then doing it while the complainer is still in the club makes a positive impression on the member and sets a tone for the staff that our guests in our house are the most important thing we deal with daily as part of our jobs.

Follow up with the member.

Personally send the member a postcard telling him the outcome of his complaint. If we could solve the situation, tell him what we did, when we did it, and how we solved it. If we are still working on the problem, tell him what we are doing and what the expected outcome will be. If the issue can't be fixed, tell him as nicely as possible why. A card should go out within 24 hours of receiving a complaint. This is obviously retro and this should be done in conjunction with an email or a post on the social media site, but going retro does not have a downside.

Post the member complaint card on the member service board and post the complaint and how it was handled on the gym's social media site.

The club should have a member service board displayed somewhere in the main traffic flow so members can stay in touch with what's being done to improve the member service in the club. Regardless of the outcome, post the member complaint cards on the board and write in red ink in the action section what the club did in response. It would be great to see 20 to 30 of these up at one time. Keep them up for about 30 days and then replace old cards with

---

Member Complaint Card

The complaint: _____

_____

_____

Date: _____

What needs to be done to solve this issue: _____

_____

_____

Suggestions for improvements in other areas of the club: _____

_____

_____

Taken by: _____

Action by club: _____

How to use this card

These cards should be kept at the front desk at all times. The staff should be trained to hand a member a card every time the member has a complaint or even a strong suggestion. Yes, this is retro, but it does get the problem dealt with immediately instead of pushing it off to an email that might never get returned.

Sample script the staff person could use with this card

The member: I really think you should do something about the class schedule. I can never get into that cycle class.

The staff person: Thank you for letting us know about the problem. To make sure it's taken care of properly and in a timely manner, could you please take a moment to fill out this card. It helps us serve you better and makes sure none of the member suggestions and ideas get lost.

Special note

All problems should be addressed within 24 hours. Members will stop giving you realistic suggestions and complaints if they know you don't respond, so take each complaint seriously, even if it is an old issue and there is no immediate solution. If you have an electronic newsletter in the club, list the suggestions for the month and the club's responses or solutions, and if it is an issue that lends itself to social media, then post the comment from the client and the solution immediately—either on your website or your social media site.

Figure 19-1. Member complaint card sample

new ones. Yes, it does encourage other members to fill out cards, which service. You can also occasionally list improvements or responses to issues on the social sites, but always keep it positive and always thank the members for the suggestion.

It is always important to blame the member in a good way. For example, if you add a new service, such as weekly payments, blame the members. Use something such as this to introduce the service but to also be able to reach back to past members or misses in sales. This script could also be modified and sent as an email blast to every past member in the system and to everyone who visited the club in the past as a guest but didn't become a member at the time:

> We have an important announcement for all of our members:
> Effective immediately, we are now able to offer
> weekly payments for all memberships. We appreciate
> the suggestion from our members and we apologize for not
> being able to offer this sooner, but it is here now and any
> member can take advantage of this new service today by
> simply stopping by the front desk.

Step Three: Interview the Entire Staff

The front-line staff members, such as the check-in staff and the counter people, are the only staff members in the club who really know everything. This group of employees hears all the rumors, knows all the scandals, and is always the first people in the gym to hear the complaints. However, the owners and managers are the last to know anything because the staff never really wants to pass bad news uphill. It is a poor way to do business, but an inexperienced or immature owner will often shoot the messenger and it is only a mature, more sophisticated operator who actively seeks complaints, knowing that the more he know, the better he can meet the needs of the membership.

If you want to know what's really wrong in a business, go to the folks who know the whole scoop. Front-line staff members are the first to hear a complaint and they constantly chat with the members and catch everything that's wrong in the gym, even if it's passed on to them in a very offhand manner. And the members are more likely to complain to someone at the bottom of the food chain than at the top due to access and the fact that many people who complain feel they might be rebuked or blamed for raising an issue. Blaming the client for the problem is a sign of an aging, stagnant business that is entrenched in what always worked and is not likely to change its method of operation to meet the complaint of a client. In their reality, it is easier to blame the client for not understanding the system than it is to admit you might be dated and need to change.

To stay in touch with members' feelings about the staff and the gym, try formally interviewing each staff member on a monthly basis. The following is a sample questionnaire that could be adapted to most clubs.

Front-line member service questionnaire

This questionnaire should be used by management as a technique to gain information from the front-line staff before implementing any member service program and then monthly after that to keep in touch with the members' current impressions as to what's happening in the club.

Interview the staff in person and write down the answers yourself. Don't make this into a handout and just give it to the staff to fill out. You will learn more about your club and your staff by asking questions and then patiently listening to the answers without interrupting. Personally interviewing staff members and asking about what they hear and what they think is also a good way to start building a more cohesive team. Simply asking about what you heard and what do you think about that issue elevates the staff person and makes him feel he is contributing at a higher level and that what he thinks is important to the business. The following are a few questions that can be used in the survey, although you can add others that might be more pertinent to your business:

- What compliments do you most frequently hear about the gym?
- What do you think our members like best about doing business with us?
- Where and when do misunderstandings with members most frequently occur?
- What member problems do you encounter most frequently?
- What systems or policies do we currently have in place that need to be corrected to help members?
- Where do you feel you lack the authority to help a member? What is your recommendation to fix this problem?
- If you had to name one thing that would make the members happier in this gym, what would it be?

Listen just as hard to what makes the members happy as well as unhappy. When we start these programs, we tune in only to the negative, but we also need to listen to our successes too because what we do right may be our biggest edge in the marketplace and learning what makes our clients happy and doing even more of it also helps develop a more comprehensive service plan.

Step Four: Interview Members Through Surveys and Individual Key Member Interviews

Here's a classic quote from a frustrated member: "You were so busy selling me, you had no time left over to listen to what I really wanted from you in the first place."

The only way to get and stay close to what the members are thinking is by constantly getting in their faces and we do that through surveys and individual key member interviews.

There are many ways to survey and interview, but all our tools should be based on asking the same question in a number of different ways. This question is: "Would you be likely to recommend our business to a friend, and if not, why not?"

What do the members really consider to be great service? How would they define the service they desire? What would it take to keep them as members of the gym—and paying—for years into the future? What would a member feel is great performance from our staff? We have our own definition as fitness professionals, but it's possible that how we define performance and what we expect from staff actually gets in the way of good member service to an ever-evolving membership base.

Obviously, gathering this type of information from members gives us a tremendous advantage over the gyms that don't take the time to do this vital task. A lot of owners don't like to ask these questions because they don't like to get any type of bad news. Worse, it is sometimes arrogance that keeps an owner from reaching out to his membership: "I have been in this business for more than 20 years and I know better than any of my members what they want and need to be happy." But when you're developing a member service program, the bad news is sometimes the good news because we may learn something that will help our businesses grow in the future, and it seems that for many owners, the longer you are in business, the more out of touch you are with what this year's membership wants from its gym. Staying current is hard work and it takes a dedicated owner who is willing to ask the members for guidance and to also attend workshops and seminars year after year and then constantly use this new material to update the business plan.

If we ask, listen, and respond to our members through surveys and individual member interviews, we should be able to spot the bad trends happening in the club before they become a big problem. We should also be able to capitalize on the good trends, know what actions we need to do and in what order, and be able to set short-term and long-term goals for the gym, our staffs, and ourselves.

Sample questions for putting together a member questionnaire

Clubs with 600 or fewer members should try to get out about 25 questionnaires a month. If there are more than 600 members in the facility, try to get out about 50 surveys a month. This is enough to get a real pulse check on what's happening in the business without making it a mind-breaking task for the staff and management. Be sure to do the surveys at various times of the day so you can get a thorough cross-section of the members.

Useful survey questions include the following:
- What equipment would you like to see us add to the gym? Your list could include new equipment or duplicates of what we already have in the facility.
- What do you think our biggest weakness is when it comes to equipment?
- What services, programming, or amenities would you like the gym to offer? Don't forget the little things we can do to keep you happy as a member.
- Please list three things you believe the gym does well and should do more of in the future.

- Please list three things the gym could do better.
- What new products would you like us to add to the pro shop?
- What was the number one reason you chose our gym?
- What new trends or programs have you read about or seen that could be added to the gym?
- Your guests are very important to us. What could the gym do better to attract and service your special guests? Please check all the points you think are important.

  __Free T-shirt for you for bringing a guest in to the gym

  __Free gift certificate to local businesses for bringing in a guest

  __Three free personal training sessions

  __One free month added on to your membership for every guest that joins

  __More guest passes available to you on a regular basis

- Please give us your thoughts on guest incentives for you and your guests. How can we better attract and serve your friends?
- Please rate how our staff treats you during your visits to the gym?

        Fair   Good   Excellent

        1...........2...........3...........4...........5...........6...........7

- How would you rate the club on cleanliness?

        Fair   Good   Excellent

        1...........2...........3...........4...........5...........6...........7

- We want to continually improve our customer service to you. How can we improve our service to you personally in this gym?
- Your comments are important to us. Please take a few moments to give us your thoughts on any aspect of the gym you feel is important.
- What were the three most important factors to you in your final decision to join this gym?
- What are the strongest points in our marketing that appealed to you as a potential member?
- What turned you off about our advertising or might have made you hesitate about becoming a member of this club?
- Was there anything that surprised you about the gym once you became a member? For example, did our gym match your preconceived ideas about the business—either positively or negatively?

Owners and senior managers should do at least 25 key one-on-one personal interviews a month, asking the members these questions. The manager interviews a member and then writes down the answer as the member gives it. Conducting these interviews in person allows you to stray from the questionnaire if a good topic comes up and lets the members know their opinions are important to the club. It also gives the interviewer a chance to watch the expression on the member's face, in case there is more to an answer and it needs to be drawn out of the member.

Step Five: Have a Third-Party Call and Interview at Least 25 Former Members Every Month

These are members who are at the end of their memberships and decided not to renew with us. We need to know why we had them and now we don't. You would expect to hear a lot of bad news from this group, but most of them are already into something else in their lives and won't give you much except nonthreatening answers.

However, every once in a while, you'll get that rare opportunity to talk with a member who was unhappy with the gym. That's what you're looking for in this survey: those one or two people who give you the real story and help the gym grow another notch.

We've found over the years that using a real or pretend third-party interviewer will get the best results. When you call as a gym representative, no one really wants to unload and get into the real issues. But if you're calling as a third party—a person a member doesn't know personally and is not afraid of hurting that person's feelings—his answers are usually better and more complete.

It does help to have someone that is at least somewhat familiar with your business do the interviews. If the member starts discussing a certain topic, a person who has an understanding of your business can talk the person further into the subject, where the most helpful information usually lies.

A sample former member phone survey

Use the following survey to gather information from past members. Don't bother sending anything. You seldom get anything back, even with stamped, self-addressed envelopes. You can also set this up as an ongoing email program and you will get back a surprising number of responses, but also do the phone calls because you are looking for that one perfect member who will tell you everything.

If the former member takes the time to participate in the survey, offer him a free month to come see the changes you've made since he has been gone and to let him know that you've taken his suggestions seriously.

> Greeting: Hello, my name is _____. I've been hired by _____ (gym name) to do a survey of former members. Would you please take a few minutes and answer a couple of questions for me?
>
> 1. Why are you no longer a member of the gym?
> 2. What three things could the gym do to improve its member service?
> 3. What did you like least about doing business with this club?

4.   What one thing could the club do to significantly improve its product?

5.   What did you like best about the club?

Closing comments: (Member's name), thank you for taking the time to answer my questions. Because you have been so helpful, may I send you a free one-month membership to the gym to come back to see the changes it has made since you've been gone?

Sales and marketing drive new members, but service is what keeps them. For too many years, the industry has only practiced the sales part. For the industry to grow and mature and to shake its sleazy, high-pressured sales image, the growth must be toward providing the consumer a better level of customer service, which ultimately improves our business by having more members stay longer and pay longer.

We are also stuck on perceived product quality, as in the "Our gym is better than your gym" mentality. Product quality is what the member gets, how the product is delivered is service quality, and that's what will set us apart from our competitors in the coming years.

Member service doesn't just happen. It's not a spontaneous act by staff. Member service has to be planned and developed over time. For most clubs, it will take at least a year to get a good member service program in place.

The steps listed in the following section are a guide to help you think about the implementation of a plan and about how detailed you have to get to make member service work. Do the steps one at a time, and once a step is part of your operational plan, move on to the next step. Take your time and complete each step correctly.

As the overall quality of gyms improves in the coming years due to the large investment needed to start one and the addition of real businesspeople to the industry, member service will become even more important because it will be all that separates one club from another. The perception of member service in your club by a prospective member will be all that separates you from everyone else in the market.

The 11 Points of Member Service

- *This is my house and these are my guests.* Create the image that the clients are guests who visit us each day for something special. We are respectful to our guests, we treat our guests as friends, we are courteous to our guests, and we dress for our guests each day. Respect the guests of the house each and every visit.

- *Live by the mission statement "We change lives!"* What we do matters and we are in the business of changing lives. This should be on the walls, on the backs of shirts, and in all the gym's advertising.

- *Answer your phone live by the third ring.* Never, ever depend on answering machines or voice mail hell as your first impression.

- *Use a welcoming statement, such as "We are having a great day at the Workout Company," when members walk through the door.* This is their time and their space and we need to greet them with a positive statement each visit, and no, this does not get old to the member.

- *Use all means possible, such as the gym's software flashing names, to get to the point that every member is known by first name.* We will learn names. We will use a computerized check-in system with his picture and name displayed prominently so we can cheat, but we will use his name. And we will find him on the floor and use his name. And our group exercise instructors and trainers will learn their names too. And the janitors need to give names their best shot too. There is nothing more important than recognizing someone who is giving you money to be in your business.

- *Thank every member after every class and training session and as he leaves the gym.* Every single member is thanked every single time he leaves the house. "Thank you for coming in today. We appreciate your business." It doesn't have to be harder than this. Use these words exactly. Don't use "Thanks, man." Don't just nod and wave. Say thank you like you understand who really does pay for the bills in this house. If you have staff members who can't do this or who find it embarrassing, fire those people and get new staff. The guests in this house are far more important than a few self-conscious staff idiots with social issues.

- *Clean daily and go for the total deep clean, not the standard lazy method of only wiping down the tops of surfaces.* Your club is never as clean as you think it is. Get a cleaning staff that can get it done, but keep these staff members moving during their shifts. We don't expect the staff to stay after work cleaning this place. We will get a professional crew or a retired couple to clean, but we do expect all staff to walk through the club throughout the day to keep the house clean for the guests. Staff will give equipment a quick wipe. Staff will pick up crap off the floor. Staff will take care of the locker rooms every 30 minutes. Our house is always clean because if not, this is one of the main reasons our guests quit us for other clubs in the area.

- *Dress for the guests of the house.* Your uniform should be at least one step better than your gym. Respect the people who pay you each day by dressing as a professional team.

- *Use magic words.* "Yes, we can do that." "I would love to help you with that." "Thank you for stopping by today."

- *Deliver service when the member wants it—at their convenience—not just when it's convenient to us.*

- *Be accessible at all times to members.* If you're the owner and you're in the gym, then you are fair game and have to be open to members. They will wear you out, they will be obnoxious at times, and they often have no idea as to what they are talking about, but if you own a business where you charge people to come visit, then you have to be part of the service experience.

Sample Training Games and Meeting Formats That Raise Member Service Awareness Among the Staff

Good news/bad news game

Give each staff member $10 to $25 in an envelope depending on the size of your gym and staff. Tell them there is good news and bad news. The good news is that the cash is a bonus for good performance in the club. The bad news is that they have to spend the money at an outside business by the next meeting and document the experience.

How were they treated in the store? Did they leave smiling after the sale or did they feel they were imposing on the salesperson's time. Were people friendly and did they spend time or were they rushing the person out of the store? The staff member then has to relate his adventure in the next meeting and how what he learned relates to the club and the member service the team is now offering.

Learning the competition game

Send each staff member to visit another gym and get pitched. This is an old game, but we probably never looked at it from the member service viewpoint. How does the competition present member service—if at all? Does what it claims in its tour match what the staff person sees in the club? For example, a club can talk about member service, but when you go into the locker room and it's dirty, then that's how that club and its staff really feels about customer service.

Learning the competition game—team style

Try the team approach as an alternative for large staffs. Split the staff into member service teams and assign a team to one of the competitors in the area. One team member works out, one gets pitched, and one makes a phone call as a prospective member and then they all give an overall view of the visited club. The goal is to steal one good idea we can use in member service and to also prove that the competition isn't so tough after all.

Breakfast club game

A staff member is assigned to get bagels and coffee for the weekly staff meeting. The only rule is that a staffer can never go back to the same place twice. Each meeting starts with a review of the buying experience and the customer service received at that week's location. If a staff member gets unusually good member service from someone, then steal him as an employee. This game keeps the team focused on customer service each week and is also a good way to recruit new staff members who already understand the fundamentals of service.

Problem-solving game

Ask the staff one tough question during the meeting, such as what new products could be added to the club that would improve member service, and give everyone one hour to come up with solutions. Be willing to let go here. Be willing to try strange suggestions if they won't hurt the business. Many of their suggestions will be positive and most will, at the worst, be neutral. By trying their suggestions, they begin to think like a team and that they're a real part of the company.

February 1, 2014
Your life comes down to one thing.

Your life always comes down to just one thing: Did you make a difference? Did you change someone's life for the better? Did you leave the world a better place? People just starting careers seldom think about this, hoping to get to the important work in life later, but living a life that has meaning is not a project. It is a way of living. And there really is no degree of play here either. You either live every day with the goal of making the world around you better or you live every day internally worrying only about you and what you want. Many of you who read this are in the business of change, but there is a huge difference between seeking physical change and being the person who goes that extra distance and creates better people. You will not be remembered for the money you have, the house you live in, or car you drive. You will only be remembered for the lives you made better because you cared enough to make a difference. Start the week with only one thought: The world will be a better place this week because I will make it that way.

February 19, 2014
Stop the damn whining.

Stop the damn whining about the weather and every other small thing in your life. It feels like someone declared this time of year the official "Whiny Season of North America" when everyone takes an entire month to endlessly complain about small things that shouldn't matter to anyone. Try this tomorrow. Get up and buy a regular old-fashioned newspaper. Turn immediately to the obituary section. Read all the names of the people listed there who died that week. If your name isn't on the list, then shut up and stop whining about small things because if you're not on the dead list you are going to have a good day, or at least better than those people. How many of those people listed on that obit page would give anything they ever had to be in your place just one more day? Look out the window. If it is snowing, go walk in it, come home, drink a hot tea followed by a glass of wine with a friend in front of the fireplace. If your business isn't working well, then learn something new and fix it and stop bitching. If your kids are miserable, get a sled, get out of the house, and drag their whiny butts through the park for an hour and wear them out. Start looking every morning in the obit section first and remember that if you aren't there it's going to be an amazing day.

About the Author

Thomas Plummer has been working in the fitness business for more than 35 years. He founded the Thomas Plummer Company in 1990, which eventually became the National Fitness Business Alliance (NFBA) in 2003. The NFBA is a group of industry vendors and suppliers banded together to bring advanced business education to all fitness business owners operating anywhere in the world. He also created the NFBA Institute, the industry's first certification body for the business of fitness and training. Currently, the NFBA offers over 30 seminars a year all across North America and is the largest provider of education for the fitness business owner in the world. The NFBA teaching team is also featured at over 20 additional seminars and workshops yearly as featured speakers for most of the major fitness organizations in the world.

Plummer is in front of more than 10,000 people a year through numerous speaking engagements as a keynote speaker, event host, and private consultant. Recently, he has been featured as a keynote speaker at the World Golf Fitness Summit, the Jewish Community Centers' annual convention, Leisure Industry Week in England, the ACE Symposium, FILEX in Australia, Perform Better's Functional Training Summits, and the Fitness Together annual convention. Most recently, he was a featured speaker for Reebok/CrossFit International.

He has authored six books on the business of fitness, which have remained the bestselling books in the industry for over 15 years, and several of the books are currently used as textbooks in numerous college programs as their source for fitness business education.

Due to the over 100,000 people who attended his seminars during the past decade, coupled with the continuing popularity of his books that have sold over 150,000 copies worldwide since first being introduced in 1999, many industry experts feel that Plummer is the most influential person working in the fitness industry today. He is perhaps best known for helping young fitness professionals understand and master the business side of the gym business.

Plummer has also served on the IHRSA Silver Anniversary Commission and is currently serving on the Titleist Performance Institute Advisory Board. In recent years, Plummer has also become a wide-ranging industry consultant and personal coach and has worked with many industry icons such as ACE, Titleist Performance Institute, World Gym, Gray Cook and Lee Burton and their FMS system, Mark Verstegen, Mike Boyle, Alwyn and Rachel Cosgrove, and Todd Durkin. He also works with many of the chain organizations and nonprofits as a consultant and business advisor.

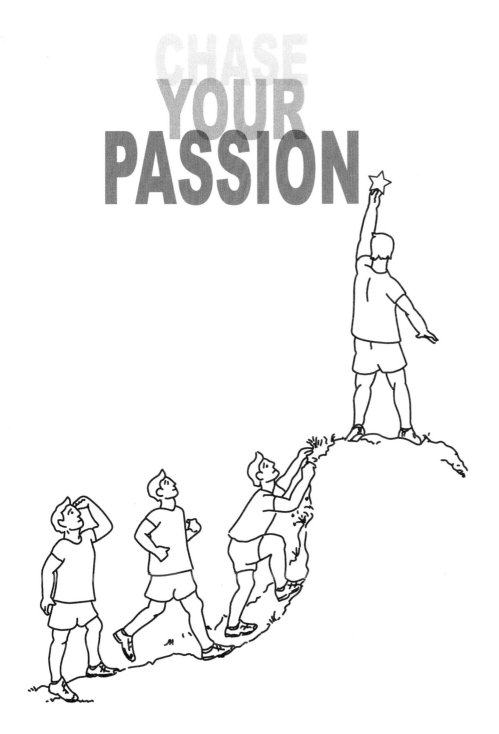

CHASE YOUR PASSION